HOW TO CHOOSE
VOCATIONS
FROM THE HAND

BY
WILLIAM G. BENHAM

WITH 66 ILLUSTRATIONS AND CHARTS

British Library Cataloguing-in-Publication Data
A catalogue record for this book is available from
the British Library

Palmistry

Palmistry, or 'chiromancy' (from the Greek *kheir* meaning 'hand' and *manteia* meaning 'divination'), is the claim of characterization and foretelling the future through the study of the palm. The practice is found all over the world, with numerous cultural variations, and those who practice chiromancy are generally called palmists, palm readers, hand readers, hand analysts, or chirologists.

Palmistry generally consists of the practice of evaluating a person's character or future life by 'reading' the palm of that person's hand. Various 'lines' (heart line, life line, etc.) and 'mounts' (or bumps), purportedly suggest interpretations by their relative sizes, qualities, and intersections. In some traditions, readers also examine characteristics of the fingers, fingernails, fingerprints, and palmar skin patterns (dermatoglyphics), skin texture and colour, shape of the palm, and flexibility of the hand. A reader usually begins by looking at the person's 'dominant hand' (the hand he or she writes with or uses the most, which is sometimes considered to represent the conscious mind, whereas the other hand is subconscious). In some traditions of palmistry, the other hand is believed to carry hereditary or family traits, or, depending on the palmist's cosmological beliefs, to convey information about past-life or karmic conditions.

Though there are debates on which hand is better to read from, both have their own significance. It is customary to assume that the left hand shows potential in an individual, and the right shows realized personality. The basic framework for 'Classical' palmistry (the most widely taught and practiced tradition) is rooted in Greek mythology. Each area of the palm and fingers is related to a god or goddess, and the features of that area indicate the nature of the corresponding aspect of the subject. For example, the ring finger is associated with the Greek god Apollo; characteristics of the ring finger are tied to the subject's dealings with art, music, aesthetics, fame, wealth, and harmony.

There are three main lines on almost all hands, generally given the most weight by palmists: 'the heart line' (representing love and attraction), 'the head line' (representing the person's mind and the way it works, i.e. learning, intellectualism and communication), and 'the life line' – perhaps the most controversial line on the hand, believed to represent the person's vitality and vigour, physical health and general well being. The life line is also believed to reflect major life changes, including cataclysmic events, physical injuries, and relocations. Contrary to popular belief, modern palmists generally do not believe that the length of a person's life line is tied to the length of a person's existence.

Palmistry has a long history, and is a practice common to many different places on the Eurasian landmass; it has been practised in the cultures of India, Tibet, China, Persia, Sumeria, Ancient Israel and Babylonia. According to some, it had its roots in Hindu Astrology (known in Sanskrit as 'Jyotish'), Chinese Yijing ('I Ching'), and Roma fortune tellers. Several thousand years ago, the Hindu sage Valmiki is thought to have written a book comprising 567 stanzas, the title of which translates in English as *The Teachings of Valmiki Maharshi on Male Palmistry*. From India, the art of palmistry spread to China, Tibet, Egypt, Persia and to other countries in Europe.

From China, palmistry progressed to Greece where Anaxagoras practiced it. Aristotle (384 - 322 BCE) discovered a treatise on the subject of palmistry on an altar of Hermes, which he then presented to Alexander the Great, who took great interest in examining the character of his officers by analyzing the lines on their hands. Aristotle stated that 'Lines are not written into the human hand without reason. They emanate from heavenly influences and man's own individuality.' Accordingly, Aristotle, Hippocrates and Alexander the Great popularized the laws and practice of palmistry. Hippocrates even sought to use palmistry to aid his clinical procedures.

During the Middle Ages the art of palmistry was actively suppressed by the Catholic Church as pagan superstition. In Renaissance magic, palmistry was classified as one of the seven 'forbidden arts', along with necromancy, geomancy, aeromancy, pyromancy, hydromancy, and spatulamancy. It experienced a revival in the modern era however, starting with Captain Casimir Stanislas D'Arpentigny and his publication of *La Chirognomie* in 1839. The 'Chirological Society of Great Britain' was founded in London by Katherine St Hill in 1889 with the stated aim of 'advancing and systematising the art of palmistry and to prevent charlatans from abusing the art.' Edgar de Valcourt-Vermont (Comte de St Germain) founded the 'American Chirological Society' in 1897.

A pivotal figure in the modern palmistry movement was the Irish William John Warner, known by his sobriquet, 'Cheiro'. After studying under gurus in India he set up a palmistry practice in London and enjoyed a wide following of famous clients from around the world, including famous celebrities like Mark Twain, W. T. Stead, Sarah Bernhardt, Mata Hari, Oscar Wilde, Thomas Edison, the Prince of Wales, General Kitchener, William Ewart Gladstone, and Joseph Chamberlain. So popular was Cheiro as a 'Society Palmist' that even those who were not believers in the occult had their hands read by him. The skeptical Mark Twain wrote in Cheiro's visitor's book that he had '...exposed my character to me with humiliating accuracy.'

Criticism of palmistry often rests with the lack of empirical evidence supporting its efficacy. Scientific literature typically regards palmistry as a pseudoscientific or superstitious belief, and skeptics often include palmists on lists of alleged psychics who practice cold reading. Despite this skepticism, palmistry is a practice and branch of human endeavour with an intriguing history – and whether it has any truth or not, provides a fascinating window into folkloric and religious beliefs more generally. We hope the reader enjoys this book on the subject.

TO

S. B.

AND THE CHILDREN

CONTENTS

Contents

ILLUSTRATIONS

THESIS

The need is great. Rising generations seek vocations for which they are best fitted. The waste of education in the past must be prevented in the future. Parents must be able to tell their children what they can do best. The answer is within the covers of this book.

THESIS

THE big problem of the present and the future is our children.

Millions of them.

When the sun rises each day a horde of new arrivals have come into existence, and each succeeding day a new horde appears.

Each one that lives must make his way in the world—he must find a place where he can cope with the economic conditions that exist.

He must find where he can earn his daily bread.

With his hands or his brain he must hew a way for himself through competition, selfishness, and the struggle of the human race for the survival of the fittest, and in this struggle millions die or become incompetent, many fail and are ground to pieces in the battle for existence, and untold thousands become criminal from lack of ability to meet the situation.

Many of these children are unwelcome and are allowed to shift for themselves. Thousands come into families unable to support or educate them. And other thousands are born to parents who would like to have them succeed but who do not know how to advise them properly as to their future callings.

In this way, many children even of well disposed parents never rise above mediocrity.

The age of machinery is making it constantly more difficult for the human machine to compete for a livelihood. No child will stand a chance in the days to come who is not prepared from his childhood for the task for which he is best fitted; so that when the time comes for him to take up his fight against the combined forces which he will have to overcome in his struggle for existence, every resource of his brain and hand is highly trained and ready for a definite position in a definite field of endeavor.

Already, out of steel and iron aided by electricity, they are building Robots who can do the work of men; and with science and discovery leagued against him, the child of the future cannot be reared in the haphazard manner of the past, he must be started from the cradle to prepare for his future work in life. We must know soon after he is born the occupation for which he is best fitted and he must be put in training from the days of his childhood, to fill a position into which he can step at maturity with a good chance of overcoming the obstacles that will lie in his path.

Here is a statement startling but true.

6,000 children emerge from adolescence every twenty-four hours.

When adolescence ends, maturity begins.

6,000 new children must face the world and find a place for themselves every twenty-four hours.

See how the problem multiplies.

The number who emerge from adolescence prepared by a proper training for the task ahead of them is infinitesimal.

For the rest there is only a pellmell struggle to get along by hook or crook. To *find* positions without qualifications for those positions. To *fill* positions for which they are in no wise fitted. To struggle each day with a mass of new applicants for their positions who are that day emerging from adolescence.

6,000 of them.

And the next day 6,000 more.

The parents of the world have not realized these facts.

It is time they should.

A vast army of parents are trying to meet this situation for their children.

Schools and colleges are filled with students, and their numbers are increasing each year.

From 1890 to 1926 enrollments in colleges and universities increased 529 per cent. When the college year of 1928 opened in the fall, one thousand American colleges opened their doors and enrolled 250,000 freshmen. The total college students at this time was near a million. It is computed that 100,000 will drop out before graduation, but the most of them will continue through their sophomore year.

In the elementary schools at the same time, a million and a

quarter children went from the elementary grades to high schools, and the public schools with this increment contain about four and a quarter million pupils.

These figures speak eloquently of the effort many parents are making to fit their children for the struggle before them.

The significant thing about it all is this:

That of all the army of young men and women who are being turned out by schools and colleges each year,

AN INFINITESIMAL NUMBER HAVE ANY IDEA WHAT THEIR FUTURE CALLING IS TO BE OR WHETHER THEY HAVE ANY QUALIFICATIONS FOR THAT CALLING.

Not one of them all positively *knows one thing* for which he is best fitted.

The youth of the world is entering the serious business of life GUESSING but never KNOWING.

This is not the fault of the schools and the colleges.

Everything necessary to know in order to be fitted for any position or walk in life, is being taught in the schools.

The whole trouble lies in the fact that young men and women do not know what they should be fitted for, and their parents cannot help them to decide.

A MOMENT WITH THE AUTHOR

In a recent article widely published in the press, a prominent Professor of Education of a prominent college said:

"We have in our secondary schools all over the country many misfits, youths who are neither apt for nor interested in what is offered them. They see—and often see clearly—nothing in it of value to them. Their accomplishments as revealed by the most scientific measurements that have been devised are pitiable. In half-heartedly attempting to learn such subjects as higher mathematics and foreign languages they not only fail to attain any mastery but they also develop attitudes so hostile that these important fields are henceforward neglected, in school and out. . . . Every thinking person recognizes the need of some means of separating, not the sheep from the goats, but the sheep who should be fed in different pastures."

A MOMENT WITH THE AUTHOR

THE sole purpose of this book is to show parents in a very concrete way, how they may select the occupations for which their young children, and those ready to enter colleges, are best fitted; at the time of life when all their training and education can be directed toward preparing them for these occupations.

It is couched in simple language, in order that parents of ordinary intelligence may apply it to their children.

When the Messrs. Putnam published my *Laws of Scientific Hand Reading* in 1900, it attracted the attention of Dr. Canfield, at that time President of Ohio State University, and afterwards Librarian of Columbia College. He urged me to use the information I had gathered about hands, adapting it solely to choosing for young children, and those of college age, the occupations for which they were best fitted; his experience having shown him that few if any young people or their parents had any idea what their vocation in life should be. Thus there was wasted annually, he said, a vast amount of effort in the pursuit of education which in no way contributed to their success.

In response to this suggestion, I have, for the past thirty years, engaged in adapting all the known and newly discovered facts revealed by the hand to the choosing of occupations for young children and those of college age; my zeal for this work having been greatly increased by the discoveries made by scientific men during the period, concerning the brain and its connection with the hand.

It is now known that when a child is born it has not an idea. Its entire brain, which is divided into the right and left hemispheres, is a blank. And it is known that all the child knows afterward is what some outside source records in *one* of the hemispheres. And science has discovered the exact area on the hemisphere selected as the seat of future intelligence, which controls sight, hearing, touch, smell, the movement of arms and

legs and eyes, and the exact area that controls speech; on which
is recorded, as the child grows older, his entire vocabulary.
And possibly the greatest discovery of all, is the fact that one
of the hemispheres *alone* is the seat of his entire intelligence,
and that the other hemisphere is *forever* blank and unintelligent; and that the two hemispheres are not interchangeable.
If an injury occurs to the hemisphere which is the seat of the
child's intelligence, the other hemisphere cannot function for it,
his mind will be a blank forever after.

The question naturally arises: if only one hemisphere of the
brain records the intelligence of the child, controls the operation of his senses and his faculty of speech by means of which
he acquires knowledge, as well as controls his movements:

How is this hemisphere selected?

How is it determined which hemisphere shall be the seat of
intelligence, and which shall be blank?

Fortunately we have the answer to these questions in *Brains
and Personality* by **Dr. W. Hanna Thompson, M.D., LL.D.**,
from which we quote:

"The endowment of one hemisphere with the gift of speech
was not owing to any original or special fitness of that hemisphere for such a function, but solely because it was the hemisphere related to the most used hand in childhood. In all right-
handed persons it is in the left brain that the speech centers
are located, while in left-handed persons they are found ex-
clusively in the right brain. Two conclusions inevitably follow
upon these facts, *first:* that brain matter as such does not originate speech, for both hemispheres would have their speech
centers, and *second:* that either of the hemispheres is equally
good for speech, if something begins early enough in life to
use it for that purpose. That something is the most commonly
used hand by the child at the time when it is learning everything, for self education always begins in our race with the
stretching forth of the hand, as any one may note in the first
purposive act of an infant, the hand which is then most used
to learn by, determined which of its two brain hemispheres
should know speech, and which hemisphere should remain
wordless, and therefore thoughtless for life."

Quoting further I find:

"The faculty of speech is located in the hemisphere which governs the hand which is most used; hand and brain are therefore physiologically connected."

"It has been found that injuries which produce the various forms of mind deafness, occur only in the left hemisphere of right-handed persons, or in the right hemisphere of left-handed persons, in other words they show how these mental functions strictly follow the hand most used in childhood, just as the speech centers do."

"The primary connection of the hand with the fashioning of the word mechanism in the human brain is conclusively settled by the location of that mechanism in the right hemisphere of left-handed persons. Whence, therefore, the impulses mostly proceed for using the particular hand in question, and settles both to what cerebral places words are to go, and from what places they are to come."

If it is true, which we cannot doubt after such testimony, that the hand of a baby is potent enough to choose the hemisphere of his brain in which all his future knowledge is to be stored, at a time of life when it is his unconscious act, it proves that the choice was that of the hand and not of the brain, for we know that at this time of his life the entire brain is a blank, it could not direct the choice. This almost leads to the conclusion that the hand is a seat of intelligence as well as the brain. At any rate we know that the hand is physiologically connected with the brain, and an active agent in the matter of choice as to the future operations of the child, otherwise it could not choose the seat of his future intelligence, the storehouse of all his future knowledge, as we have seen it does. And accepting all these proven facts as true, which I have done, we are certainly justified in relying upon the hand for information as to the occupation for which a child is best fitted.

After many years of study, I have found that the seven types of people furnish us this information, and with the tests which we make to determine the quality of the child, I have no hesitancy in saying that all Dr. Canfield hoped for in the study of the hand has been accomplished.

One of the most prominent men in the United States in a recent address to the graduating class of a college said:

"The misplacement of human beings is one of the greatest tragedies. Young people frequently start out quite aimlessly. They either drift from one place to another or, having taken a place unsuited to them, have not the initiative or courage enough to lift themselves out of it.

"The years go by and in the minor jobs they do the work well enough perhaps to get some progressive increase in earning power. Each year makes it more difficult for them to move and one day they wake up to the realization that there is nothing ahead for them in the line into which they have drifted and they are then too old to be accepted in another. This, as I have said, is one of the greatest tragedies of modern life. Be careful not to misplace yourselves."

This book is a sincere effort to prevent such tragedies.

WILLIAM G. BENHAM,
2 West 45th Street, New York City.

EXPLANATION

You will find a chart at the end of each chapter. When you have compared the hand of your child with the descriptions in the chapter, and with the illustrated plates as noted by the numbers in the chapter, fill in the chart with the indications found, the type identified, and the result of the tests. By referring each item on the chart to the paragraph on that item in the chapter on the primary type, you will find its meaning fully explained, which will enable you to read the chart correctly. With a little practice you will find it as easy as reading a newspaper.

EXPLANATION

I N the study upon which we are about to enter, we shall use the word *child* throughout, meaning, wherever it is used, young children of both sexes, and young men and women as well, up to college ages. Each recommendation for occupations applies equally to all of these, even though only the word *child* is used. This use of a single word to include all of these young people is to prevent verbiage. The book is for the use of young men and women about to enter college, as well as for those who have the care and guidance of children.

We shall use the word *he* throughout, meaning at all times children of both sexes, and young men and women. We find this necessary as a matter of generic assistance in preparing the text.

In our selection of the occupation best suited to a child, using the word as explained above, we shall base our opinion on the identification of his Mount type from his hands.

It is our firm conviction, based upon many years of observation and study, that the Mount types of people embody all the qualifications necessary to the successful operation of the universe, and experience has taught us that once the type of a child has been determined, we know the occupation for which he is best fitted.

Every child born into the world belongs to one of the seven types, and if an occupation is selected which belongs to his type, there is an easy and pleasant pathway to success open to him.

As the parent is the one who has the child in charge at the time when his future is being decided, it is the parent who must, if it is done at all, place the child where he belongs. This can be done after the Mount type has been identified, after which it is only a matter of educating and preparing him for his future occupation.

It is necessary in all cases to determine the grade of the child, as his grade will be the deciding factor as to whether

he can be placed in positions of responsibility in given industries, or whether he must occupy the middle or lower grades
of positions in the same industries. In establishing the matter
of grade, the hands furnish a number of tests, which give us
all the information we need, and after we have identified the
type and determined the grade of the child, we know exactly
what position he can occupy.

You will note that our recommendations are in each case
specific. We wish to call attention to the fact that this is the
only system of choosing occupations for children that does
not deal almost entirely in generalities. In the following pages,
recommendations are made for definite positions in definite industries or divisions of trade and industry, as well as the grade
of position the child should occupy in that particular industry.
A recommendation, to be of value, should be exact, and in
this lies the importance of this method of vocational choice.
We believe that this is the first and only time that definite
and concrete recommendations have or could be made as to the
exact occupation for which a child is best fitted.

In the chapters which follow, we deal with each type separately, first placing before you a complete mental picture of
the type and its qualifications, afterwards adapting this information to the various occupations for which the child may
be trained, then applying the tests to determine the grade of
positions the child can occupy in the industries recommended.

The system can be applied by anyone with ordinary intelligence.

These are the seven types.

1. The Jupiterian.	The leader.	Plate 8
2. The Saturnian.	The balance wheel.	Plate 46
3. The Apollonian.	The artist.	Plates 48–49
4. The Mercurian.	The business man.	Plate 50
5. The Martian.	The fighter.	Plates 52–54
6. The Lunarian.	The writer.	Plate 56
7. The Venusian.	The lover.	Plate 58

These are the tests.

1. The texture of skin.	For quality-grade.	Plates 10, 11.
2. Color of hands.	Vital force.	
3. Flexibility of hands.	Elasticity of mind.	Plates 12, 13, 14, 15
4. Consistency of hands.	Energy.	

5. Three worlds.	Mental, business, lower.	Plates 17, 18, 19
6. Knotty fingers.	Analysis, mental, material order.	Plates 20, 21, 22
7. Smooth fingers.	Artistic qualities.	Plate 23
8. Long fingers.	Minutiæ—detail	Plates 24, 25
9. Short fingers.	Impulse—quick conclusions.	Plate 26
10. Finger tips.	Idealism, art, system, originality.	Plates 27, 28, 29, 30
11. The thumb.	Will power, reason, character.	Plates 31 to 45

Here are listed the seven types which form the basis of our work, and the tests we apply to determine the grade of the child. To a consideration of all the detailed qualities of the types as applied to children, and to the tests as applied to their grades, we now invite you.

THE CHART

In order to simplify the choosing of an occupation for a child, and avoid memorizing, we have prepared a chart, which contains all the information necessary to enable us to be accurate. In hospitals, a chart is kept which records the hourly temperature, pulse, administration of medicine, and other information. From this chart the doctor, when he arrives, can tell at a glance the condition of the patient. Our chart should be prepared with the same care. It should show the type identified and the result of the tests. In preparing this chart, the type should first be determined, and the tests applied as given in the chapter on that type. This information should be noted on the chart. When completed, the chart can be read; the type qualities showing the occupation for which the child is best fitted; and the tests showing the grade of positions he can fill in that occupation. This chart makes it easy to apply the subject matter of each chapter to the child, and is a distinct advance in the method of hand reading.

IDENTIFYING THE MOUNT
TYPES

It is really quite easy to identify the Mount types. In the chapter that follows, every indication that will identify a type is given. Only a little practice is needed to enable you to do it quickly and easily. In a short time you can do it at a glance.

IDENTIFYING THE MOUNT TYPES

How to do it without trouble. A reference chapter, with which you can identify any Mount type, without need for memorizing.

THIS chapter has been prepared with great care for detail, but do not let that alarm you. It is a reference chapter, to which a parent can turn whenever a difficult case presents itself. It is not expected that anyone will memorize the means of identification here given, nor is it necessary. But we have felt it necessary that there should be no method of identification of the Mount types that was not fully explained, and with this idea in mind, no pains have been spared to make the chapter as complete as possible.

A careful reading will give the *general idea* of Mount identification, after which as each child is examined, you can turn to the *portion of the chapter which treats of the markings* found in the hand and recorded on the chart, and easily identify the Mount type to which the child belongs as well as the secondary type.

MAP OF THE MOUNTS

The Mounts are located in the palm of the hand, four of them at the base of the fingers, and one at the base of the thumb. One is located at the upper part of the base of the thumb, and two on the side of the hand called the percussion.

The complete geography of the Mounts is presented in Plate 1, with which it is necessary to become familiar, so that the boundaries are immediately apparent as soon as you look into the palm. It will be necessary for you to judge whether one of the Mounts laps over onto another, or is in any way deflected from its proper position, or whether all the Mounts are within their boundaries. This is easily done from Plate 1. It will be best to examine a number of hands in comparison with the map, until you become perfectly familiar with the geography of the Mounts, before you attempt to identify the Mount types. This need take only a few moments time.

The Apices of the Mounts

A close examination of the skin in the palm of the hand will show that its surface is covered with convolutions, and it has been found that there are no two hands in the world wherein these convolutions are alike. These facts have been known for centuries, but it was only within recent years that they have been utilized in the identification of individuals by means of thumbprints. In our study, we use these convolutions, or a part of them, in the location of the Mount types.

A close examination of the skin covering the four Mounts under the four fingers, will show a triangle on each, formed by the convolutions of the skin, either on the tops of the Mounts or somewhere on their surface.

In hands where the skin is coarse, this apex is easily seen, but in hands where the skin is very fine, it will require the aid of a small magnifying glass to locate it.

In order that you may see clearly what is meant by the triangle or apex of a Mount, we present an excellent example in Plate 2. Preliminary to its use in identifying Mount types, and as a matter of practice, it will be well to compare this plate with as many hands as possible, so as to become familiar with the apex in different locations, and with skin of various degrees of fineness.

Then with the geography of the Mounts clearly in mind, and the apices well understood, you are ready to begin type determination.

Size of the Mounts

The first thing to look for in identifying types is the manner in which the Mounts bulge when the hand in held toward you with the palm uppermost.

As the Mounts are balls or pads of flesh rising in the hand, some of the balls are quite prominent and stand out from the rest, in which case these prominent pads identify themselves as the leading Mounts. Plate 3 will visualize some high Mounts for you.

In other hands the Mounts will be perfectly flat (Plate 4), in which case a number of tests will have to be applied in order to identify the Mount type to which the child belongs. In some hands, the Mounts will be actually deficient, and depressions will be seen where Mounts should be (Plate 5). In this case you will have to rely upon other things than bulging Mounts for the identification of the type.

HELPFUL MARKINGS

There are a number of markings which strengthen a Mount, and when the Mount itself is prominent, the presence of these markings make the identification of the type more certain. In the first place, the apex of the Mount is a great help (Plate 2), for when you find it located *centrally* on the Mount, it adds strength to the certainty that this is the primary Mount type, and if in addition it is located *high* on the Mount, it is still further confirmation.

A well cut vertical line on the Mount is another evidence of strength, and a single line is an indication of greater strength than two lines or a number of lines. The more vertical lines there are, the more they dilute the strength of the marking and the less strength they give the Mount.

If the Mount is one which lies under one of the fingers, the length and size of its finger must be noted. If the finger is long and large, it will add much to the strength of the Mount, and in cases where the Mounts are flat or deficient, the presence of a large finger on one of them will identify this one as the Mount type.

CONSISTENCY AND COLOR

Consistency of the Mounts must be examined, for often you will find one of them much *harder* than the others. In this case, the hard Mount will be the primary Mount if the others are soft or flabby. Elastic or hard consistency add to the strength of any Mount.

Color will also play a part. In some hands you will find one Mount pink, and another white, which will indicate that the pink Mount is the stronger of the two. Red will be still stronger, and yellow color will show a tendency toward the bad side of the Mount.

Normal Length of the Fingers

As the size and length of a finger will often determine the type of the child, it is necessary to be well posted on the normal length of each finger. We will consider this subject, basing the consideration on a hand where the fingers are of normal length (Plate 6).

On every normal hand, the finger of Saturn is the longest, and the normal length of the fingers of Jupiter and Apollo are determined from it. The finger of Jupiter should reach so that the tip of the first phalanx comes to the middle of the first phalanx of the finger of Saturn, and this will also be the normal length of the finger of Apollo. The finger of Mercury, when of normal length, reaches to the first joint of the finger of Apollo, and in all cases, when the fingers are shorter than these measurements, it will show that the Mount on which the short finger is placed is deficient in the qualities of the Mount. In like manner, if any finger is longer than these measurements, that Mount will be the strongest one.

The Three Worlds

In estimating the strength of a Mount, the three worlds as shown by the three phalanges of the fingers (Plate 1) will show you in which world the qualities of the Mount will operate. If the first phalanx be longest (Plate 17), on a finger which is also the longest finger, it will show that the qualities of that type will operate in the mental world. This child should be started in an occupation in which the mental qualities of that type are first considered, as we know that it will be the mental qualities of the type in which he will be strongest.

In like manner, if the middle phalanx is best developed (Plate 18), it will show that he will succeed best in an occupation in which the practical or business side of the type can be utilized, and if the lower phalanx be best developed (Plate 19), he should be placed in the more ordinary occupations of the type where not so much mental development is required.

You will often find that two of the phalanges are better developed than the third, in which case it should be determined which of the two is the leading one, and this one must be used as the key to the strongest world; the next longest phalanx should be regarded as the supporting one. A little practice in this sort of analysis will enable you to determine these facts quickly, and apply them correctly.

We would urge you, before making a decision as to the occupation to which you are going to devote your child, that you make frequent application of the tests herein outlined, to *children other than your own*, not with a view of determining their occupation, but of gaining practice for yourself. You will find that with a child *you do not know* as well as you do your own, you will be much more free to apply the rules to the markings you find, and it will be much better practice than with one you know too well. Do not let your impression of a child cause you to deviate from a strict application of all the rules as herein indicated, for the rules are right, and your impressions are very likely to be wrong.

FINGER TIPS

The finger tips must be considered carefully in the estimate placed upon a Mount, for the square tip (Plate 29), and spatulate (Plate 30), will strengthen a Mount, and the conic (Plate 28), and pointed (Plate 27), will decrease its strength.

In an effort to determine the leading Mount, a spatulate tip on the finger of a Mount will be stronger than any of the other tips, and everything else being equal, this will be the leading Mount. The square tip will be next, and the conic and pointed in this order.

When Mounts are bulging and the leading indications not obscure, you will not have to go to any length to identify the leading Mount, but it is often the case that Mounts are low and apices not well placed. Then it is that the tips and all other indications will have to be called into play to determine the type.

The Mounts which do not have a finger, viz., Mars, the Moon, and Venus, will have to be determined by their size, and the extent to which they bulge into the hand, also by consistency and color and by the lines upon them. In the case of these Mounts, it will be found that these markings are generally sufficient to identify them easily, and you will not have to resort to as close a scrutiny of all possible indications as with the Mounts below the fingers. You will not find apices on these Mounts as we do with the Mounts below the fingers, but despite the lack of many indications, Mars, the Moon, and Venus are generally the easiest Mounts to identify and their relative strength is seldom hard to determine. In the separate chapters on the Mounts, we will give you a description of the appearance of each of the types in their pure state, and this helps materially with the three just considered.

Length of Fingers Helps Identify

Length of fingers will influence the operation of a Mount to a marked degree. Each of the types has a different set of qualities, and with some of them short fingers would be more favorable than long, and with others the opposite would be the case. So when examining to determine the leading Mount, if one is found *where short fingers are most favorable,* and the finger of the Mount *is short,* it will indicate this to be the leading Mount, and further examination should be made to see if other indications, such as apex and the size of finger, confirm this estimate.

Likewise, where a long finger is found with a Mount on which *long fingers are most favorable,* that will be a leading Mount and the process will be the same as to confirmation.

On a hand where the Mounts are *flat* (Plate 4), the length of fingers will often give you the clue to the leading Mount. Where the distinction is very close, it will be well to consider the child as partaking of *some* of the qualities of *several Mounts,* and a much weaker situation develops than if one Mount is strong. In such a case the long or short finger qualities will be very important if present.

Remember the qualities of short fingers (Plate 26), "quickness of thought and action, impulse, impatience at detail, and desire to deal with subjects in their entirety, also a strong desire to achieve big things," and *apply them* to the Mount you find *best developed.* See if its reaction to these qualities would be favorable to the best operation of this Mount. Often you can locate the leading Mount on a hand with flat Mounts in this way.

Also remember the qualities of long fingers (Plate 24), "love of detail, slowness, suspicion, care in small things, and the instinct of going into the minutiæ in everything," and apply these in the same way, by which method you can use them equally as well to locate the leading type on a hand with flat Mounts.

KNOTTY FINGERS

Knotty fingers add a serious aspect to the Mounts. The philosophical qualities of knotty fingers, if both knots are developed (Plate 20), add to the strength of the Mounts and give assurance that order and system both in mental and material matters will give the Mounts a stable quality, so that a child with this development may be placed with safety in occupations requiring the use of the best side of the Mount types.

If only the knot of mental order be present (Plates 1-21), it will be best to consider occupations where the mental side of the Mounts will be most required. Thus with a Saturnian Mount well developed, the knot of mental order will add to the studious qualities of this already studious type, and he can safely be assigned to the study of philosophy, physics, psychology or intensive laboratory research.

A Mercurian, with the knot of mental order developed, and at the same time with the first phalanx of his fingers long, can be assigned to a study of the law. He can be especially successful in pleadings to a jury, hence a good criminal lawyer. We cite these cases to show the manner of application of the knot of mental order to these two types. It can be applied with equal success to the other types by taking their known qualities and placing back of them the qualities of the knots of mental order as a developing force. If the knot of mental order be found on only one finger, and the rest be smooth, this will assist you to identify the primary type of the child as that of the finger on which the knot is found. This is made more certain if the finger is large and the apex centrally located.

If only the second or knot of material order be developed (Plates 1-22), the order and system will be expended in the home, the office, the farm, in dress, in business, and in all practical things. The result of this development will be, that whatever the type, it will operate best on the material plane. To determine which is the best direction for the efforts of a child with such fingers, you will find the tips of great assistance. First you should note whether all the fingers of the hand have knots of material order or only one of them. If only one be found, it will indicate that the finger on which it is seen is that of the primary type, to be confirmed by other indications already explained, and no matter how many fingers have this knot, the tip should be noted to determine the strength of the indication.

The spatulate tip will show the greatest strength, the square next, the conic next, and the pointed last, so if you find the single finger with the knot of material order and a pointed tip, it would not be a strong enough indication for you to decide this to be the primary Mount.

But if you find a spatulate or square tip you can safely do so. These tips will also show you the best direction in which the Mount type qualities can operate when influenced by the knot and the tip found. It will not be difficult to make an accurate estimate if the Mounts be high, but you will find many hands in which the Mounts are flat and even deficient. In these cases the knots of both mental and material order, and the tips, will often help you to a determination which would otherwise be impossible.

Many times you will find both the knots of mental and material order developed, in which case the child can be placed in a greater variety of occupations. He will be studious, careful, slow, orderly, practical, and persistent, especially if he has a strong thumb; and if this formation be found on only one finger, it will be almost certain that this is the primary type, especially so if spatulate or square tips be found.

If this be the case, your next move will be to take the qualities of the type, and estimate what effect mental and material order and system will have on the operation of the type qualities present, and this will give you the answer to the best occupation for the child. With both knots developed you will find a much larger field of operation possible than if only one of the knots be found. The effect of this combination of both knots is not the best for all the Mounts, for instance: with the Jupiterian, Apollonian, Venusian and Martian. These types need more spontaneity than is given by the knotty fingers, but this may be said in this connection, that knotty fingers are not often found on these types.

Smooth Fingers

When smooth fingers are found (Plate 23), it will be largely on the hands of Jupiterians, Apollonians, Venusians, and Martians, as these types are governed by inspiration to a greater extent than the other types. You will find a great many smooth fingers, and sometimes they will be found on Saturnians, Mercurians, and Lunarians. There will be no difficulty in applying them however if you will bear in mind that wherever found, the child will act by inspiration, impulse, and intuition, rather than by analysis.

This is the reason we find smooth fingers on the four types mentioned above, as these types do not analyze but take things for granted and trust to intuition. They are the types that are popular with their fellow men, who enjoy life, are filled with the spirit of good cheer, and are most often successful by reason of the fact that people like them and help them along. Consequently, they do not seclude themselves from their fellows and spend their time in study and the analysis of profound subjects. Smooth fingers on these four types will open a great many more channels to the child, they will be found in greater plenty and will achieve their ends with less effort than will knotty fingers.

Smooth fingers will not help you to identify a type, their presence is not unusual enough, and the qualities they represent are not forceful enough to make them a guide in type determination. It is only when they are found on the types *to which they do not distinctly belong* that they attract our attention, and to find smooth fingers on a Saturnian would not be a sign of strength, it would show that the Saturnian would operate in a manner unusual to his type, and would raise the question whether it could be done successfully; we would not think of identifying a primary type from the presence of a smooth finger on a Mount of Saturn. It is however very necessary to give them full consideration wherever found and to apply to the type on which they are found the full measure of smooth fingered qualities.

Long and Short Fingers

A similar condition exists in the estimate of long and short fingers in connection with the types. Long fingers play a conspicuous part in the identification of the types, and are often the determining factor in a close decision, for if all other indications seem of equal value, the length of a finger will determine the primary type.

The qualities of long fingers will also be a big factor in the operation of any type, for their slowness and their great love of detail would in the case of the spontaneous types such as the Jupiterian, Apollonian, Martian, and Venusian be a retarding factor which might have much to do with diminished operation of these types; but a long finger found on any of these Mounts would, if all other indications were of equal value, identify the Mount on which it was found as the primary Mount.

Long and Knotty Fingers

If with long fingers we also find knotty joints, we have a combination that must be carefully considered, for the knotty fingered analysis added to the slowness and love of detail of long fingers, if found on the wrong type, would be unfavorable. On the spontaneous types it would be too great a retarding factor to produce the best results. Such fingers on the Saturnian or Lunarian would not be unusual, and would be favorable in their operation.

With other indications, long fingers produce some fine results for a Mercurian. For instance: if the first phalanx of the finger of Mercury be long, with knots, and a long finger, the child will have great ability in the law, he will be a forceful speaker who will prepare himself for every occasion with pertinent and well digested facts, and he will be highly successful.

Short Fingers

Short fingers (Plate 26), will not assist you in the identification of a type, but they will have much to do with the operation of the types. They belong to the spontaneous types and produce their best results in combination with them. Short fingered people are those who want to do big things, who think quickly and act quickly, who do not analyze, who abhor detail, and whose first impressions are their best. By resort to second thought, they make most of their mistakes. Such a

combination with Saturnians or Lunarians would produce poor
results, but with the other types, provided they have good
thumbs, they produce brilliant people.

Many prominent business men, lawyers, doctors, architects,
and those in other important occupations, have short fingers, but
in combination with the proper type: but they also have good
thumbs, consistency, color, flexibility, and nails, and the right
worlds developed; from all of which they receive the proper
support for their type.

Long fingers may restrain a type and keep it from going
too fast, they may furnish support to a type, may identify a
type, but they do not need support *for themselves*. They *give*
support but do not ask it.

Short fingers *give* their *qualities of impulse* to a type, but
they do not restrain, nor support nor identify, often they
themselves have to be restrained and supported. They are most
important in their influence upon a type, but we must be on the
watch to see that a too spontaneous type does not have too
much impulse from short fingers, or a brilliant child may be
ruined by an excess of desirable qualities.

Even Mounts, The Balanced Hand

On many hands you will find the Mounts so evenly developed
that it will be hard to determine which is the leading Mount.
This does not refer to flat Mounts alone for often the condition exists with Mounts that are high and well formed. Nor
does it refer alone to those Mounts that are deficient.

This is the *well-balanced hand* that we are referring to here,
and in such a hand the fingers are set even on the palm, and the
Mounts are of even height, so that no excess or deficiency of
the Mounts is evident (Plate 7). This balanced hand will be
the one that will test your skill, for it is not so hard to
identify a Mount type on a hand where there is a marked excess or deficiency, these things make the type self evident. But
with the balanced hand, you must apply all the known tests
and among this number you will always find *the one* that is
the *deciding factor* as to the primary type.

First examine the apices carefully in order to see if any
one is more centrally located than the others. You will often find
in a case of this kind that one apex will be centrally located,

and the ones on each side will lean toward it. Then you will know that the centrally located apex is the primary type and that the ones that lean toward it are the supporting types. You will also note that in these supporting types the one whose apex leans toward the primary Mount *most* is the *weaker* of the two, and one that *does not lean so much* is the secondary or *stronger* type of the two.

In such a case, the less an apex is deflected from the center of its *own Mount* the stronger it is. The height at which an apex is placed *on* a Mount is also a matter for consideration, for if an apex is found high on the Mount and centrally located as well, it is the strongest indication that can be shown by the apices, and such a formation would indicate the primary type in most any sort of a balanced hand.

Next you have the vertical line mentioned earlier in this chapter to assist you with the balanced hand. Even if the apices should be so evenly placed that you are not able to determine the primary type from them, you may find on one of the Mounts a well cut vertical line which is not on the others. If such is the case, this will be the primary Mount. Or you may find this vertical line on one Mount and on the other Mounts, or on one of them, two lines, or a crossing of lines, vertical crossed by horizontal lines, a grille as it is called, in which case the Mount with the single vertical line will be the primary Mount.

As a general rule, all lines which cross a Mount are a detriment, and when there are many of them, it amounts to a great interference with the good operation of the Mount qualities. Such a marking will nullify even a well developed Mount. In any close decision always look to see if any of the Mounts are filled with cross lines, or if, even worse, the lines form a grille as explained above, in which case the Mount so marked may be eliminated from a possibility that it may be the primary Mount.

After having examined the markings as above, you should note the fingers, first as to size, for if one finger on the balanced hand is conspicuously longer and larger than the rest, this will be the primary type. If they all seem to be the same size, begin and consider them separately as to whether they are long or short, smooth or knotty, and the kind of tip found on each finger.

We have explained which of these indications give the most strength to a Mount, and which weaken it. It often happens that each of the fingers have a different tip, in which case you will remember that the one with the spatulate tip is the strongest, the square next, and the conic and the pointed in this order, and with this information you will decide that the one with the spatulate tip is the primary Mount, and you will place the square tip as the secondary Mount.

If one finger be long and the other short, the long finger will identify the primary Mount. In only one case will the short finger identify a Mount, and that is when one of the spontaneous types has a short finger. *As the qualities of the type and of the finger* are such that *one supplements the other,* this is a strong combination, and will justify the classification of the Mount with the short finger as the primary type. In no other case does the short finger aid you in locating the primary type.

Knotty fingers will identify a type, if one finger alone is found to have them, or if all the fingers have the knot of material order except one which has *both the knots;* the finger with *both knots* will identify the primary type. The balanced hand is often encountered, and it is for this reason that so many tests are given. This hand shows an even temper, broad mindedness, generally better health, and a balance of characteristics which make it desirable to use all the good qualities possible in the choice of an occupation. In order to do this we must locate the proper type.

You will never find a case in which you cannot find the primary and secondary types by the use of the tests which we have just enumerated. *Some one of the tests* will bring it out so clearly that you cannot mistake it.

MORE ABOUT THE APICES

We have spoken many times of the apices of the Mounts and their importance in locating the primary types, and we wish to call your attention to their importance again and ask that you make them a special study until you become able to locate them without difficulty. It will be well to supply yourself with a small magnifying glass as there are many cases in which you will find it helpful, especially in the judgment of skin texture and the apices.

In judging a Mount which bulges, it is not always the top of the bulge that is the apex of the Mount, though many make the mistake of so regarding it. No hasty judgment should be made in this matter, great care should be used, as the time taken for a thorough examination will be well expended. In every case, locate the apex of the bulging Mount even if you have to use the glass, and at the same time the apices of the other Mounts as well.

Every variation of the apex *toward* another Mount will show that the Mount toward which it leans is the stronger of the two, and the extent to which it is deflected from the center of its own Mount will show how much of its own strength it *gives up* to the other Mount. In many cases you will find the deflection, while apparent, still slight, which will show that this secondary Mount is almost as strong as the primary, in which case the child will have a combination of the strength of both Mounts. In like manner, you can get the *degree* of strength of *every* Mount from properly located apices, and in the end will know just what forces may be charted to the credit of the child.

Excess Development of the Mounts

While all of the Mounts have their good side, they all have their defects as well, and you must be on your guard so that these defects will not escape you.

In the first place, remember that excess of even good qualities is a defect. Too much ambition in a Jupiterian may make him unsuccessful, too much of the gloomy side of a Saturnian may destroy his studious qualities, excess in an Apollonian may make him vain, boastful, self centered; and excess may turn the shrewdness of the Mercurian into greed and dishonesty. The good qualities of Venus may become the low passions which produce jealousy and murder. Too much Martian quality will make a bully and common brawler, and excess of the Lunar type will most likely end in insanity. So you must be watchful for excess developments which may result in trouble, and first you must see that the Mounts do not bulge in a manner out of proportion to the rest of the hand, and that the color is not one which will mean excess, and the emphasis of bad qualities.

High bulging Mounts with extreme redness will produce excess, and extreme whiteness will be excess in the other direction. Yellow color brings some of the worst combinations that we encounter.

BAD SIDE OF MOUNT TYPES

You will find as you study each type that some of them are naturally bad, and from these types come most of the really criminal. The Jupiterian, Apollonian, and Venusian are not criminal types, and you will rarely see yellow color on any of them. When they do criminal things, it is not from a criminal instinct, but because they are too often led astray by stronger characters, without criminal intent. Very often they are creatures of circumstances. But these types do not plan criminal operations and carry them out with their eyes wide open.

The Mercurian is not distinctly a criminal type, but he lives constantly very close to the line where shrewdness ends and dishonesty begins. You will find yellow color in the hands of many Mercurians. The Martian is not a criminal type in the sense that criminality is usually regarded. He is, if in excess, a violent type, and does what are classed as criminal things. He loses his temper and assaults his fellow man, and often he kills him. And his excess of strength sometimes causes him to overcome a fellow creature and take his belongings, but he must have a very bad development of his type before such things occur. A balanced Martian of good quality would never think of or countenance such things.

The Saturnian which numbers some most famous examples among the men of history is of itself a criminal type, and you will seldom find pink or red color in the hands of a Saturnian. Yellow or white will almost universally be found.

White or yellow is the color of the Lunarian, and his imagination will often lead him into dubious ways. He is the most susceptible to untruth of any of the types. So in looking for defects of the types you must bear in mind which are the good types and which are the bad.

THINGS THAT EMPHASIZE TYPE DEFECTS

Anything that emphasizes the *disagreeable* side of a type is a defect. For instance, short critical nails will be bad on a violent Martian, and they will emphasize the bad side of the Saturnian or the Lunarian; stiffness of hands or thumbs will add to it.

Lines distinctly cut on the Mounts are either a favorable or an unfavorable marking in accordance with the manner in which they run. Vertical lines, especially a good single line, will be a favorable indication. Two vertical lines less so, and when a great number are seen, decreasingly so as the number increases. Horizontal lines are decidedly a detriment to a Mount and when found they must be classed as a serious defect. The more of them that cross the Mount, the greater the defect. Vertical lines crossed by horizontal lines forming a grille is the most serious defect of all. A Mount with such a marking will show the bad side of the Mount to be present, and a study must be made at once to discover all of the favorable indications present which will tend to counteract the defect. A strong thumb will be the most favorable indication that can be found.

EXAMINE BOTH HANDS

In every examination for Mount determination both hands should be examined. Usually the apices of the Mounts are located in the same place in both hands, but there will be variations in the length and shape of fingers and other markings. If there is any doubt which is the primary Mount, you will find some marking we have described, quite prominent in one of the hands, and maybe not so prominent in the other; something that is so different that it attracts your attention. By reference to the paragraph in this chapter, which deals with this marking, you will find that it identifies the primary type. For instance: if all the apices are located in the same position on the Mounts but one, which is located in a different position, this differently located apex will identify the primary Mount. The same method applied to long and short fingers, knotty fingers, the tips, and size of the fingers, will show some one thing in one of the hands different from the rest, which will identify the primary Mount.

WHAT IT IS NECESSARY TO LEARN

In order to be completely successful in identifying the Mount type to which your child belongs, only a few things are necessary for you to learn. These are: the location and geography of the Mounts, the normal length of fingers, when fingers are larger and longer than normal, how to locate the apices, how to identify long and short fingers, knotty and smooth fingers, the three worlds, and the tips. All of these subjects are carefully treated in this chapter, and excellent illustrations of all these markings are shown. *In an hour's time,* with the hands of your own family or a few friends to practice on, together with the illustrations and descriptions in this chapter, you can fit yourself to correctly judge all these matters and prepare a chart that will enable you to fix definitely the vocation for which your child is best fitted. In Chapter Eight we show you how easy it is to read a chart and read one for you.

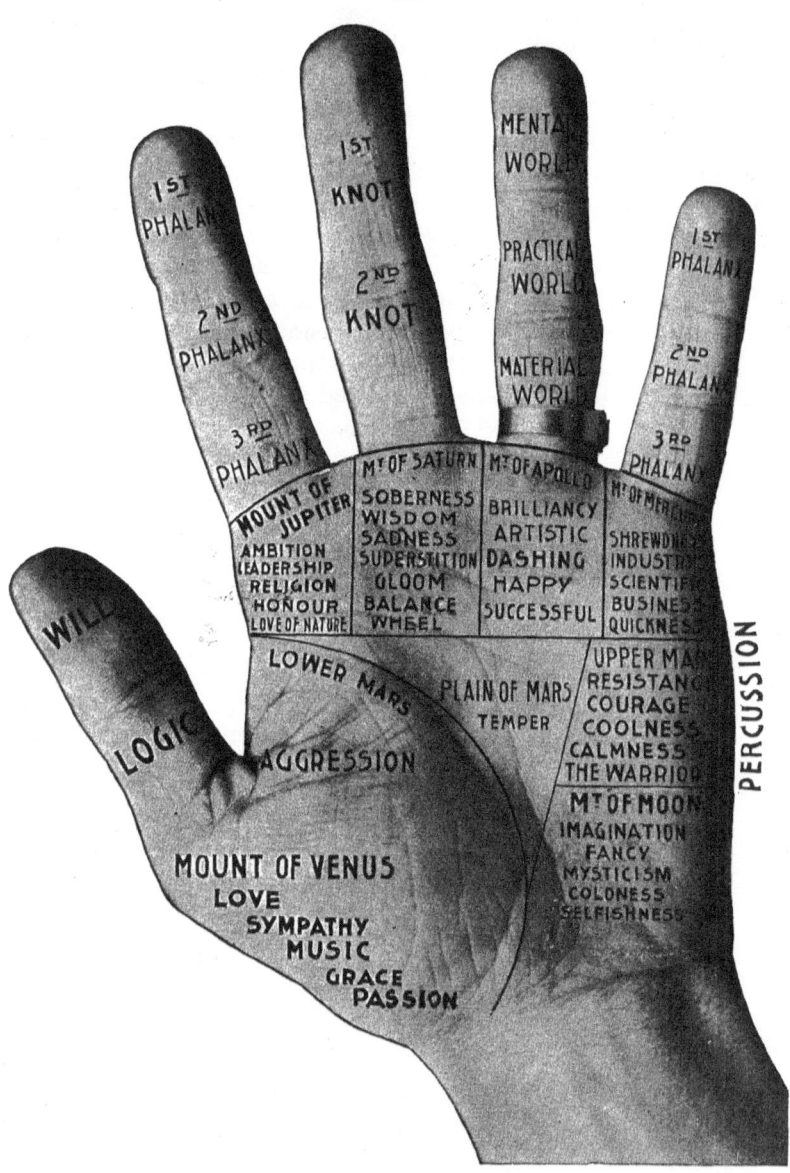

No. 1.   Geography of the Mounts. Knots on Fingers. Three Worlds.
Phalanges of Will and Logic

LII

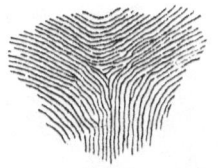

No. 2. Apex of a Mount

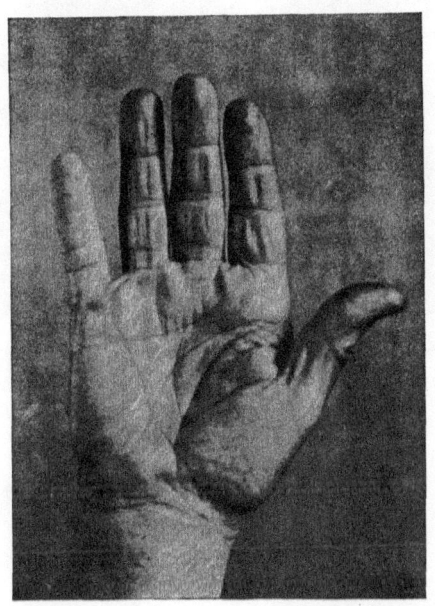

No. 3. High Mounts

LIII

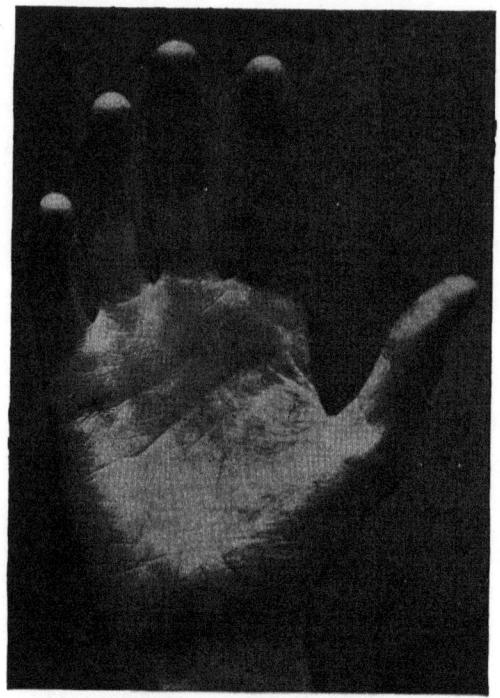

No. 4. Flat Mounts

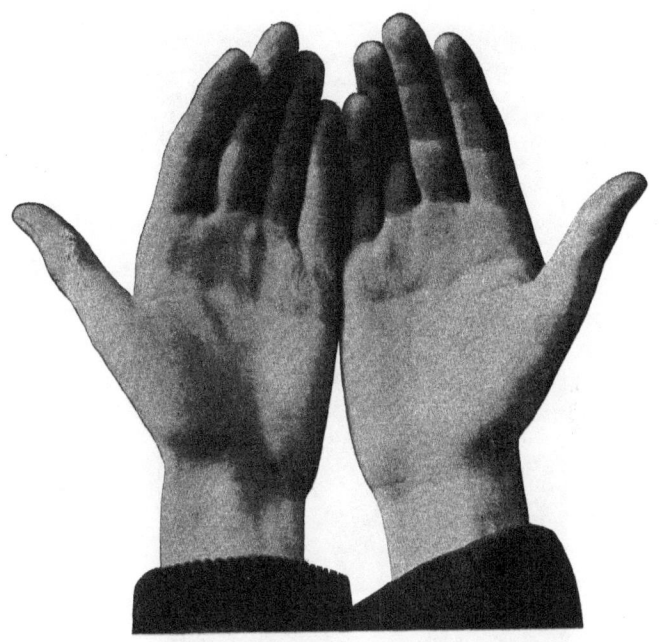

No. 5. Deficient Mounts

LV

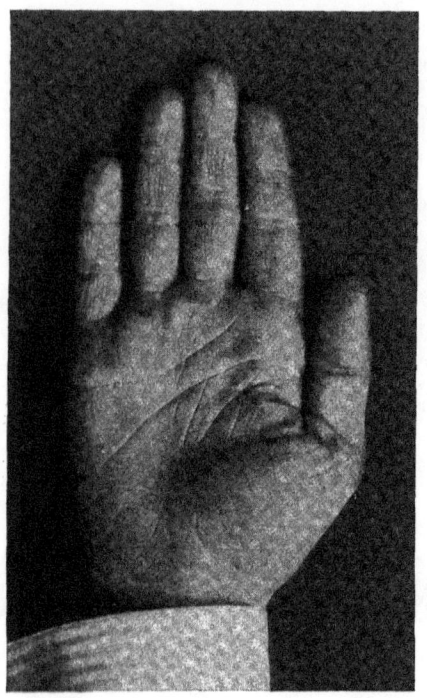

No. 6. Fingers of Normal Length

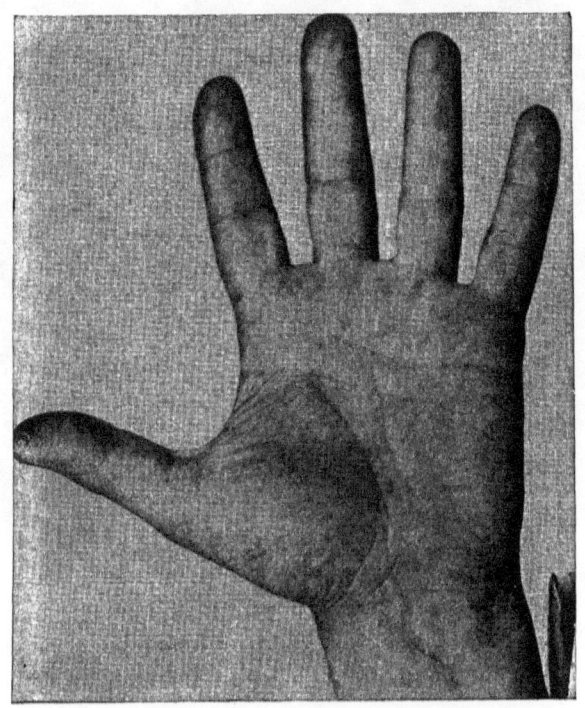

No. 7. Fingers Set Even on Palm

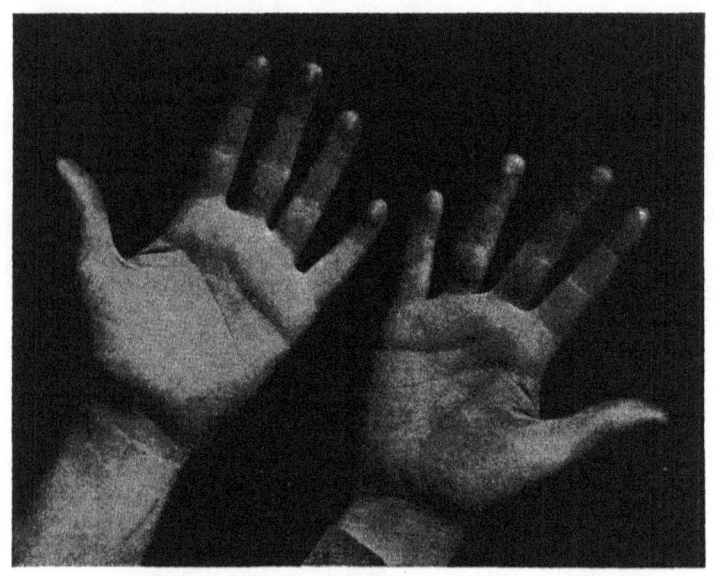

No. 8. A Jupiterian Hand

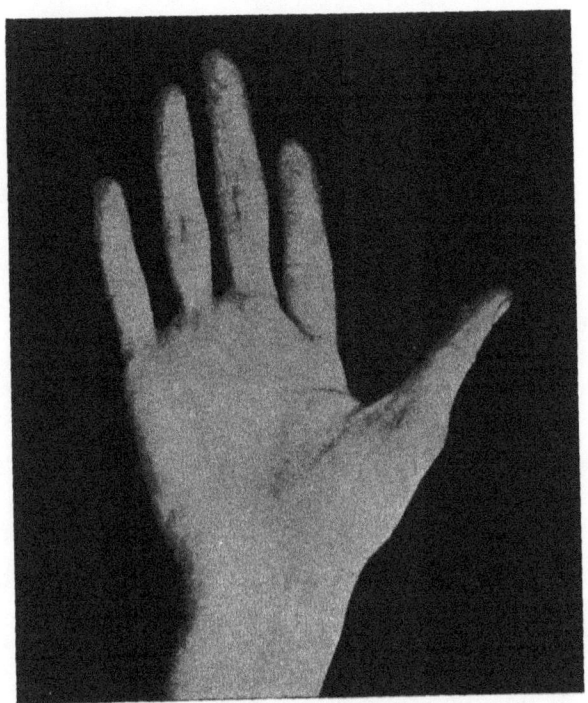

No. 9.   Mount of Jupiter Deficient

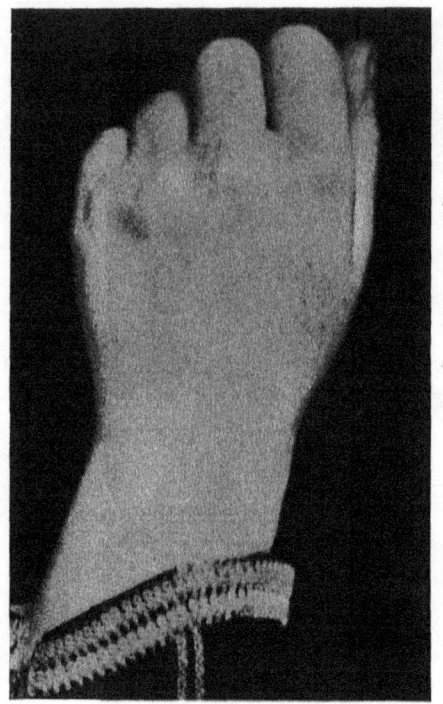

No. 10.   Fine Texture of Skin

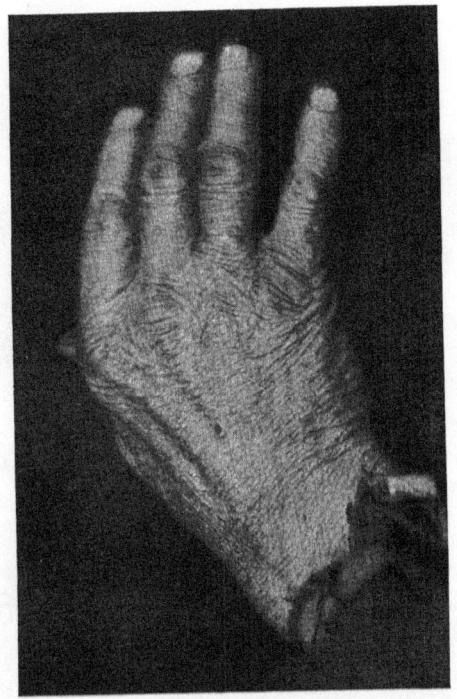

No. 11. Coarse Texture of Skin

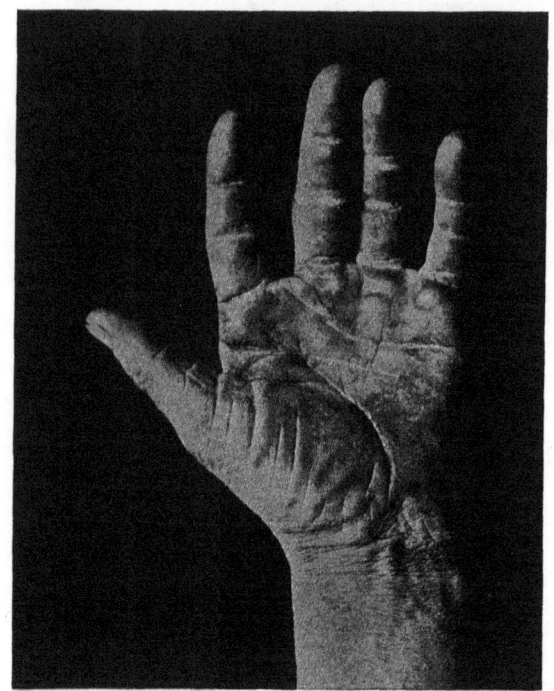

No. 12.   A Stiff Hand

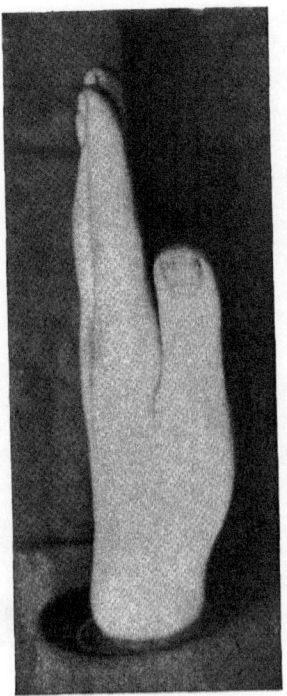

LXII

No. 13. A Straight Hand

LXIII

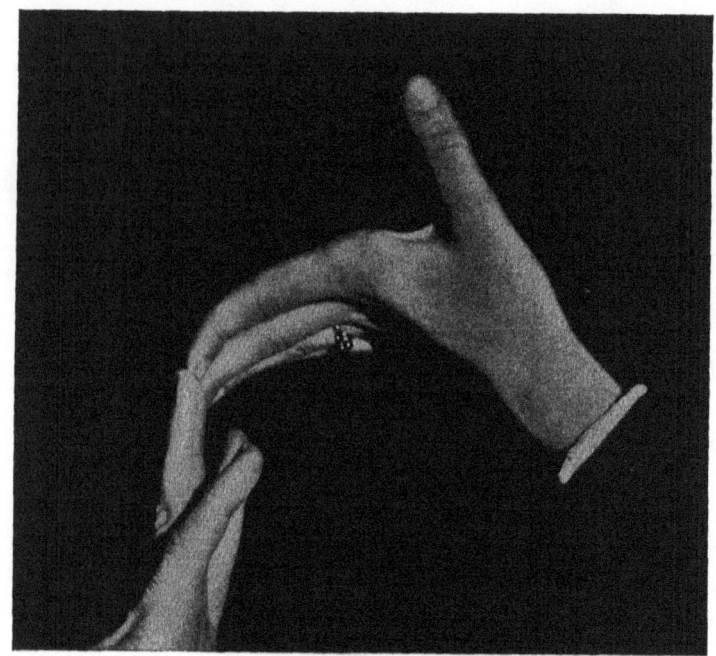

No. 14.   A Flexible Hand

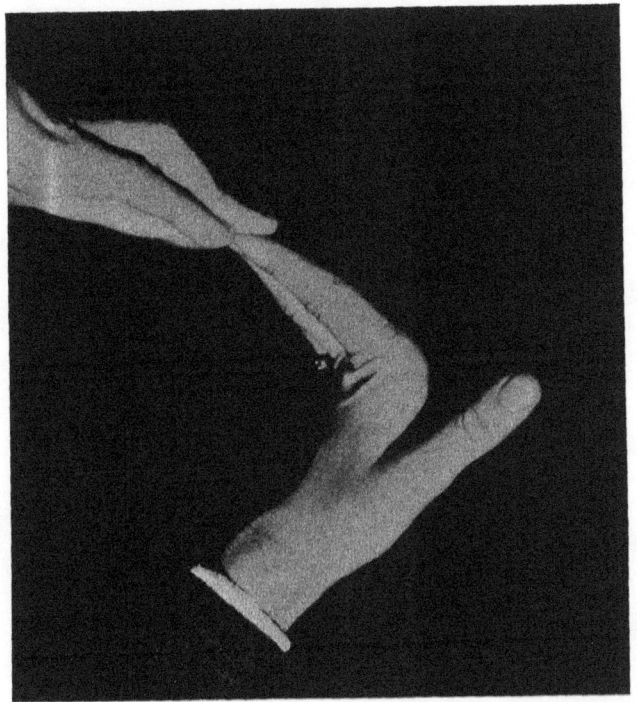

No. 15.   A Super Flexible Hand

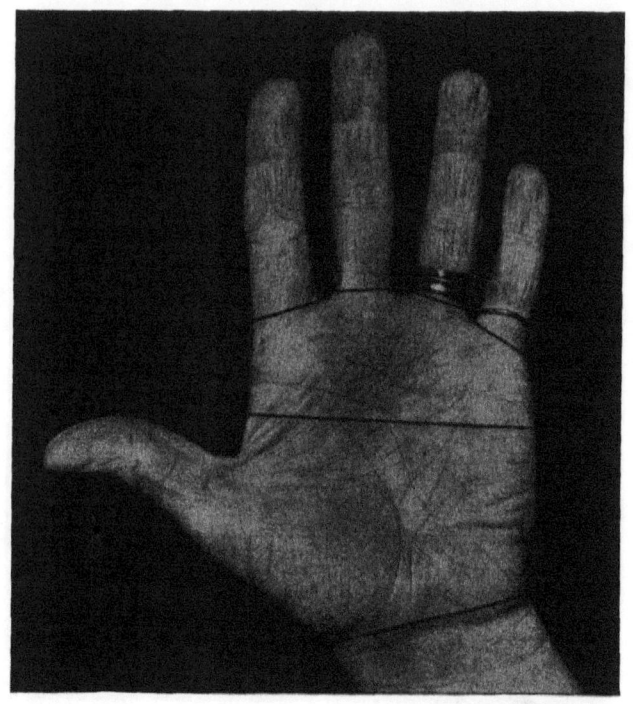

No. 16.   Mental, Middle, Lower Worlds, Hand as a Whole

LXVI

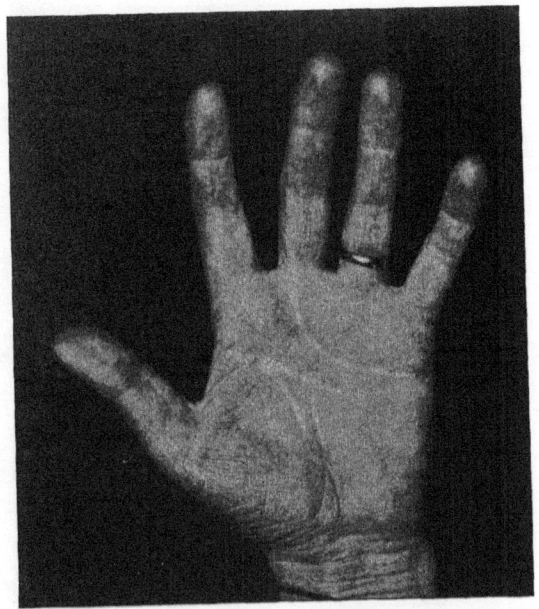

No. 17. Mental Phalanx Long

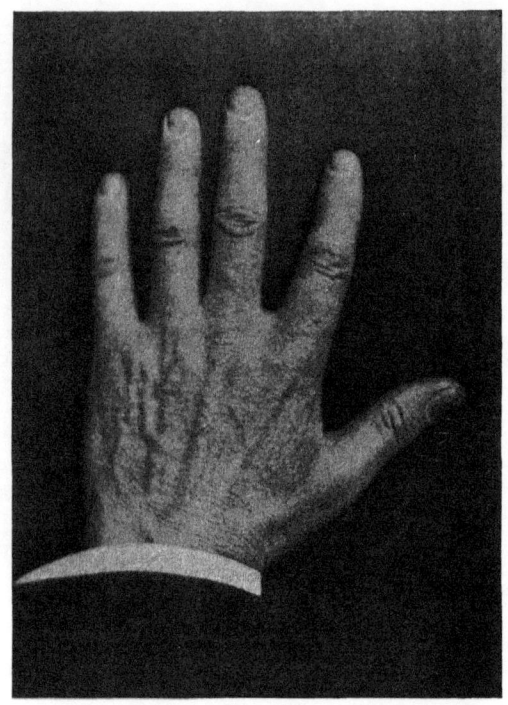

No. 18.   Middle Phalanx Long

LXVIII

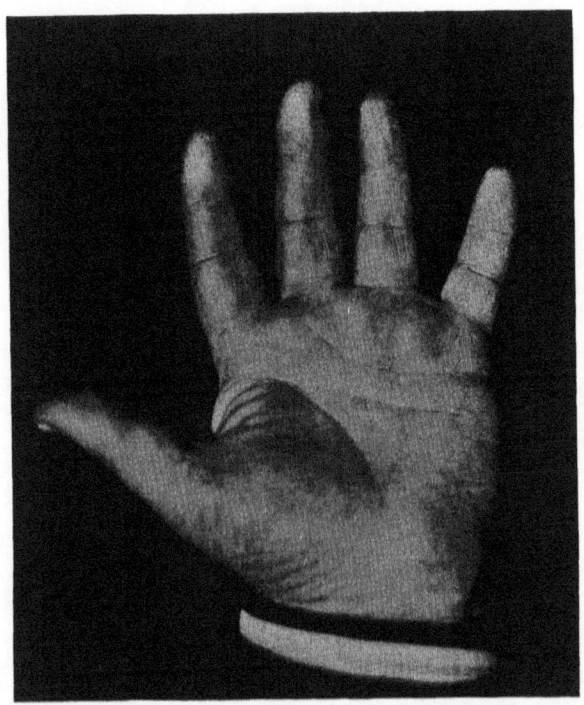

No. 19. Lower Phalanx Thick and Long

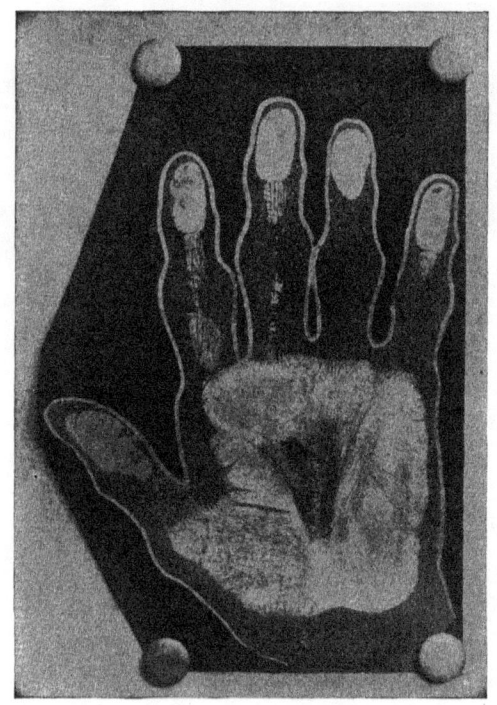

No. 20. Knotty Fingers

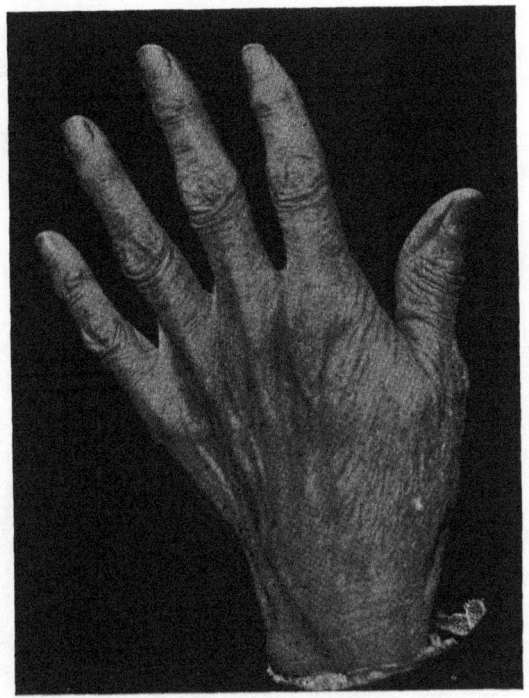

No. 21. Knot of Mental Order

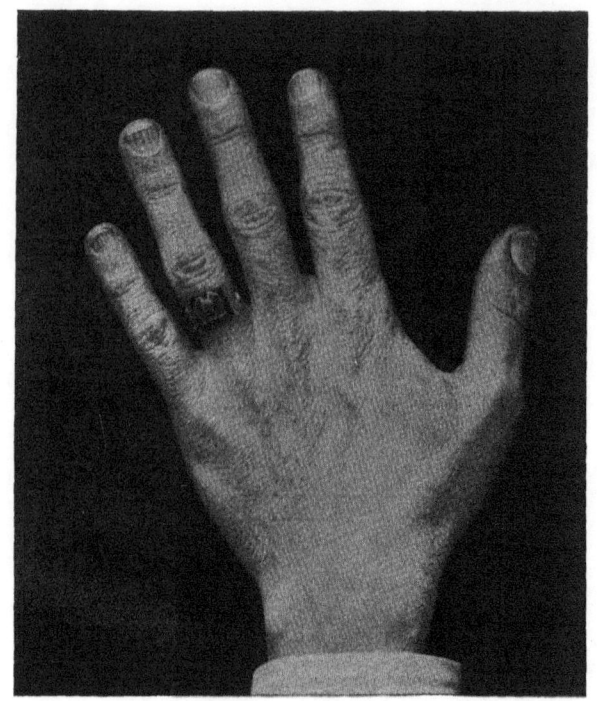

No. 22. Knot of Material Order

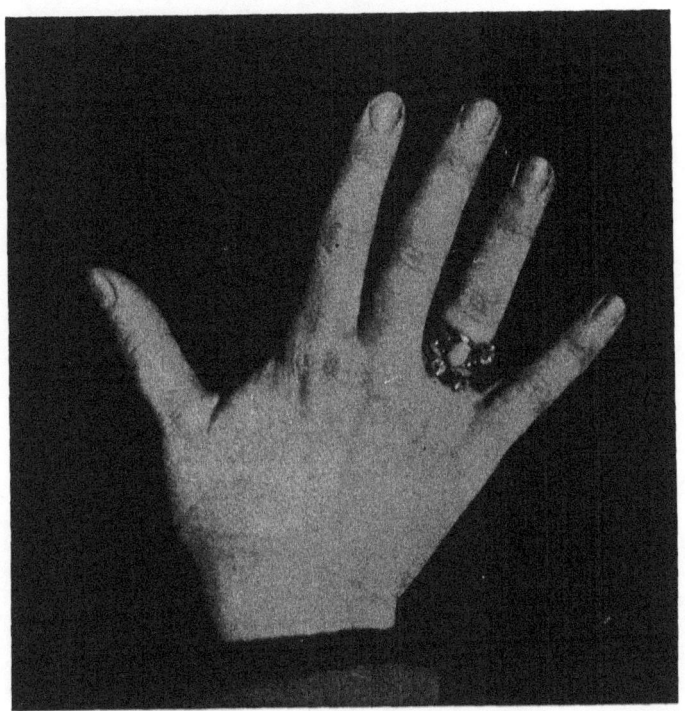

No. 23. Smooth Fingers

LXXIII

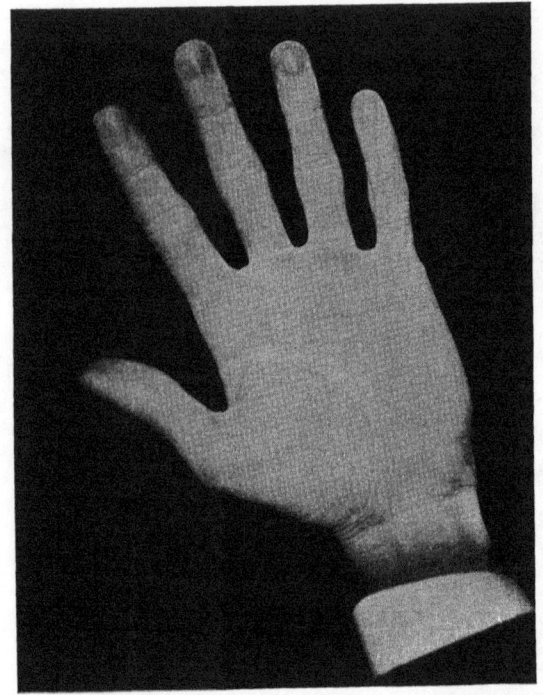

No. 24. Long Fingers

LXXIV

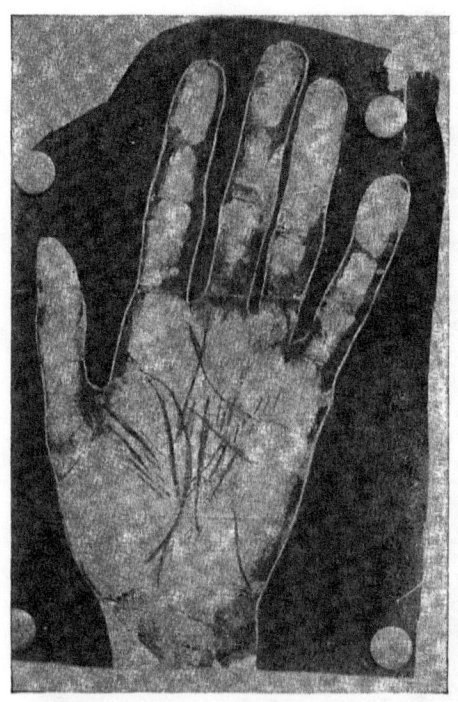

No. 25. Extra Long Fingers

LXXV

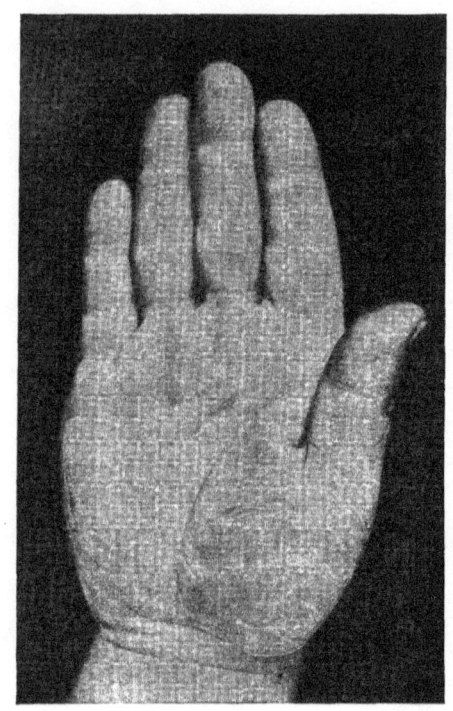

No. 26. Short Fingers

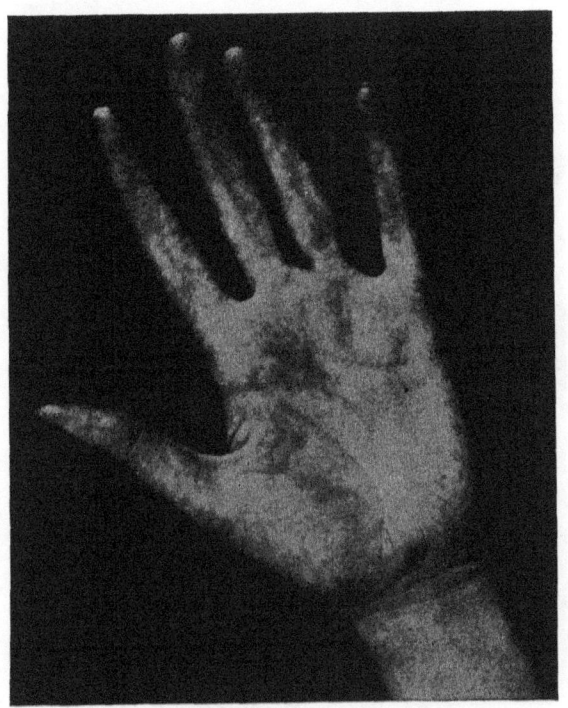

No. 27. Pointed Tips. Pointed Thumb

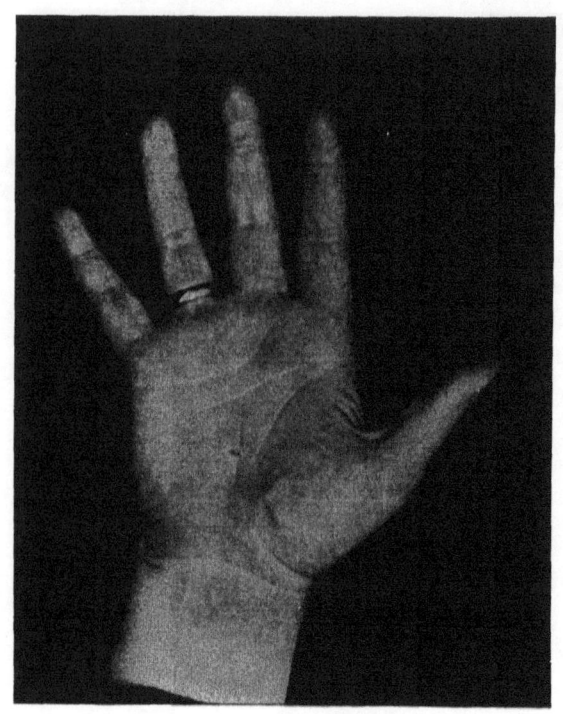

No. 28. Conic Tip

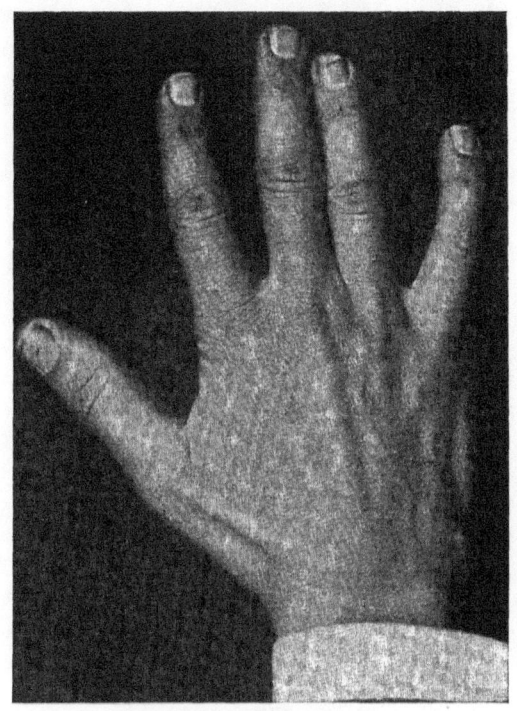

No. 29. Square Tip

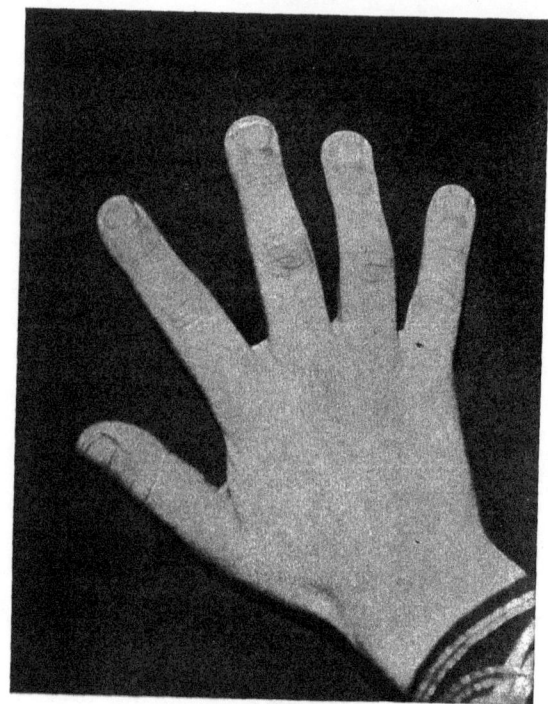

No. 30. Spatulate Tip

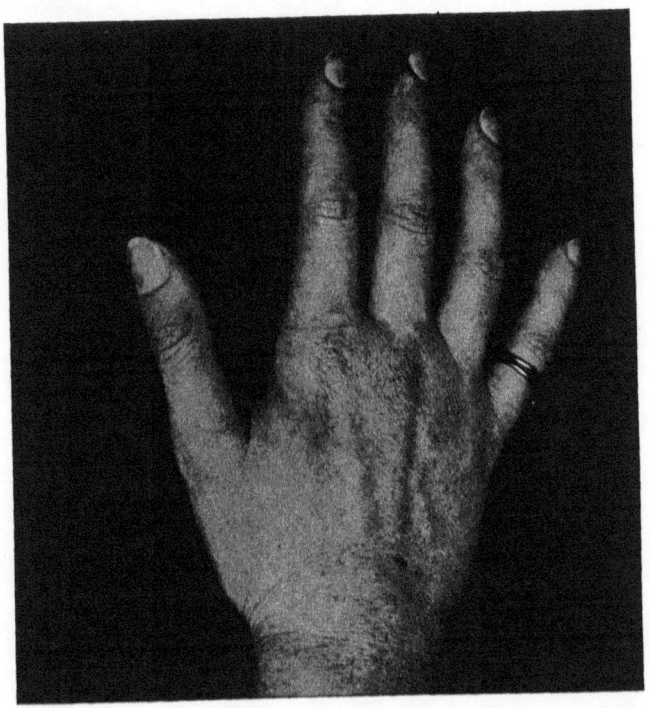

No. 31.   Large Thumb

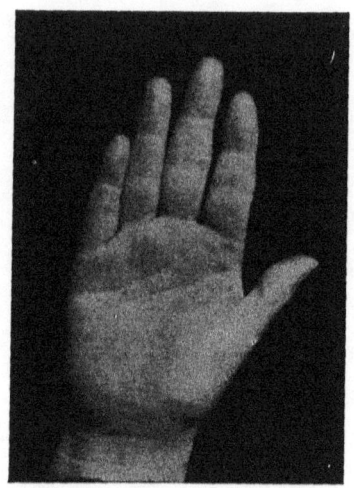

No. 32. Small Thumb

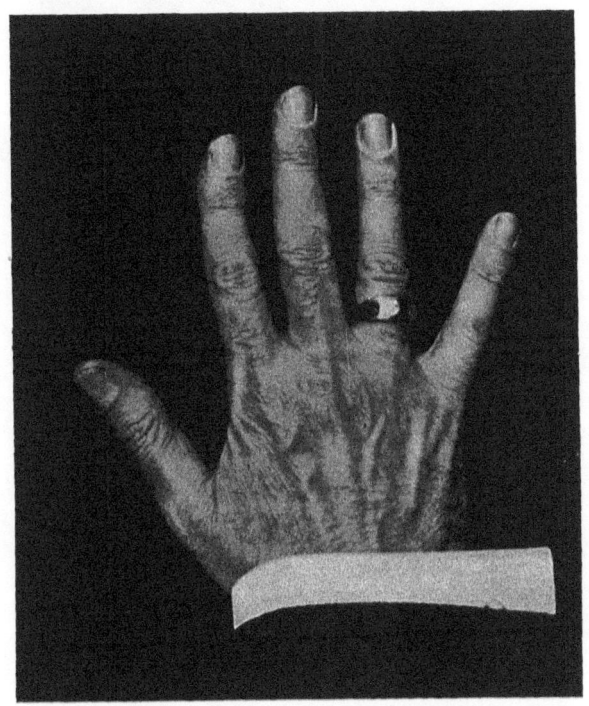

No. 33. Thumb Erect Away from Hand

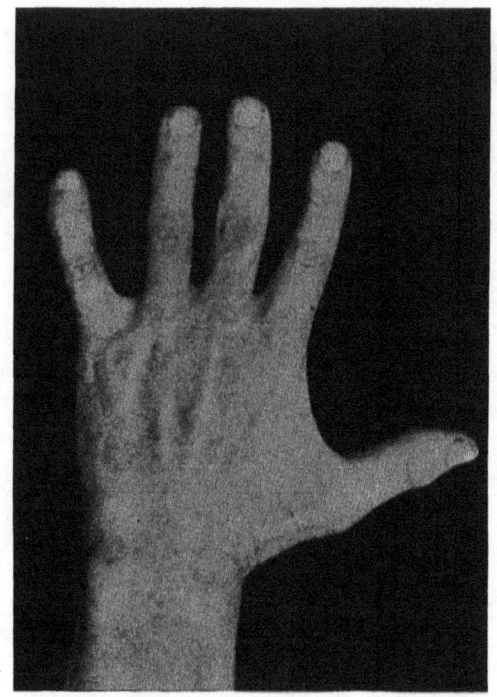

No. 34. Low Set Thumb

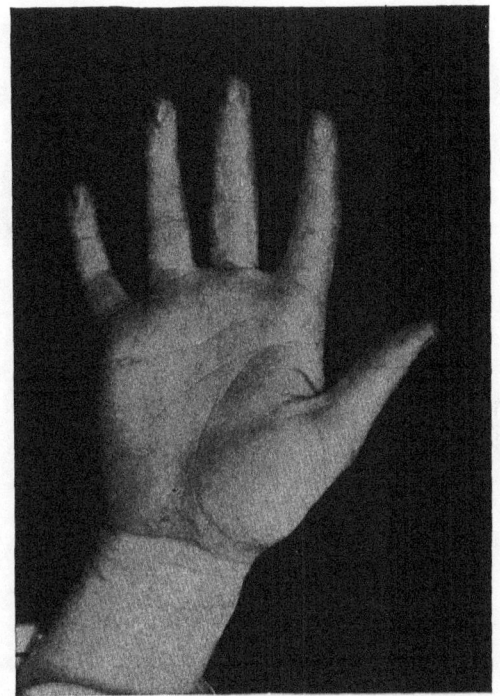

No. 35. Medium Set Thumb

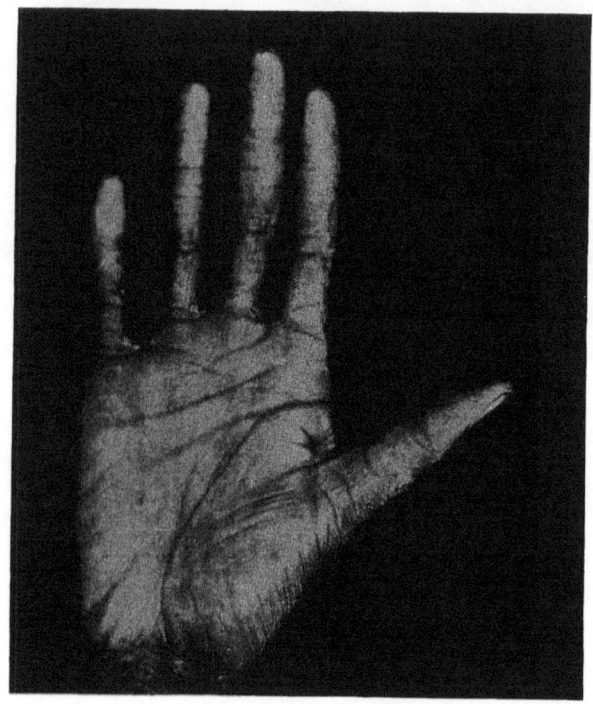

No. 36.   High Set Thumb

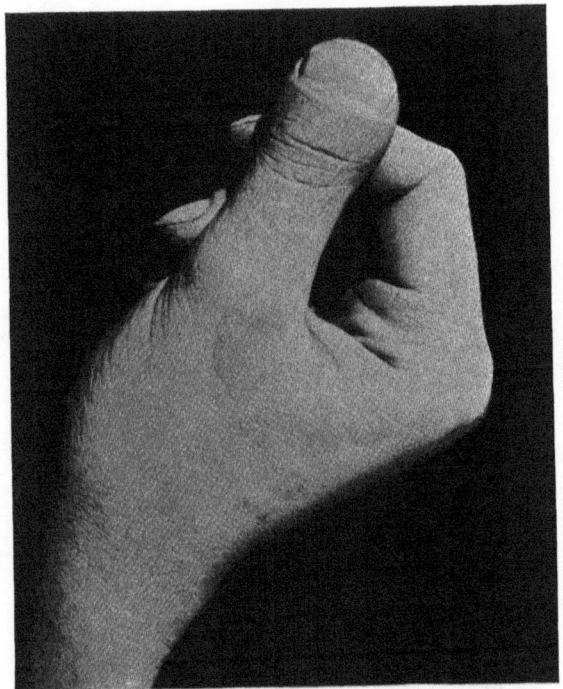

No. 37. Bulbous First Phalanx

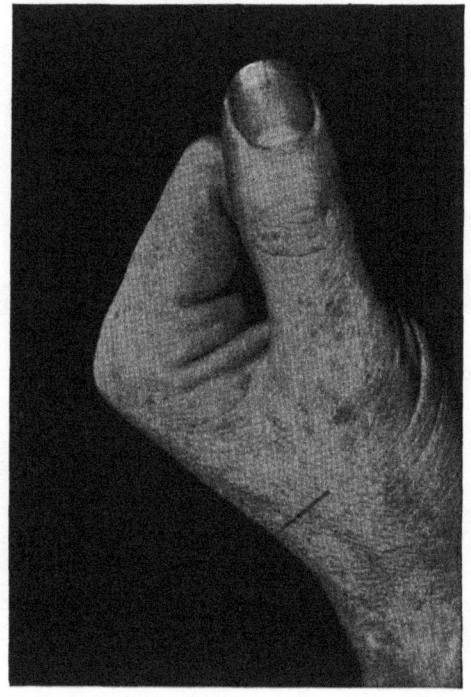

No. 38. Well Formed Long Phalanx. Balanced Phalanges

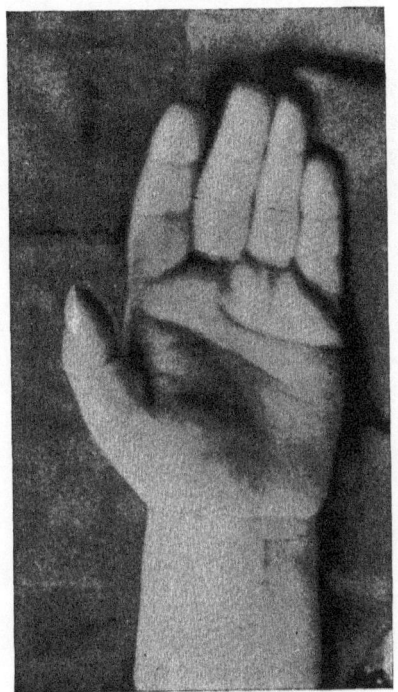

No. 39. Will Phalanx Shorter than Logic

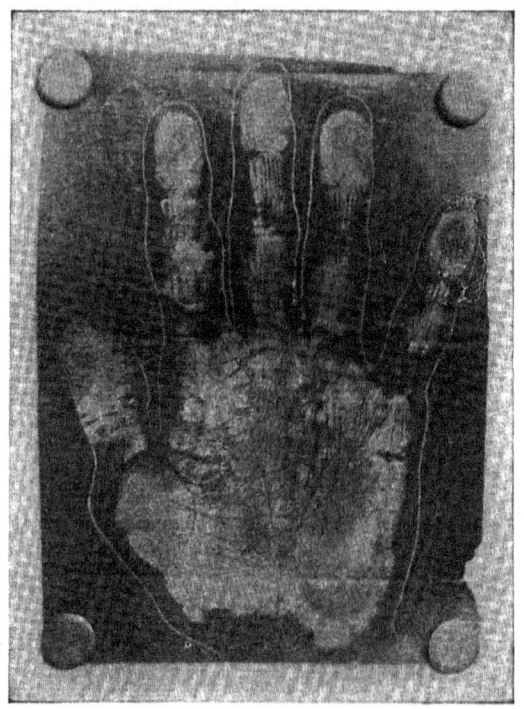

No. 40. Logic Phalanx Shorter than Will

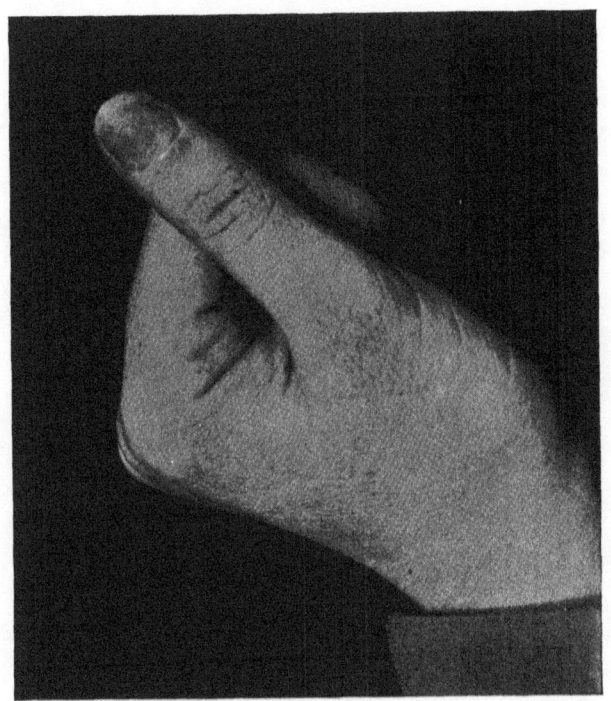

No. 41. Fine Will Phalanx

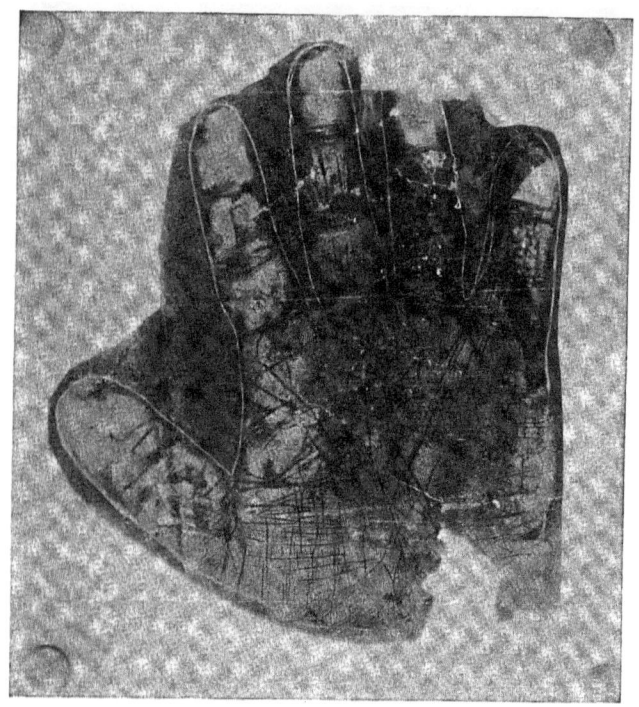

No. 42.   Elementary Thumb

XCII

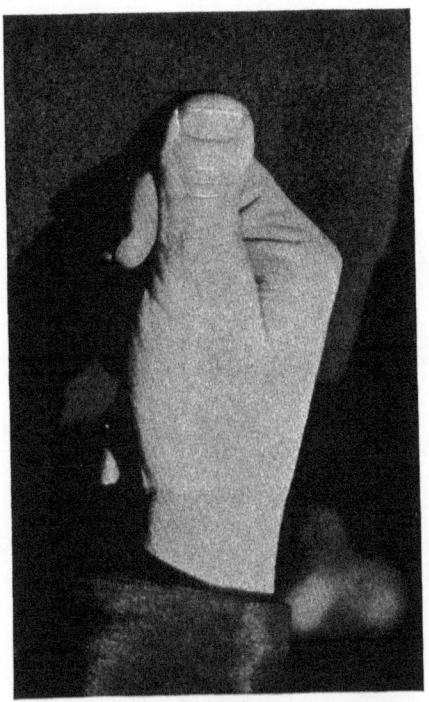

No. 43. Spatulate Tip on Thumb

XCIII

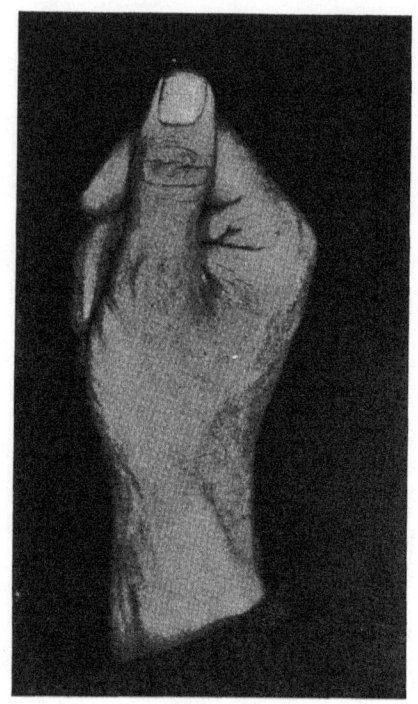

No. 44. Square Tip on Thumb

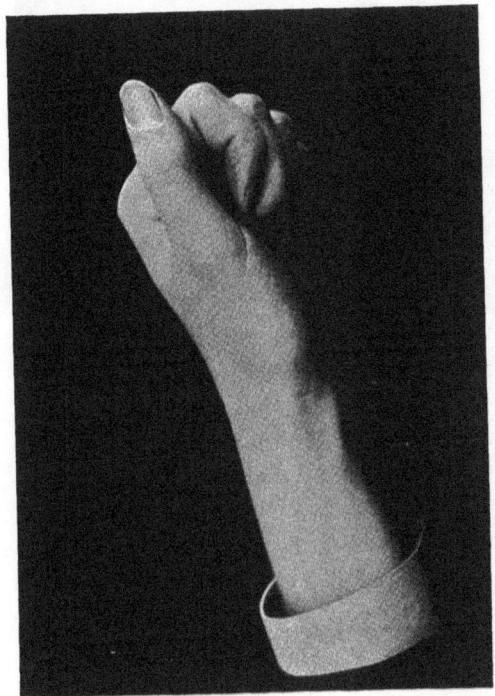

No. 45.   Conic Tip on Thumb

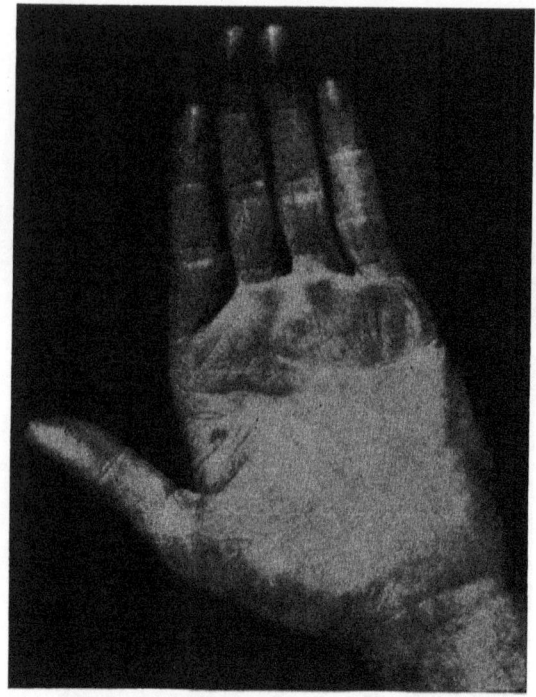

No. 46. A Saturnian Hand

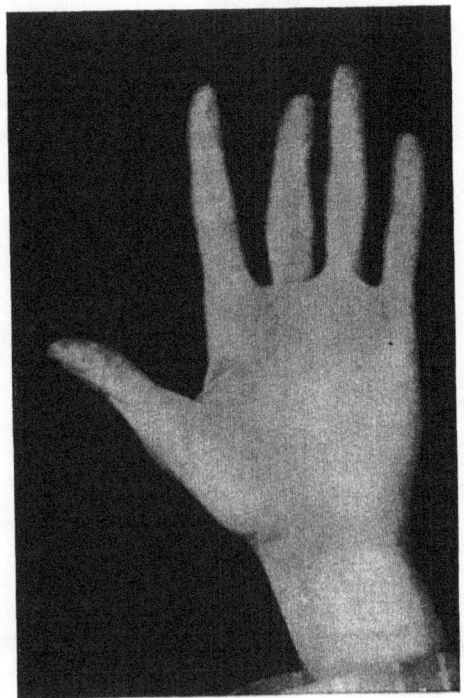

No. 47.   Mount of Saturn Deficient

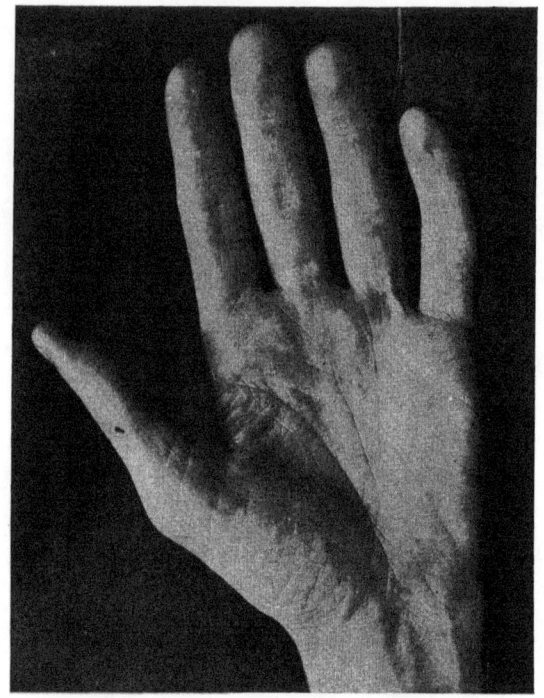

No. 48.   An Apollonian Hand

XCVIII

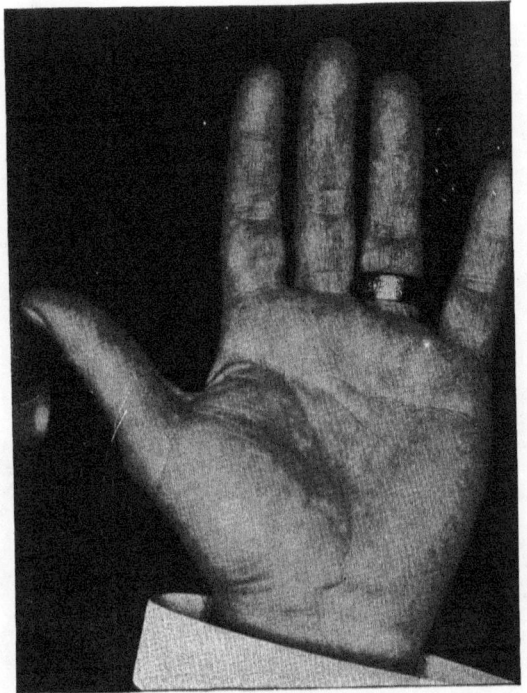

No. 49. An Apollonian Hand

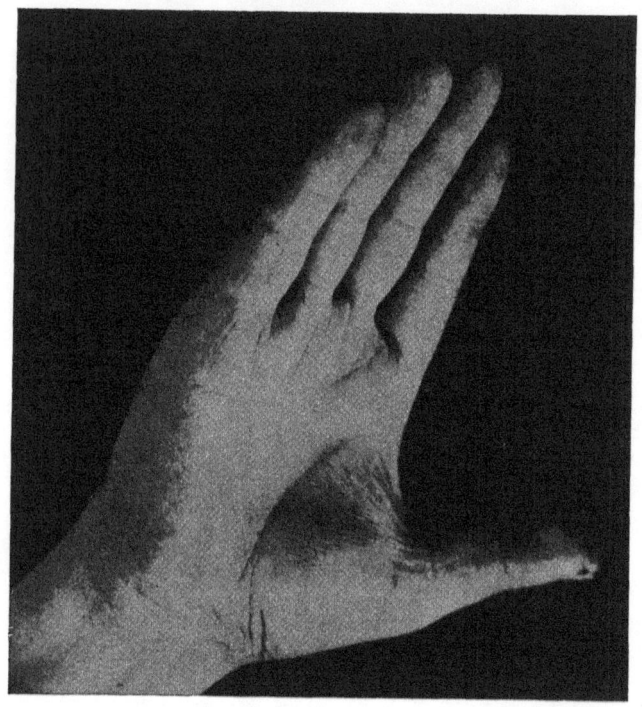

No. 50. A Mercurian Hand

C

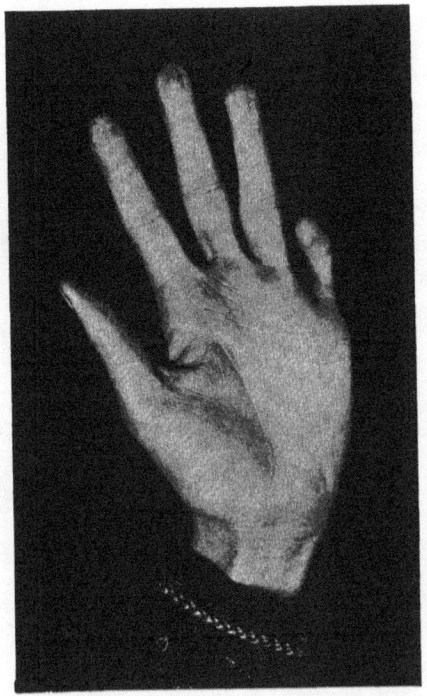

No. 51. Mount of Mercury Deficient

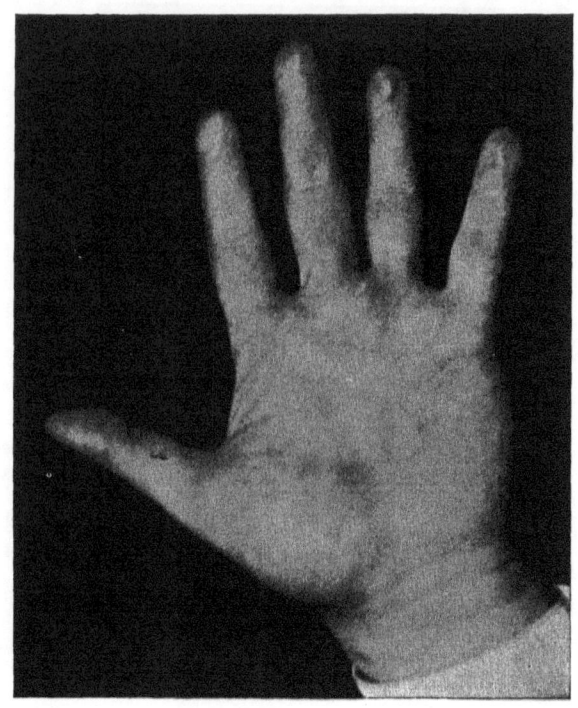

No. 52. Upper Mount of Mars

CII

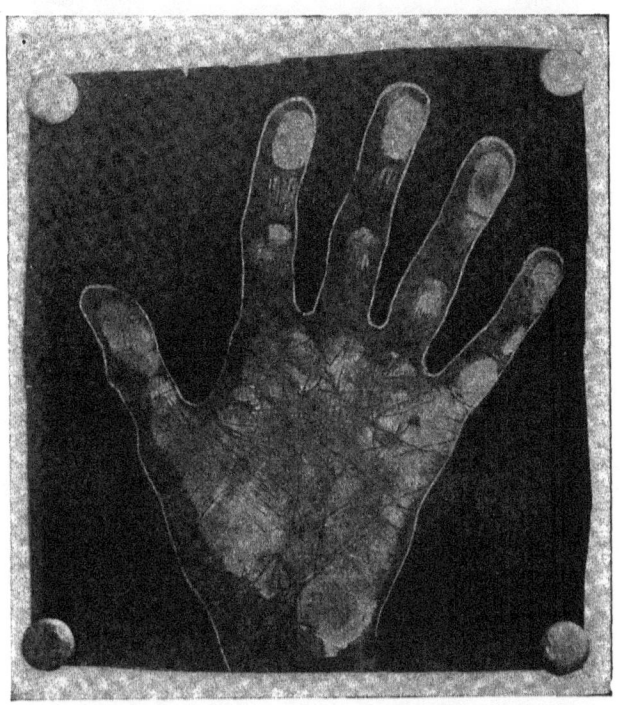

No. 53. Upper Mount of Mars Deficient

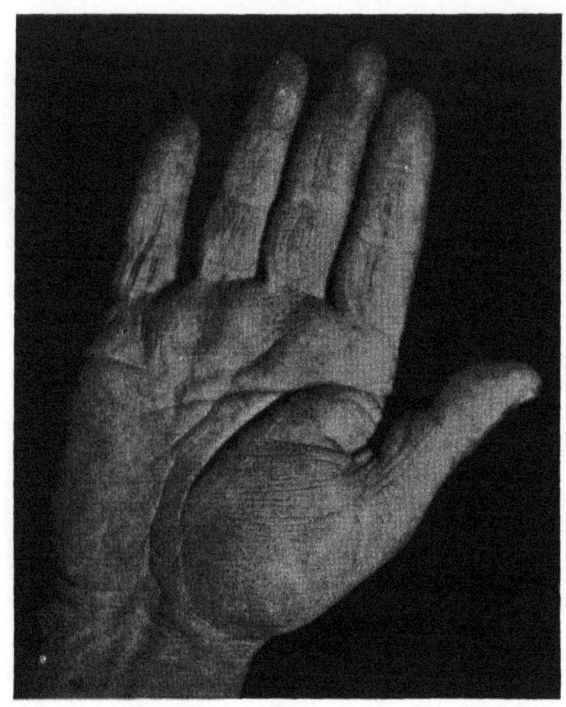

CIII

No. 54. Lower Mount of Mars

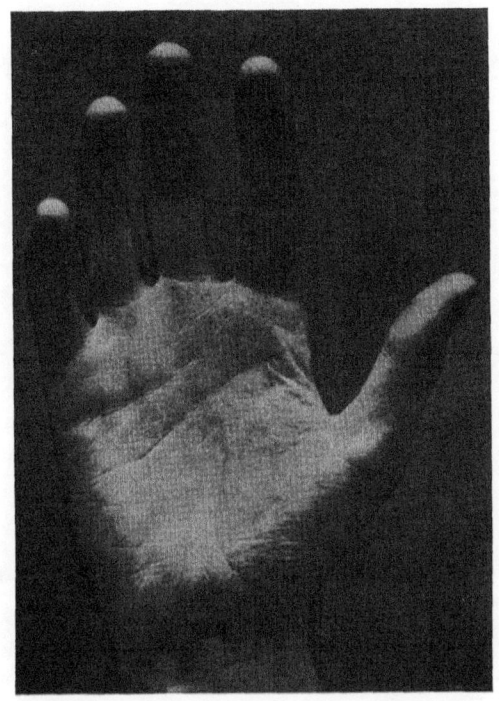

No. 55. Lower Mount of Mars Deficient

CV

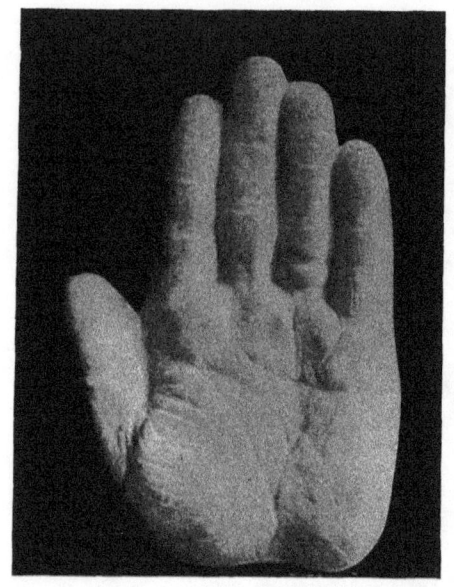

No. 56. A Lunarian Hand

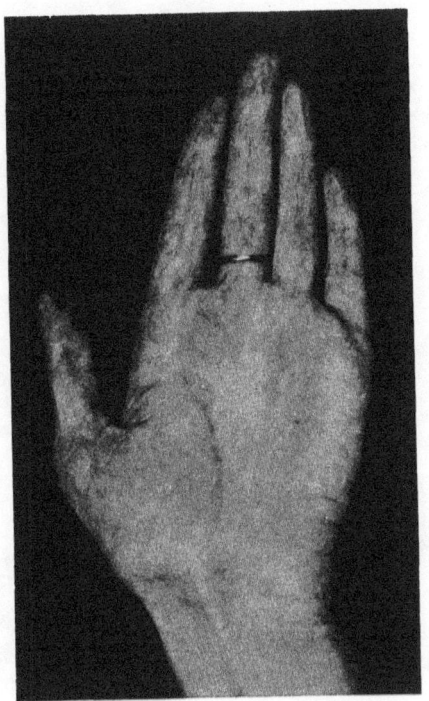

No. 57.　Lunarian Mount Deficient

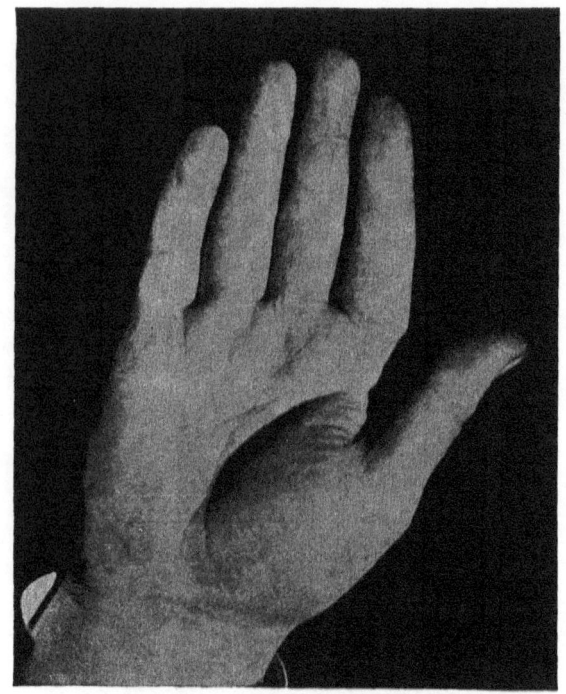

No. 58.   A Venusian Hand

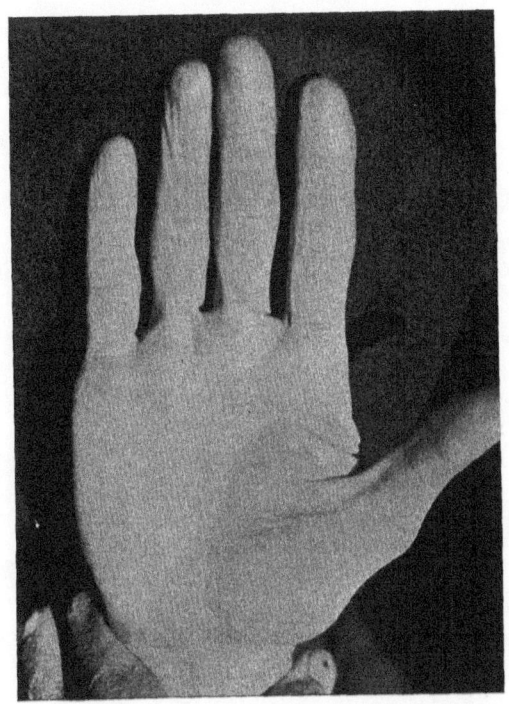

No. 59. Mount of Venus Deficient

CHAPTER ONE

THE JUPITERIAN MOUNT TYPE

The Leader

Let no one be discouraged. Every child can be successful. Some in high positions, some as subordinates, some quite successful and happy at manual labor. In one of these spheres every child must work. Success waits for each, in the vocation for which he is best fitted. This book and a willing parent can bring the child and success together.

HOW TO CHOOSE VOCATIONS
FROM THE HANDS

CHAPTER ONE

THE JUPITERIAN MOUNT TYPE

THE Jupiterian is the first of the Mount types which we will study, the map showing location of the Mounts being shown in Plate 1. We will begin our study of this Mount type by supposing that the child under examination is a pure specimen of the type, and for the purpose of understanding the type thoroughly, an adult male. The Jupiterian, as we first speak of him, is an effort to place before you a mental picture of the type. The Jupiterian occupations, when we begin to speak of them and use the word child, mean that a Jupiterian child will be fitted for them when he is grown. The type is also plentifully represented among the female sex, and the general description and attributes of the female follow very closely those of the male.

THE JUPITERIAN HAND

In order that you may visualize a well developed Jupiterian hand, we are inserting at this time a beautiful specimen in Plate 8. The subject from whose hands this plate was made is one of the best known women in America, and her life has been a splendid example of success arising from the use of the highest side of Jupiterian qualities.

Please note in this plate the high Mount of Jupiter, with the finger standing straight and independent and all of the other fingers leaning toward it. In such a case as this, you do not have to go into any detail to determine the leading Mount, it stands out clearly, and in the consideration of this Mount type please bear in mind the appearance of the hands in Plate 8 as a perfect specimen of Jupiterian development, and judge

3

other hands from it. We also show you in Plate 9 a perfect specimen of the complete absence of Jupiterian development, and from these two extremes you should be able to judge
the degree of development of any hands with which you come
in contact.

In the present book, we are giving our entire attention to
the hands of children, and young men and women of college
age, and no child has reached the full adult development of
hands such as are shown in Plate 8 at the time of life when
we wish to give him his first examination. But his hands *will*
show soon after birth, by the apices centrally located and the
way the finger is held, to which Mount type he belongs, and the
full development of his hands confirming our first opinion will
come later. His character will take on the Jupiterian qualities
in proportion to the degree of development of his hands, as his
age increases. By the time the child has reached maturity
his description, appearance, and characteristics will tally
closely with the description of the pure type given in succeeding pages and knowing from the *very beginning* that this will
be the case, and having bent our efforts from his earliest years
toward the development of his Jupiterian qualities, he is ready,
as soon as he reaches the age of maturity, to make the most
of them and achieve the success to which his type qualities
entitle him.

Describing the Jupiterian

The pure Jupiterian is of medium height. He is not the
tallest of the seven types; that distinction belongs to the
Saturnian; neither is he the shortest, for this honor belongs
to the Mercurian. He is, however, a large man, very strongly
built and inclined to be fleshy. His flesh is solid and not fat,
nor does it partake of the spongy softness of the Lunar type.
His bones are large, strong and well able to support his weight.

He has a smooth, clear skin which inclines to be fine in
texture, pink in color, and healthy looking. His eyes are large
and expressive, the pupils are clear and dilate under the play
of emotions.

The eyebrows are arched and the hair grows evenly, giving
the brows a clearly defined outline. The nose is straight and well
formed, tending to be large in size, and often Roman in shape.

The legs and feet are shapely and of medium size, but

strong and firm. The walk is stately and dignified. The hair is brown or running into chestnut.

The chest is well developed, and his lungs are bellows from which is forced a rich, musical voice, which is just the voice to give words of command, or speak to or influence a multitude; helping to make the Jupiterian the natural leader that he is.

JUPITERIAN CHARACTERISTICS

The Jupiterian is a strong type physically and he is just as strong in characteristics, belonging to the good types and those which are known as spontaneous. The leading characteristic of the Jupiterian is *AMBITION*, and in fine children the ambitions are for advancement in the best grades of occupations, the aspirations are lofty and the type qualities assist them to realize these ambitions and be successful in them. Even in the coarser developments of the Jupiterian type, he still has great ambition, and if he is only a digger in trenches, he will be the leader in his group and will wield an influence with his companions. In nearly every case this influence will be for good.

As a result of ambition, the Jupiterian child has the quality of *LEADERSHIP*, which is the second strong characteristic of the type. This faculty of leadership will extend from the most exalted positions to those of the day laborer, but in each strata you will find the Jupiterian child leading the rest with no great effort to do so. It is the inherent type quality that he has, which seems to communicate itself to those around him in an unconscious manner.

His third important characteristic is that he is naturally *RELIGIOUS*. Examples of this type are to be found in exalted places in all the churches, both as members and as clergymen, and they are very successful in the ministry and in all occupations relating to religious efforts. Many conspicuous members of the type have been bishops and missionaries of a high order of ability.

The fourth conspicuous quality of this type is a high sense of *HONOR*. This is very marked and extends through all the ranges of degree in fineness or coarseness. So we find the Jupiterian child highly trustworthy, making him a confidant in whom you can rely and fitting him to be custodian of sums of money, or an ambassador in charge of important secrets.

The fifth prominent characteristic is a *LOVE OF NATURE*. Here he seems to find expression for all the other qualities, for it is commonly agreed that he who has a love of nature has a love of all that is good.

The sixth leading quality of the Jupiterian is *PRIDE*, which in the proper quantity, is a great force for good, for it makes one anxious to succeed, anxious to realize ambitions, and so becomes a spur to effort which results in bringing out the extreme strength of any child.

DIGNITY is the seventh strong characteristic of the Jupiterian and well becomes his type with its strength, its fine appearance, its size, and its qualities.

As he expends a large part of his effort in making a good impression on his associates, dignity becomes an asset of value, and often silence and dignity will make an ordinary man seem like a philosopher; thus dignity will enable a Jupiterian child to attain an end that would not be possible without it.

The great forces inherent in the Jupiterian type, when marshaled, are found to be:

> Ambition
> Leadership
> Religion
> Honor
> Love of Nature
> Pride
> Dignity

These contain within themselves the possibilities of a happy and successful life which may extend itself into many fields of activity.

THE JUPITERIAN AND MARRIAGE

The Jupiterian has very definite views on marriage. His ambitious nature expresses itself in his choice of a wife. For him to be happy he must be exceedingly proud of the one he chooses, and she must have a commanding presence, physical beauty, charm of manner, and intelligence. In most cases he makes his choice from one of his own type or one of the Venusian type, these two types embodying more of the qualities he desires than any of the others, and if his choice is well made he is happy in the marriage relation. But if he chooses one who becomes slovenly, careless in appearance, or who does not use taste in dress and strive for charm of manner, his pride is wounded and he becomes tired of her.

JUPITERIAN HEALTH

Each one of the types has health peculiarities, and a predisposition to be attacked by certain diseases, and the Jupiterian is no exception to this rule. As we have seen, he is a vigorous individual, with a large frame and great energy. Thus he requires a considerable amount of food which he enjoys and which he consumes in immense quantities. As a consequence he suffers from the sin of overeating and his health defects are those which arise from a disordered stomach. Indigestion often affects the action of his heart, producing vertigo and apoplexy in extreme cases. He is also subject to gout, eczema, various rashes, and often weak lungs.

JUPITERIAN QUALITIES

There are many things about a Jupiterian of pure type, such as we have described above, which strongly influence his career. He cannot help but feel his strength, and this makes him self confident. He relies upon his own judgment and seldom asks advice. He feels his influence pervading those with whom he comes in contact, he hears the richness of his own voice, he blusters a bit, he is not free from vanity but he is kindly and warm hearted, all of which qualities aid him to acquire leadership which he ever desires.

He is an aristocrat, is independent, but his sense of fairness often leads him to be the champion of the plain people in politics which endears him to them and makes him a very successful politician. He keeps his friends, is a general favorite of all classes who often force him into desirable positions. All of these qualities are favorable to a career in the Church, and as the Jupiterian child is inherently religious, he inclines to enter the ministry in which calling he succeeds admirably. His speaking voice gives him a great advantage, and his presence and desirable qualities bring him the confidence of his fellows. No one succeeds in politics better than a Jupiterian. Whatever his grade he is a "vote getter" and always a capable political

"Boss." Ambition causes him to seek important offices which he fills with credit to himself and his party.

In business he is found in high places. If he is started on a business career when he is young, his qualities will take him to important offices which he can fill with distinction. A well educated Jupiterian child is versatile enough to adapt himself to circumstances under nearly all conditions.

THE JUPITERIAN ENTITY

There is contained in the above description of a Jupiterian and his qualities, the complete picture of an individual beginning with his personal appearance, and going through his leading characteristics, his marriage relations, his health peculiarities, and a list of attributes concerning his relations with his fellow men. It must be plain, that having identified one of this type who is a pure specimen, we have a very intimate knowledge not only of his personality, but of his thoughts upon important questions, his likes and dislikes, and his attitude toward his fellow creatures. In other words, how he is going to use his talents in his journey through life.

We claim, that having this knowledge we can make life much easier for him, much happier, for we can see to it that he has a chance to do the things he can do best, to live the life that will bring him the greatest success and happiness.

THE SECONDARY TYPE

We now start upon a study which will give us a complete understanding of the Jupiterian child.

We must find out which of the types is *secondary* to the primary Jupiterian type, and how strong this secondary type is, for here we will learn what forces from other types are to assist the child to achieve success.

SATURN SECONDARY TYPE

Next to the Mount of Jupiter stands the Mount of Saturn, and first we examine it to see if Saturn is to be the strongest force behind the Jupiterian child. If we find the Mount of Saturn leaning toward Jupiter, the apex leaning in the same direction, it will show that Jupiter is stronger than Saturn. If in addition we find the finger of Saturn also leaning (as in Plate 8), it will be a further strong indication that this is the secondary Mount, and if no other Mount shows stronger evidence, we may conclude that our decision must be given to Saturn.

When this is the case, the soberness, wisdom, and all the various balancing qualities of the Saturnian will support the Jupiterian child and he may enter the fields of research, notably in mineralogy, soil analysis, and food values; in laboratory experiments, in chemistry, physics or astronomy, many of the sciences, and he can make an excellent teacher in all the grades from the elementary schools to the head of a university, especially of philosophy and literature. Saturn has also, in addition to his scientific ability, great aptitude for all occupations relating to agrarian pursuits and mining, which will enable the Jupiterian-Saturnian child to occupy important positions in clay, stone, and glass industries, such as brick yards, tile factories, marble quarries or potteries. In plants manufacturing or working in such products, the fine grades of Jupiterian children can be the executives, and as the grades decrease in fineness the positions he occupies must be reduced in importance to fit his grade, such as mixers, molders, blasters, or blowers. The positions which a Jupiterian-Saturnian child can fill, extend through all the range of office positions in fine grades, into the factory and manufacturing departments with lower grade children, even down to the common labor which does the rough work in the plants. If a child is of a grade where he cannot be assigned to anything better than day laborer, he will be more successful and happy if he is connected with an industry for which his type has aptitude.

The Jupiterian-Saturnian child can engage successfully in brick molding, in terra cotta factories, lime, cement, sand and artificial stone factories, or marble and stone yards. He can also be successful, owing to the Saturnian Mount, in fertilizer factories, paint and varnish factories, powder mills, cartridge, dynamite, fuse and fireworks factories, and soap factories. In all of these occupations the Saturnian has ability which as the secondary Mount he imparts to the Jupiterian-Saturnian child. There are a vast number of positions in factories of this character where all grades of children can be successfully employed. The Jupiterian-Saturnian child will be a student, he has the ability to understand the most abstruse problems, he can write a profound treatise on philosophy with great understanding and can have great success as a professor of philosophy in a large college. He can be most successful as a teacher in schools or academies on such subjects as history, literature, composition, both prose and poetry; he can make a most successful president of a college and can teach music in all its forms, harmony, theory, counterpoint, or with proper training can be successful as a pianist or violinist, presupposing in all these cases that his grade is fine.

APOLLO SECONDARY TYPE

Often we find the Mount of Apollo (Plates 48, 49) as the secondary Mount, in which case the artistic qualities of the Apollonian will be added to the Jupiterian child and he can succeed in many forms of artistic endeavor. According to his grade this will take him from a house painter, a worker in stucco, an interior decorator, a designer, on through portrait, landscape, and miniature painting to sculpture. The practical side of all of these artistic employments will be aided by the Jupiterian qualities. Saturn as the secondary Mount is not as natural a combination for the Jupiterian child as Apollo.

The artistic ability of the Apollonian as the secondary Mount will greatly aid the Jupiterian child in all artistic occupations. He may be at the head of companies, or an officer in corporations engaging in the manufacture of artistic goods, such as tapestries, lace curtains, embroideries, silks, or period furniture, or he can be successful in the sales departments of these companies if his grade be fine, or he can occupy positions in all the departments down the line as his grade decreases, such as weavers, cabinet-makers, finishers or packers. He may be a window dresser, draper, carpet, curtain, or rug designer, or salesman, or if of lower grade, hold positions in the factories manufacturing these products. He can be successful in stores selling curios, antiques, and novelties, as owner, buyer, or salesman, according to his grade. Or in the same capacities in dry goods, fancy goods, or novelty stores, five and ten cent and variety stores, or as owner, buyer, or salesman in jewelry stores, furniture stores, florists, or in stores or factories in the following lines: costumes for sale or rental, Jap goods, ladies tailors, gift shops, and they will be very successful in sales promotion in all these lines and as owner and teacher in dancing schools.

MERCURY SECONDARY TYPE

Sometimes we find Mercury as the secondary Mount (Plate 50), and this will accentuate the business side of the Jupiterian child. The shrewdness of the Mercurian added to the friend-making qualities of the Jupiterian child will make a very strong combination for a career in the business world, and such a child can make a success in salesmanship, ranging all the way, according to grade, from a house to house peddler in the coarse grades, to the head of a national sales organization.

Many Mercurians also make excellent doctors and lawyers, and a secondary Mount of Mercury can make the Jupiterian child a success in either of these professions. It will be more likely to do so if the first phalanx of the finger of Mercury be long, the finger well developed, and the medical stigmata on the Mount of Mercury well marked.

The addition of the Mount of Mercury to the Jupiterian child can enable him to be successful, according to his grade, in stores or manufactories in the following lines (if of fine grade, in executive positions, and in the lower grades in the less important positions): gloves, hosiery, ribbons, radio, as program producers and announcers, in women's apparel, vending machines, shirts, silks, beverage, as clothing manufacturers, and they can be most successful as bridge instructors, caterers, promoters, in shopping service, as a lecturer and in a lecture bureau, as a market analyst and counselor, as insurance agents or officials, in real estate, department stores, clothing and men's furnishing stores, cigar stores, and banking in all the positions from the president down to the doorman.

MARS SECONDARY TYPE

A very natural combination is to find either of the Mounts of Mars as secondary Mounts to a Jupiterian child. In this case the Mounts of Saturn, Apollo, and Mercury will be found to be flat and the Martian Mounts will be full and well colored (Plates 52-54). We have found more of the upper Mounts of Mars as the secondary Mount than of the lower, in which case we find that the courage, coolness, calmness, and the power of resistance of the upper Mount of Mars will make the Jupiterian child determined, daring, and hard to overcome, and such children make excellent soldiers, diplomats, missionaries, explorers, and aviators, all of which are pursuits where courage and daring are required. They are especially capable where resistance is needed.

With the upper Mount of Mars secondary, the Jupiterian child will, according to his grade, be successful in factories manufacturing automobiles, in foreign trade, as a builder, concrete construction contractor, manufacturers' agent, dealer in power plant equipment, as claim adjuster, bridge builder, salesman of heavy machinery, mill supplies, as a ship broker and builder, in railroad equipment either as manufacturer or salesman; as salesman of building material, for commercial agencies, collection agencies, as agricultural implement manufacturer, as bank savings solicitor, as dealer in automobiles, as owner or employee of armor car service, as head of detective agencies, as detective, appraiser, in marine salvage companies, in baggage transfer, timberlands development, or street railway operator in all grades from president to tracklayer.

In all of these activities, the Jupiterian-Martian can be successful.

If the upper Mount of Mars is not so well developed as the lower Mount, and this lower Mount is identified as the secondary Mount, the Jupiterian child will have great aggression and his already strong qualities will be intensified. This is not the best combination for a Jupiterian child and nullifies a good many of his favorable qualities. The aggression of the lower Mount will make him push too fast and much of the diplomacy of the Jupiterian child will be neutralized and as he gains many of his advantages from a diplomatic approach, he will lose by too much Martian aggression.

This combination will be likely to force the Jupiterian-Martian child with the lower Mount secondary, unless he be of exceptionally fine grade, to occupy less important positions. His lack of tact will throw him into the positions of foreman or superintendent if of good grade, and if of lower grade, into positions as workman. He can be successful in such vocations as a stock yard operator, manager of a trucking company, steeple jack, warehouseman, sand blaster, railroad conductor, masseur, mover, road making contractor, animal dealer, bill poster, coal dealer, tanner, life guard, swimming pool instructor, in traffic service, or as wrecking contractor.

Or he can be successful as a fruit grower, nurseryman, lumberman, or in blast furnaces, steel rolling mills, car and railroad shops, brass mills, saw and planing mills, or if of very fine grade he can be successful in any of the occupations recommended for Jupiterian-Martian children with the *upper Mount* secondary.

LUNARIAN SECONDARY TYPE

The Mount of the Moon (Plate 56) is not often found as the secondary Mount in the hand of a Jupiterian child, but when it is, it will be when the other Mounts are flat and the Mount of the Moon stands out in a prominent way. It can always be recognized when such combination exists.

In this case, the coldness and selfishness of the Lunarian will affect the spontaneous qualities of the Jupiterian child and he will not attract people as in the pure type, or with Apollo, Mars, or Venus as the secondary type. He will not succeed in many of the occupations possible with the other combinations. But he will make good as a short story writer where imagination is needed, and he will have a fine command of language and a large vocabulary.

The addition of the imaginative faculties of the Lunarian, which takes place when the Mount of the Moon is the secondary type, adds greatly to the strong qualities of the Jupiterian child, who is inclined to be very matter of fact and little given to flights of fancy.

He can succeed in the conduct of a letter writing service, as an advertising counsel, in outdoor advertising, in poster and radio advertising. In all of these he has special talent. He can also succeed as an art publisher, in concert management, as a translator, an author especially of heroic tales, in teaching lip reading, in the conduct of a book store, in publishing art calendars, in conducting a school of languages, as a magazine publisher, conductor of a clipping bureau, as a librarian, a writer of movie titles, a proof reader, in conducting an information bureau, a publicity service, an entertainment bureau, as a news dealer, a publisher's representative, as conductor of a travel agency or bureau, a literary agency, a teachers agency, or a subscription agency. All of these will furnish occupations in which the Jupiterian-Lunarian child can be successful with proper preparation and if of fine grade. The inferior positions in these occupations must be filled by Jupiterian-Lunarian children of a lesser degree of fineness.

Venus Secondary Type

If the Mount of Venus (Plate 58) is the secondary Mount, it will be very high and full, and in this case the Jupiterian child will be extremely fond of women and will attract them to him. According to his grade, his love affairs will be ideally spiritual, or a display of low passions. He will be very attractive in looks, gracious in manner, and, though often superficial, he will make friends who will help him on his way. He will be extremely fond of music and can be a composer, generally of light and tuneful music.

When Venus is the secondary Mount, it brings to the Jupiterian child love, sympathy, music, grace, and passion, which soften the character of the primary Mount, and lead him into new avenues of endeavor. He can do a number of things which he could not in his pure state. So we can place this child in amusement enterprises as manager, owner, or as performer, and he can be successful in the conduct of art schools. He can be successful as a dealer or manufacturer of artificial flowers, or in conducting a boarding house, as a buyer of carpets, curtains, and rugs; he will do well as a music publisher or song writer, or as a china decorator, in clay modeling, as a clergyman, or a secretary of clubs.

He will do well with concessions at expositions and the business of concessionaire is a respectable and lucrative one for the right person. He can conduct an upholstery shop, or a large upholstery business if his grade be fine. He can be a weaver, a designer of window displays, a dealer in tapestries, he can conduct a theater ticket agency, or deal in theatrical shoes, draperies and effects, toilet articles, and can conduct a school for music, be a piano tuner, run a sightseeing bus, work in a social settlement, or be a worker or dealer in stained glass. He can conduct a store for millinery, be a perfumer, a radio dealer, a play broker, deal in house furnishings, lamps, shades, supplies, and frames. He can be a dealer in precious stones. In all of these occupations the Jupiterian-Venusian child can do well, and a child may be started to fill positions of all kinds in these various lines of business with full assurance that he will be successful. His grade will determine whether he will be at the head of the enterprises or occupy the subordinate positions.

THE TESTS FOR GRADE

By this time, if you have given close attention to the text, you have a good idea of the Jupiterian type and of the support the child may expect from the other types in combination. Our work from now on will be to place the Jupiterian child in his proper grade, as upon his grade will depend whether he holds the best, the medium, or the inferior position in the industries we have recommended.

FIRST TEST—TEXTURE OF THE SKIN

The texture of the skin is the first of the tests we use to determine whether the child is fine or coarse. To judge in this matter we examine the back of the hand where we either find skin smooth, velvety, and soft, or coarser in grade, until we come to some child who has the extremely coarse skin shown in Plate 11.

If the child is of fine grade he will have skin of a fine texture (Plate 10), in which case he can be placed in the better positions in a great many industries in which we have found that a Jupiterian child can succeed. As his skin grows coarser in texture, the child cannot fill the better positions in these same industries, and it is not fair to him to assign him to them. He will however have greater success if he is placed in positions in accordance with his grade, in industries for which his type has special qualification. Between a very fine textured skin of which the hand of a baby is the best example, and the very coarse skin shown in Plate 11, there are many degrees, which with a little practice it is not hard to become familiar. When the skin is of fine grade and the rest of the tests the same, a child can be prepared for the highest positions in the industry chosen for him. He can be president of his corporation, vice president, treasurer, manager, and fill other executive positions, while a child with coarser skin and tests can only fill positions as foreman or superintendent, and as we find children whose grade is still coarser as shown by the tests, they must work at the looms, or run the presses, or work on the assembly line, or be the porter, watchman, timekeeper or fill other positions of similar grade. And when we find one whose skin is as coarse as that shown in Plate 11, he must shovel the coal, dig trenches, and perform the lowest class of manual labor. In other words, the type shows us *which industry* the child should select, the skin and other tests the *kind of a position* in that industry which he can fill. The Jupiterian child will always have the qualities of his type no matter what his grade; he will be ambitious and want to lead the men in his department, and will have all the good qualities that belong to his type, even though he must operate them in lower strata of positions.

Second Test—Color of the Hands

The color of the hands will tell us a great deal about the virility of the child and also a great deal about health conditions.

White Color

White color, which is shown in the palm and under the nails, is not often found in the hands of a Jupiterian child. It does not belong to this type, but it will be found occasionally. This child will not be energetic nor forceful, nor will he be dominant in his relations with others. With white color, the Jupiterian child will allow himself to be led more often than is natural to the type, and when we find it, we must modify to a great extent our estimate of the qualities of the type. Such a child cannot be placed in as prominent a position as he could with a better color. We must find positions for him as clerk, stenographer, stockkeeper, bookkeeper, cashier, or similar positions where he has only routine work to do.

Pink Color

Pink color is natural to the pure specimen of Jupiterian child. Here he has a warming influence which brings out all of the strongest qualities of the type. He will, though a strong type, operate with moderation; there will be no lack of force, but there will not be excess. Pink color will mean a healthful physical condition and this will mean that the attractiveness of the type will be present and in operation. Children with a well developed Mount of Jupiter, fine texture of skin, pink color, and with the first phalanx of the finger of Mercury long, can be placed in the professions, either of law or medicine and wherever a good quality of mental effort is required. They will succeed in the insurance business as general agents, in the brokerage business especially as stock broker, and they can be successful customers' men. They can succeed in the air transportation business, as organizers of chambers of commerce, in conducting a night club or as manager of a restaurant.

Red Color

Red color is found in the hands of Jupiterian children whose grade is not as fine. When red color is seen it is the beginning of the coarsening of the type and much attention should be given to the grade of the skin which will usually show, by its increasing coarseness and roughness, the progressive stages in the descent from a very fine child to one that is coarse. When red color is seen it will at once warn us that the child will be a strong specimen of the type. He will push his ambitions vigorously and as he becomes coarser in grade will become obstinate and tyrannical and, if ignorant, extremely disagreeable. He can be successful, however, in the sale of camping supplies, as a business broker, bridge builder, in the conduct of a hat and coat check room service, as an amusement director, in the conduct of a resort or recreation park, in the conduct of a garage, or in the wholesale or retail lumber, coal or ice business. It will never do to place this child in the finer employments recommended for fine grades of Jupiterian children.

Yellow Color

Yellow color is not often found in the hand of a Jupiterian child. It does not belong to the type, and when it *is* seen, it will be an indication of a health defect. Children of the Jupiterian type who have yellow color, will not do so well in occupations requiring great mental effort. Even if everything in their hands indicates the possession of the better side of Jupiterian type qualities, they must not be assigned as difficult tasks as if the color were pink. They will not have as great powers of concentration, as clear judgment, or as much application with yellow color, nor will their standards be as high. They can be successful as clerks, record keepers, as a nurse in hospitals, or as a ticket taker at theaters, a ticket broker, a house detective in a hotel, a railroad conductor or brakeman, superintendent of a cemetery, superintendent of a park, in the conduct of a vegetable market, a delicatessen or as a combination news, cigar, and novelty dealer.

THIRD TEST—FLEXIBILITY OF THE HANDS

Flexibility of the hands will be important in the hands of the Jupiterian child, for they will show whether a flexible or a stiff mind will rule him.

The Stiff Hand

Beginning with the lowest grade in the scale of flexibility, as shown in Plate 12, a Jupiterian child with stiff hands will be common and coarse, he will be stubborn, ignorant, and no amount of effort will raise his standard of intelligence. Still he will dominate the circle in which he moves and such a child can be the leader of a gang of some sort, often only a social club, many times a gang in the underworld. None of the high ideals of the refined Jupiterian are known to this child and his occupation must be in a common grade of labor in the industries recommended for the Jupiterian child. He can be a press feeder, wash the automobiles in a garage, be a cleaner in a market or butcher shop, work in a rolling mill, drive a truck, be a laborer in an incineration plant, an attendant in an institution for insane or mentally defective, a longshoreman, or work in a stockyard or a fertilizer factory.

The Straight Hand

The straight hand, Plate 13, will be one which cannot be bent backward, but does not cup, and will show a mind that while not brilliant, is still not necessarily coarse. A Jupiterian child with a straight hand will not be dense, but he will not have great adaptability to a large variety of tasks. He can, however, take on a considerable amount of education, and his ideas can be broadened by contact with educated and refined people. Thus he can be fitted for the ministry or work into a ward organization in politics. He can also be prepared for a teacher in a primary school. As a minister, this child will not be above the ordinary; he will be one of those who do not make much stir, but if that is all there is in the child, it will be better for him to be that than something he cannot do as well. It is only because the primary Jupiterian type is religious that he should choose that field. Besides the vocations mentioned, this straight handed child can succeed as a title searcher, a mortgage broker, an exterminator, a dealer in optical goods, field glasses, microscopes and drawing instruments and supplies for engineers, or as a dealer in supplies for gymnasiums such as sport shoes, boxing gloves, punching bags, and the many devices sold by such stores, such as trapeze, turning bars, rings, and exercise horses. It will depend to a great extent upon his thumb how far this child goes in these enterprises, for even if his ambition is aroused by his Jupiterian Mount, unless he has enough will power he may not be persistent in his efforts to improve his mental equipment and go as far as he could.

The Flexible Hand

Finally, we reach the flexible hand as shown in Plates 14-15, and here we find an elastic mind, flexible, and adaptable to all circumstances; brilliant, and ready to make the most of the higher side of the Jupiterian qualities. A child with this flexible hand can be placed in a variety of occupations, and in the higher brackets of many of the Jupiterian callings. He represents the highest grade of the Jupiterian type; his ambitions will be to reach the top in everything he undertakes; he will make a trustworthy leader, whether in religious callings, politics, or business, and he can be assigned to positions in any of the classifications. He can succeed in the ministry and it will not be an indifferent success. He can take an education, and as a scholar and theologian will have few equals. His fine appearance and melodious voice will attract people to him, and he can fill pulpits in the most prominent locations. A Jupiterian child with these flexible hands should have the best

preparation and training for a career in the ministry. If
Mercury is the secondary Mount, he can succeed in medicine if
the Mercury finger be long and the medical stigmata well
marked on the Mount, or he can succeed in the law if the first
phalanx of the finger of Mercury be long. Here again he can
have a distinguished success. Or he can succeed as an actor,
or in moving pictures in principal parts; he can have great
success as a writer if the Lunarian be the secondary type, or
he can be a leading salesman in life insurance, automobiles, advertising, or succeed as a promoter.

Fourth Test—Consistency of the Hands

It is quite important to know whether the Jupiterian child
is lazy or energetic and for information on these questions we
turn to the consistency of the hands.

A large part of the success of a Jupiterian child comes
from the fact that he is not hampered by a weak constitution,
but that he has strength to carry forward the plans necessary
to realize his ambitions. Cases are found, however, where laziness
interferes with the development of his most favorable qualities,
and if we find a lazy Jupiterian child we will have to plan a
way to overcome the inertia which otherwise will ruin his
chances.

Flabby Hands

If his hands are flabby in consistency, which means that
they crush in your grasp and offer no resistance, he will have
the highest degree of laziness and while this consistency is not
often found, still there are cases where it is present with an
otherwise splendidly marked hand, in which case all of the
fine qualities of the type will amount to little unless we can
arouse ambition, the desire for leadership, and his love of praise
and adulation sufficiently to overcome the deadly influence of
the flabby hands.

Soft Hands

Soft hands, which do not crush easily and offer resistance
to your grasp, will not be as bad as flabby, for there will be
more energy present and it will not be as hard to arouse ambition and get this child into action. This will have to be done

by the same methods as outlined for the child with flabby
hands and the effort will more often be successful.

Elastic Hands

The most favorable consistency is the elastic, which is firm,
and as you press it has resiliency and does not give way as
do the flabby or soft hands. Here there will be a sufficient
supply of intelligent energy which will bring out the strongest
qualities of the child. On a pure type this combination will
produce the finest results, for whatever his mental attainments, he will have the force to make the most of them.

In positions of trust this child will be more accurate and
reliable, and he can be placed in positions of greater responsibility with an assurance of faithful performance. No matter
what the secondary type may be, he will utilize the best qualities
of that type, and bring them to the support of his Jupiterian
qualities.

Hard Hands

Hard consistency which does not give at all as you press
it, will often bring too much energy to a Jupiterian child,
especially if he be a highly developed specimen of the type and
we will find as his grade coarsens that the hardness will be
more pronounced. In Jupiterian children, where we find extremely red color, and stiff elementary hands, we will find them
very hard; and this hardness will tell us the grade of the
child.

When we find hard consistency, we must hunt for the grade
of employment in the Jupiterian occupations in which we are
going to place this child, and it cannot be in as fine a grade
as when we find elastic consistency.

Such a child can do well in military life, either as an officer
or in the ranks according to the grade of his hands. He can
be a distinguished top sergeant if he has this hard consistency
and also red color; or an evangelist with the same formation,
and the kind of a political boss who is pictured in cartoons.

Fifth Test—The Three Worlds

In placing a child in his proper occupation it makes a
great deal of difference whether his abilities lie in the direction

of mental activity, in practical or business affairs, or whether the lower world of animal desires which deals with the coarser side of life is his field of operation. We have for our guidance in these matters the three worlds in hand reading and we find that the entire hand may be divided into the three worlds, and that the fingers are also divided in the same way. We have found that these two sources of information are very accurate and that they verify each other. In using the whole hand, we divide it by using the fingers to the point where they join the palm as the upper or mental world, and by drawing a line across the hand from the top of the Mount of Venus to the percussion we enclose the practical world, and from this line to the base of the Mount of Venus at the wrist we have the lower or baser world (Plate 16).

The fingers we divide into the three worlds by using the first or nail phalanx as the mental world, the second phalanx as the practical world, and the third phalanx as the lower or baser world (Plate 1). Often the hands are so plainly marked in respect to the three worlds that the question is soon settled, but in other cases measurements have to be taken to determine which is the ruling world. What we learn from these worlds, is whether the child will find his best occupation in the mental world, or the practical, or the lower.

The Mental World

When we find the mental world best developed (Plate 17), we know the Jupiterian qualities will find their best expression on the mental side. Thus we seek for occupations that will require mental proficiency. Such a child will not do best in occupations requiring manual labor, or labor of any kind. His efforts will be to superintend, to direct the efforts of others, to teach, to plan, to write, to speak well, to learn the sciences and elucidate them, to plan military campaigns, to teach theology, or to be chairman of a county, state, or national committee. His ambitions will be for leadership in select callings, where his mind can be employed in furthering his advancement through directing others. Such a child can be a professor in a college of education, a teachers' college, or as a professor of literature, journalism, political economy, language, or art (with Apollo secondary),

or he can conduct a business college if Mercury be the secondary Mount. He can be a teacher of Bible history, composition,
military tactics, law, or a lecturer on any of these subjects.

The Middle World

When we find the middle or practical world best developed
(Plate 18), the Jupiterian child can succeed best in the world
of affairs and of business. He will not desire, nor will he often
take a liberal education. He will want to start into business
when quite young, but he should be placed in Jupiterian occupations where he can most likely make money. He can be
the opulent member of the family and will think his brother
of the mental world is wasting a lot of time.

The child with the middle world will be found in all the
grades of fineness and coarseness. In the finer grades you can
get him to take more education, but in the coarser grades it is
a waste of time. A Jupiterian child of fine grade with the
middle world best developed can be placed in the best positions
in the business world. He can be an executive at the head of
large corporations, railroads, and in business for himself. In
all of these places he will have the great ambition and desire
for leadership that belongs to his type and he will make the
friends who will help him achieve his desires. This child can
succeed in the department store business, especially if Mercury
be the secondary Mount, he can be the president if his grade
be fine, his consistency elastic, his skin fine and color pink, or
he can be vice president or treasurer, but cannot be recommended for secretary. He can be sales manager for a brokerage house, for investment bankers, manager of a thrift department in a bank or trust company, but he should not be trust
officer. His ability will lie in selling the thrift idea, not in
operating the trust department. He can successfully operate
a hotel, or a summer resort, or a wholesale or retail clothing
store. As his grade becomes coarser he must be placed in
positions less prominent, until with the lowest grade he must
be a porter, a night watchman, a drayman, or some position
of similar grade.

If we find the first phalanx of his fingers highly developed,
and at the same time the middle world, it is a favorable combination, for the mental qualities of the first phalanx will have

the support of the practical qualities of the middle world. Thus the child will be able to fill a vastly larger variety of occupations with credit and profit to himself. With such a combination he can succeed in the best business positions which should be sought for him, or if his tastes run very strongly to the law, medicine, theology, politics, or military pursuits, he can be successful in any of them with the proper secondary Mounts.

The Lower World

When the lower world is the strongest (Plate 19), which we discover from the fact that the third phalanges of the fingers are longest and also full, and that the lower third of the hand is full and bulging, we must class the child as belonging to the lower world, which generally means the coarser grades of the type. Generally we find with the lower world dominant, coarse skin, red color, and stiff hands. We know from the type to which he belongs that he is ambitious, but it will not be for preferment in the higher grades of employment. This child will be hard to keep in school, and seldom takes more than an elementary education, so he is not fitted for more than ordinary employment. He will be satisfied with a "job." He can be successful as proprietor of a second-class restaurant, a cheap hotel, a livery stable, plumbing shop, a cleaning and dyeing establishment, a rug and carpet cleaning company, a window washing company, a cheap auction room, a second-hand store for furniture or clothing, or an oil filling station.

Middle and Lower Worlds Combined

We often find the middle world and the lower combined, and this will take away some of the coarseness from the lower world, for here we have a practical side to the type which will tend to raise the lower world and cause it to operate on a better plane. More often we find in such a combination a refining influence coming from the middle world, and such children can occupy a higher grade of positions in politics, business, and military affairs. Such a child can succeed as proprietor of a delicatessen, a laundry, a quick repair shoe shop, a news stand, as a pawn broker (more successfully if Mercury be the secondary Mount), in running a vegetable and meat market, as keeper of a second hand book shop, a lunch stand, an auto tire repair shop, a milk or ice route, or in running an electric repair shop.

SIXTH TEST—KNOTTY FINGERS

The sixth test is knotty fingers (Plate 20), which means that the joints of the fingers are prominently developed so that they are perceptibly knotty in appearance. The knotty finger shows that the child has the power of analysis. He does not take anything for granted, he resolves everything into its parts, he probes, he searches, and in the end emerges with the facts. This development is not natural to the Jupiterian child, as these children are not analyzers, but belong to one of the spontaneous types. But we do find knotty fingers on Jupiterian children, which shows that they will be more careful than usual, they will be slower to make up their minds, and will have to have proof before being convinced. They will also act more slowly and will be unlikely to make mistakes.

We find with knotty fingers that sometimes it is only the first knot that is developed which is the knot at the first joint of the finger. This we call the knot of mental order, which shows that the child is orderly and systematic in his mental processes. He may be disorderly in his surroundings or his dress, but his mind will be stored with facts which are systematically arranged for use at a moment's notice. Such children are mental subjects and are often slovenly in person and indifferent as to appearance, but never in mental operations. Their minds are storehouses of facts systematically arranged, and always in order.

The second knot is the knot of material order. This is the joint between the second and third phalanx. If this is developed so that it is noticeable, the child will be very careful of his appearance, he will have everything orderly in his home, his office, his clothes will be pressed, but if the knot of mental order is not developed, his facts will be in disorder, he will have no mental system.

Knot of Mental Order

. If only the first knot is developed (Plate 21), it will show the child to be systematic and orderly in thought. He will act only on facts which will always be in order and he will be proficient in debate. Such children make good lawyers. They can be successful as statisticians of financial houses, banks, and with brokers ; as office managers of these same companies, as economists, as reporters for financial publications, in research departments of colleges or with foundations, as analysts for bond houses or foreign exchange brokers, and these Jupiterian children with the mental knot can be the secretaries in department stores or with wholesale or retail clothing manufacturers or dealers. They can be successful in the transfer department of banks and trust companies for stocks or bonds, or in the stock departments of automobile companies, cash register companies, or manufacturers who have many parts to look after and handle.

Knot of Material Order

If the knot of material order is best developed (Plate 22), these children can make good organizers, for they lay out the work that is to be done and plan just how it is to be accomplished ; they assign some one for each position and require full reports. Such children can be very valuable in the organization of a large sales organization, for they will not only be good organizers, but the Jupiterian is himself a good salesman.

He will also be proficient as an army man, for he will be strict in discipline and require prompt and accurate performance of duty.

There is a big field for this child in the distribution end of an automobile factory for here he needs not only organizing ability but discipline. He must organize the dealers in a large number of states, lay out their sales plans, see that they put them into operation and that correct reports of conditions all over the field are made. He must have real sales sense. This he gets from the Jupiterian type qualities and the organizing ability he gets from the knot of material order. If Apollo is the secondary Mount with this child, there is no sales organization so big that he cannot master and succeed with it.

SEVENTH TEST—SMOOTH FINGERS

Smooth fingers (Plate 23) belong to the Jupiterian type and will most often be found, by which we mean that the sides of the fingers are smooth and that there are no knots. They give to the Jupiterian child intuition, impulse and inspiration, a quick way of thinking, dash, brilliancy, and consequently will accentuate the known qualities of his type.

These children succeed best in occupations which do not require analysis or detail, such as an auctioneer, where the fine voice of the Jupiterian child, his agreeable personality and the spontaneity of the smooth fingers will make him most successful. Such a child could also succeed as an evangelist, and with training, as an inspirational orator and public speaker, as head of a dramatic school, as a press agent for public personages, actors, circuses, or movie stars. He could successfully manage singers, pianists, violinists, or lecturers, and can be very successful as manager of a lecture bureau.

EIGHTH TEST—LONG FINGERS

It will be necessary for you to judge long fingers, and for that purpose we are referring at this time to Plate 24, which is a fine example. You will note that these fingers reach approximately to the lower portion of the Mount of Venus when they are closed on the palm, and in order that you may get a better idea, we also introduce Plate 25, which shows the longest fingers we have ever seen. With a little practice and with these plates in mind, you can judge long fingers at a glance, but until you can, it is better to measure them and in this way judge the extent of the long finger development.

Long fingers do not belong to the Jupiterian type, but when they are found they slow it up a great deal. No one with long fingers is anything but slow, and quickness and dash should belong to the Jupiterian child, consequently when long fingers are found, they cannot be regarded as beneficial to the best working of the type.

Jupiterian children with long fingers will do best in positions where they need not be hurried, and where a great deal of detail is required. Such a child can be successful as a builder of skyscrapers, if his grade be fine, either as a general or subcontractor for the iron and brick work, especially on the buildings now being ornamented in the modern style where there are a great many details of material and workmanship to be looked after. He can be very successful in the trust department of a bank in looking after the detail of the securities owned by estates, their due date and the collection of interest. He can be successful as the loan clerk in a bank, and can make an exceptional private secretary for a prominent official in a large corporation, especially a railroad corporation, from which position he is bound to advance. He can be most successful as a train dispatcher in lower grades, or a maintenance-of-way superintendent.

NINTH TEST—SHORT FINGERS

Short fingers belong to the Jupiterian child for here we find quickness of thought personified. This child will think quickly and act quickly. In fine grades he will be brilliant, dashing, attractive, magnetic, and will draw followers from many of the other types who think more slowly than he does.

Short fingers are quite distinctive in appearance; in some cases they are so short that they attract your attention. We are introducing at this point Plate 26, which is an excellent example of short fingers.

Short fingered Jupiterian children plan large enterprises, build some of the biggest buildings, the most important railroads, and found the largest corporations. Such children possess a quickness of judgment that no other children have. They make up their minds while you are talking to them and have the answer ready when you are through. And their first impressions are nearly always right.

If the first phalanx of the fingers is longest, the short fingered quickness will operate in the mental world and this child can be the invincible military strategist. He can be the minister who "thinks on his feet" and with no apparent effort. In business he will decide important questions involving huge sums as if they were of no importance. And in doing these things he does not make mistakes, his judgments are sound. This child has a fine field in the public utilities. If of fine grade, he can be at the head of a company engaged in the sale of electricity, water, artificial or natural gas, or the development of oil fields. He can have great success as promoter of such companies, in arranging the financing, in the personal sale of stocks or bonds, in the merger of a number of companies, in presiding at stockholders' meetings; he can be general manager for such companies, and from such positions at the top, Jupiterian children with short fingers descend in the scale of their importance as their grade becomes coarser, until they reach the labor strata which string the wires or lay the pipes. In the public utility field alone there are places for all short fingered Jupiterian children.

TENTH TEST—THE FINGER TIPS

At this point in our type study, we consider the finger tips, which we will apply to the Jupiterian child and see what they will do for him.

The Pointed Tip

We do not often find a pointed tip on a child of the Jupiterian type, but when we do, we find the strength of the type much diminished. This tip is well illustrated in Plate 27, from which you will see that the ends of the fingers form a distinct point as well as the thumb. You will not encounter any tips which are more pointed than those shown in this plate and having seen them, you will have no difficulty in identifying them in the future on the hand of a child. Such a child must not be placed where he will be required to exert great strength of will, but he can be successful in positions where he comes in direct contact with people, such as selling positions, private secretaries, floor managers, or in the diplomatic service. This tip will not be found on the coarser grade of hands. This child can succeed as a clerk in an art department or store, in drafting or commercial illustrating; he can be a successful salesman in the jewelry department of a department store, or in the book department, or as salesman for gents' furnishings, shoes, or hats, for a tailor, as floor walker in a ten-cent store, in the package goods department of a drug store, or as room clerk in a hotel.

The Conic Tip

Conic tips (Plate 28), make the Jupiterian child artistic and if of the mental world, he can succeed as a writer, a critic of art, and as a preacher; he can be highly inspirational. He will not incline to politics, but in business can succeed in positions requiring tact and diplomacy, such as a hotel manager, retail store manager in men's and women's wear, clerk or manager of jewelry or art goods or chain stores, salesman or sales manager with firms or a corporation whose business is widely extended; as press agent, real estate promoter, advertising solicitor, advertising manager, bond and stock salesman, and in all positions where he comes in direct contact with the public.

The Square Tip

The square tip shown in Plate 29, makes the Jupiterian child exact, systematic, a lover of order, and inclines him toward technical positions. He will succeed as a building contractor, civil engineer, filing clerk, stock clerk, undertaker, social worker, patent attorney, and in the lower grades of development as a box maker, machine operator, marble cutter, book binder, barber, dyer, tire maker, brick maker and similar occupations where he needs some skill together with an exact eye and mechanical sense.

The Spatulate Tip

The spatulate tip, shown in Plate 30, will be the best on a pure Jupiterian child, for this tip brings out all the strong qualities of the type. He will be original, independent, practical, active, enthusiastic, skillful in games and sports, reliable, constant, and brave.

He can be successful in politics and hold the higher offices, in the ministry, in the army or navy, or in business. A large variety of occupations are open to him if he is of the finer grades. His love of nature will fit him for a career as an explorer, or if he wishes, as a missionary in foreign lands. He is eminently fitted for positions which bring him in contact with the public.

The Jupiterian child with spatulate tips can do many things well, such as: executive positions in electrical equipment manufacturing companies, as secretary, treasurer, or even president. Unless he is so fixed financially as to be able to control stock, he will probably have to begin in lower positions and work up, but the leading positions are not beyond his ability to fill. In the medium grade of positions in the same companies he can begin as salesman, buyer, department manager, bookkeeper, office manager, advertising manager, or advertising writer and, if his grade be coarse, in positions such as porter, watchman, time keeper, or freight delivery.

He can occupy positions, or in business for himself, as a horticulturist in which he should be most successful; or be a playwright, aviator, architect, decorator, market gardener, fruit grower, designer, teacher of athletics, dancing, a cartoonist, financial corporation manager, foreign exchange broker, credit insurance manager, investment broker, in the consular service, sales research and surveys, as a note broker, purchasing agent or radio dealer. In all the grades of fineness and coarseness which we find among Jupiterian children, there are positions in the various occupations here mentioned which will fit his grade. If he is fine he will have the better positions, and as he descends in the scale as shown by the tests, he can fill the less conspicuous but necessary positions with success.

ELEVENTH TEST—THE THUMB

No matter how brilliant the Jupiterian child may be, he will not reach his highest measure of success unless *he wills* to succeed, and strength of will we determine from the thumb.

Thumb Curled Under Fingers

Beginning at the first indication in the chart of the thumb, we see whether it is curled under the fingers or stands out boldly. Here we determine whether a strong will is in operation or whether a weak and feeble one is what we have to depend upon.

If the thumb is held covered by the fingers, we know that the will is in abeyance. We should examine for this indication when the hand is in repose and the child does not know that he is under observation. With the thumb so held, and especially if it is *usually* carried covered by the fingers, the child has a weak character and cannot be placed in positions of responsibility or where he has the direction of other people. He must be assigned to subordinate positions in industries recommended for Jupiterian children. He cannot be the president or any of the executive officers of a corporation, but can be a clerk, an assistant in various offices, or if his grade be coarse or medium, he can only fill positions such as porters or watchmen. If the thumb does not curl under the fingers but stands out boldly, the child has a strong character and can be placed in responsible positions and have the supervision of others. If his type be strongly developed and the tests show him of proper grade, the child can fill the most important positions in the industries recommended for Jupiterian children and we will know, that with this strong independent thumb the child can succeed, for he has the will to force success.

Size of Thumb

Note the size of the thumb, for we find that a large thumb (Plate 31), indicates a strong character and a small thumb (Plate 32), a weak character; and by a strong character we mean one who dominates himself and others and by a weak character one who is dominated by others. No child with a weak thumb can bring about the best operation of his type qualities.

High and Low Set Thumb

Next we note whether the child has a low set thumb (Plate 34), or a high set thumb (Plate 36). A low set thumb is much the best indication, as it shows a higher grade of mentality, stronger will, and the ability to do a larger number of things that require manual skill, thus opening to the child a greater variety of occupations. The low set thumb has a greater power in opposing the fingers, and this child can fill positions known as skilled labor which the child with a high set thumb cannot. He can be placed in occupations in which he does the work himself, such as engraving, embossing, molding, turning; he can make an expert diamond cutter, draftsman, carpenter, harness maker, machinist, railroad or stationary engineer, lithographer, manufacturing jeweler, or craftsman in wood.

Phalanges of Will and Reason

The first and second phalanges of the thumb show the amount of *will power* and the *reasoning* and *logical* faculties possessed by the child. The first or nail phalanx shows by its length and shape the amount and quality of will power and the second phalanx shows the reasoning qualities of the child also by its length and shape.

Shape of Will Phalanx

We have learned that the shape of the first or will phalanx shows whether the child is merely brutally stubborn or has an intelligent will. This is shown by the fact that if he is brutally stubborn he has a bulbous first phalanx, (Plate 37), and if he has an intelligent will, he has a well formed, long phalanx (Plate 38). The bulbous first phalanx is not the best indication on a fine grade Jupiterian child, but has a tremendous influence in coarsening the operation of his qualities and lowering his grade. The best one is the finely shaped thumb with the will phalanx well formed and long. In this case we know that a strong, intelligent will is operating to bring his best side into play.

Will and Reason Balanced

What we most desire, is to find the first and second phalanges, indicating will and reason, balanced (Plate 38), that is, that they shall be of equal length, for here we shall find will and reason in equal supply and the result will be a normal and balanced child.

Will Phalanx Short

It will be very unfortunate if we find the first phalanx the shortest (Plate 39), for then we will find a weak will, and this cannot drive the engine to its greatest advantage.

Phalanx of Reasoning Long

To have the second or phalanx of reason long (Plate 38), or at least in balance with the first, will be a happy combination, for the child will then be able to reason things out and formulate his plans and will have the will to carry them out.

Phalanx of Reason Short

If the second phalanx be *very short* (Plate 40), he will not reason at all, but will be uncontrollably stubborn. This

child must never be placed where he will have to use the faculties of logic. Thus he is condemned at the outset to coarser
occupations where he must rely upon a domineering spirit; in
others words he will be a slave driver. As foreman of railroad
construction gangs and in similar occupations he will get
along.

The Thumb Tip

The tips of the thumb indicate the same things as they do
on the fingers, and must be applied to the Jupiterian child
as we have applied all other indications, viz., What will be
their effect on this particular grade of a Jupiterian child? We
will find that a spatulate tip (Plate 43), will be the strongest
indication of a powerful will and the pointed tip (Plate 27),
will show the weakest and an impressionable will. The square,
(Plate 44), and conic tips (Plate 45), will provide system and
artistic sense. So on a strong specimen of Jupiterian child with
a spatulate thumb, we know that everything that strong will
can do will be done to develop his strongest side, and if he is of
fine grade, he can be placed in the choicest positions where
ambition and a desire to lead can have an opportunity. Also,
if we find the pointed tip, we know that he must never be placed
where he will be required to take responsibilities. In various
paragraphs in this chapter, you will find many occupations in
which the child can be successful. The tips of the thumb will
tell how much will power he will have, to force success in these
occupations.

CHART NOTE. Take plenty of time and examine the hand
critically. The entire success of our effort to help the child is
centered on the proper identification of his type and his
secondary type and the tests. To locate the type properly
means that you can place your child in his best occupation.
It is worth all the effort you could possibly make to do this.
When you have made your decision, as to his type, note it on
the chart.

TEST CHART

Types

    Primary.

    Secondary.

    Others.

Tests

    1. Texture of skin.

    2. Color.

    3. Flexibility.

    4. Consistency.

    5. Three worlds.

    6. Knotty fingers.

    7. Smooth fingers.

    8. Long fingers.

    9. Short fingers.

    10. Finger tips.

The Thumb

    11. How carried.

    How set.   High.   Low.   Medium.

Will Phalanx

    Bulbous.   Short.   Very short.   Long.

    Very long

Phalanx of Logic

    Long.   Very long.   Short.   Very short.

    Will longer than logic.   Will shorter than logic.

    Will and logic balanced.

    Large thumb.   Small thumb.

    Elementary.   Medium.   Fine.

    Tip of thumb.   Pointed.   Conic.

    Square.   Spatulate.

Age of Child   *Sex*   *Date*

CHAPTER TWO

THE SATURNIAN MOUNT TYPE

The Balance Wheel

In this book, scant reference is made to lines in the hand. The type and conformations are considered. No predictions are made as to the future, the entire attention is centered on what the child *can* do. Whether he does it or not, is his affair and that of his parents. Our duty is done when we tell him *how* he can be successful.

CHAPTER TWO

THE SATURNIAN HAND

THE Saturnian Mount type is identified by a large Mount of Saturn, the apex centrally located, the finger large, and the other fingers leaning toward it. When all of these indications are present, it is not difficult to identify the child as belonging to the Saturnian type. A high Mount is not often found, however, but in most cases the type is identified by the other fingers leaning toward it, with a strong vertical line on the Mount, and the apex centrally located. As this combination is the one most often encountered, we are using as an illustration of a Saturnian hand one which is so marked (Plate 46).

The subject from which this plate was taken was a typical Saturnian in appearance, in characteristics, in mental qualities, and in habits. He was one of the outstanding scholars of his day, the author of several books on philosophy and other subjects, and his end was typical of the Saturnian type. Plate 47 shows the hand of another subject in which the Saturnian development is *entirely lacking* and with these two plates in mind as the two extremes, you will have no trouble in identifying any child who either does or does not belong to the Saturnian type. You will also find no difficulty judging any hands which come between these two examples nor to determine the degree of Saturnian quality present.

DESCRIBING THE SATURNIAN

The appearance of the Saturnian, prepared from a number of pure specimens of the type, shows him to be the tallest of the seven types, as his finger is the longest.

He is gaunt, thin, and his skin is yellow, rough, dry, and

usually wrinkled, or else drawn tightly over his bones. He is the purely bilious type and yellow is his distinctive color. His hair is thick and dark, most often black, straight, and harsh. His face is long, his cheek bones high and prominent. The cheeks are sunken, with skin flabby and wrinkled. The eyebrows are thick and stiff, growing together over the nose and turning up at the outer ends.

The eyes are deep set and extremely black, with a sad expression which changes only when flashes of anger, suspicion, or eagerness stir his mind.

The chin is prominent and large, and neck long and lean, with muscles showing prominently like cords and the blue veins standing out under the shrunken and flabby skin. His Adam's Apple is plainly in evidence. The shoulders are high and have a decided stoop and the arms are long and hang in a lifeless manner at his sides. His step has no spring and his gait is a shambling one.

SATURNIAN CHARACTERISTICS

In the plan of creation, the Saturnian acts as a steadying force to the other types. He is the balance wheel which slows down some of the spontaneous types and keeps them from going too fast. In this respect he is a favorable influence, but is a dangerous type, for from it we get some of the wisest of men, but also some of the worst criminals.

There are many pure specimens of the Saturnian type, notably one of our martyred Presidents, who have risen to great heights as statesmen and benefactors of the human race, notwithstanding the gloomy melancholy characteristics of this type. So we must not infer upon the discovery of a Saturnian child that he will be a failure, but we must approach the study of a child of this type with a full sense of the seriousness of the undertaking.

In the present chapter, we shall treat the Saturnian as an adult male and a pure specimen of the type, though there are just as many females. As we can locate the primary Saturnian type on very young children, we will have the advantage of knowing what the child is going to look and be like when he has reached maturity and can prepare him for the problems that will confront him. When we speak of the Saturnian child in relation to occupations recommended for him, we mean that he will be fitted for them when he is grown.

The Saturnian is not one of the spontaneous types, which win their way through the world because of their attractiveness, but his very appearance and his physical condition cause him to be a repressing influence which holds the other types in check, and for this reason we have called him the balance wheel. He is first of all a cynic, and looks upon life as a none too pleasant experience. He is of all the types the most profound student and here he finds the best expression of his talents. He loves solitude where he can engross himself in his studies, and no subject is too deep to attract his attention. He loves the laboratory where he can use the latest discovery in chemistry, or bring an atom under the microscope. His first dominant characteristic is *WISDOM*.

The Saturnian views life as a battle. He has never experienced the joy of living as do the spontaneous types, so *SOBERNESS* is his second dominant characteristic. His face rarely lights with a smile, he seldom jokes, his recreations are found in his studies, he retires rather than advances himself.

SADNESS is his third dominant characteristic. This expresses itself in his writings, for he can produce many books each of which is tinged with sadness and the indefinable melancholy which at times overpowers him. His musical compositions, for he can be a prolific composer of the classics, are tinged with the same strain of sadness which is a part of his nature.

He is often the victim of *SUPERSTITION*, which is the fourth dominant characteristic. The Saturnian is inherently a mystic and studies all the occult sciences. His success as a chemist is partly owing to the mysterious workings of nature through her chemical elements which appeals to him. Often he has strange ideas about religion, he investigates many cults and all of the established religious forms and all such things as the miracles appeal to him. He fears death and observes the superstitions which tend to delay a visit from the Dark Angel. These throw him into an extremity of fear and add to his *GLOOM*, which is the fifth dominant characteristic.

As we have had under consideration a pure specimen of the Saturnian type, and one who is of fine quality, it will appear that the lower grades of the type must be very disagreeable people if the best specimens have so many depressing characteristics. This is true, for as the Saturnian descends in the scale, all of these sobering qualities turn not only into disagreeable or depressing indications, but he becomes mean, tricky, dishonest, unscrupulous and in the lowest grades, venomous. It is therefore evident that we must judge the Saturnian child very correctly and place him in his exact grade, for we cannot afford to take any chances with a subject so full of potentialities.

The higher grades of Saturnians are distinguished for their:

Wisdom
Soberness
Sadness
Superstition
Gloom
And are the Balance Wheels

The lowest grades are:

Mean
Tricky
Dishonest
Unscrupulous
Venomous
Criminal

THE SATURNIAN AND MARRIAGE

The Saturnian is not predisposed to marriage. His physical make-up is such that he inclines to coldness, he has little animal heat, he is bilious and such a thing as sex attraction plays little part in his affairs. He much prefers to live by himself, not to be interrupted in his studies, to eschew social gatherings, to avoid contact with other people as much as possible, and such an one does not readily enter into the marriage state. He does marry however and in his choice of a wife he makes many mistakes. She is all for society, is fond of dress, fond of show, fond of gayety, fond of everything which he detests. He dislikes dress, his clothes never fit him even if made by the best tailors.

If the Saturnian does not choose a Venusian, it will be a Jupiterian, or an Apollonian, each of these being his antithesis. We have never seen a Saturnian with a wife of his own type.

SATURNIAN HEALTH

The Saturnian has very positive health defects, a predisposing cause for which may be found in disturbed functioning of the liver. Here he seems to have an inherent defect, which causes him to be prone to biliousness. This in turn gives him a yellow color and brings on the train of health difficulties to which he is liable. His trouble with his liver is not merely a temporary disorder but is permanent, making him exceedingly nervous and often ending in paralysis. The extent of his nervousness can often be detected in his nails, which are fluted and ridged and very brittle. He is also attacked with what is called rheumatism, consisting of much pain in his joints, largely in his feet, knees, and hands. When the trouble goes as far as paralysis, it is generally in his legs which seem to be a constant source of weakness. He is also predisposed to hemorrhoids and other varicose veins, and to trouble with his ears.

THE SATURNIAN ENTITY

We are not dealing at length with health matters here, but are confining ourselves strictly to indications which bear directly on the matter of occupation. We deem it necessary however to explain the matter of health defects as we have, so that you may realize that the Mount types of people are definite entities, personalities in fact, with their own distinctive qualities, one of which is their liability to specific diseases. We are trying to give you the picture of a man, so that when the name Saturnian is mentioned, this picture in all of its ramifications comes at once to your mind and you visualize him, you think what he looks like, what his strong characteristics are, how he marries, his health defects, and his viewpoint on all subjects. Then you think whether he is fine or coarse and when you have done all this, you know the potentialities of the Saturnian child as they can be known in no other way.

SATURNIAN QUALITIES

None of the types show as great a lack of the social qualities as the Saturnian; he not only does not seek society, but he avoids it. Life in the cities with its noise and bustle does not attract him, he prefers the country where there are not so many people and where life is not so strenuous. So the Saturnian child can be successful as a farmer, a truck gardener, a nurseryman, a botanist, a horticulturist, and he can teach these subjects in schools and colleges with great success. He is seldom successful in business, for he has not the faculty of making friends nor of holding them, and in such positions as salesman, sales manager, or wherever he is required to come in direct contact with the public he is not so successful.

The Saturnian child has a mathematical mind, and in all the higher branches of mathematics he is not only proficient, but he can make an excellent teacher of these subjects. He has also an engineering mind, and is especially successful as a mechanical engineer. He can be an excellent engineer in chemistry, electricity, radio, automobile, or wherever an exact mathematical mind is required. He can have a prominent place in the ranks of inventors, especially in the above-named and allied industries, and any inclination on the part of a child for any of these engineering occupations should be encouraged.

The Saturnian child loves everything connected with the occult. He delves into spiritism, hypnotism, mesmerism, and in recent days he is one who is having much to say about psychology in all of its connections. He can make a good teacher of all of these subjects.

His mind is well fitted for the study of physics which he can follow through all of its intricacies and seemingly master with ease. We have known several Saturnian professors of physics in prominent colleges who have become nationally famous.

He can make an excellent physician, more renowned for his knowledge of the subject than for his affability in the sick room. His practice also interests him more for the cures he makes, than for the money he receives. The Saturnian child is a true scientist.

He can write a great deal, mostly on scientific subjects, and can be a composer of delightful music, mostly of the classical variety. Liszt was a Saturnian.

But we must not forget when enumerating all the things which a high-grade Saturnian child can do, that there are many grades below him, and we find a large number of the children we examine belong in these lower grades. These can be placed in the minor positions in the various occupations in which we have found the fine-grade Saturnian child can be successful. There are many positions in laboratories where all grades of Saturnian children can be successfully employed, also in all the farming and horticultural occupations. These extend downward in the scale to the ordinary day laborer, and as we locate, in the children we examine, the grade to which they belong, we can find them employment in their proper grade of Saturnian occupations. Here we must use all of our tests.

We must never forget the depths to which a Saturnian child can descend. In appearance he may have stooping shoulders, a hunched back, or be a cripple; often with crossed eyes, scant coarse hair, and leathery skin; such an one will be capable of almost any crime. He is malevolent and a low, mean, surly villain. Deep lines crossing the Mount forming a grille, crooked gnarled fingers, hard consistency, coarse skin, elementary stiff hands, and deep yellow color, will be found on such a child. You will only find a few of them, but there are many in the world.

THE SECONDARY TYPE

The Saturnian child we have been considering up to this point, is a pure specimen of fine quality, and a primary type. We must now consider the secondary types which will strongly influence him.

JUPITERIAN SECONDARY TYPE

The Jupiterian Mount (Plate 8), lies on one side of Saturn and should be examined closely to see if the Mount or the apex leans toward Saturn, and whether the finger of Jupiter also leans toward Saturn. If so, we should decide that the Mount of Jupiter is the secondary Mount, and that Jupiterian qualities will influence the Saturnian child. This will make him more ambitious than a pure Saturnian would be. It will result in greater effort in all his lines of endeavor. Instead of pursuing his studies for the love of the study, he will desire that his work shall be known, and that he may become famous and make money. Here his Jupiterian desire for leadership will enter and he will, if the secondary Mount be strong, wish to be a leader in his profession.

There will be no change in the things this Saturnian child can do best, many of which have already been enumerated in this chapter; the change will be in his attitude toward people and his desire to have his work known and appreciated. His writings will not have the tinge of sadness with the Jupiterian secondary Mount, nor will his music be as melancholy. His love of nature will be increased, and in his agricultural, horticultural, or botanical pursuits, he will not only be more successful, but he will take more pleasure in his work. With Jupiter as his secondary Mount, this child will be less sober, less sad, and less gloomy, and can fill more positions where he comes in direct contact with the public. So, sales positions will be open to him which are impossible to the pure specimen, and more executive positions.

If the secondary type be very strong he will be able to do more in the business world, and, according to his grade, can be placed in a greater variety of positions than can be filled by the pure specimen. The leaven of the Jupiterian secondary type will enable him to hold onto all of the things peculiar to the Saturnian type and will add to them the spontaneous qualities of the Jupiterian type. This child can become a writer of popular articles on scientific subjects, military subjects, or can be successful in the preparation of campaign literature. Thus he can be a feature writer on a large daily, or more successful as a foreign correspondent. He can succeed as a political writer in foreign or state capitals, all highly paid positions. He can successfully edit a farm paper or magazine, or prepare and lay out a seed and flower catalogue for a nurseryman or seed house. He can teach psychology in a popular way or prepare successful syndicated articles on the same subject.

APOLLO SECONDARY TYPE

On the other side of the Mount of Saturn, is the Mount of Apollo (Plates 48-49). It must be examined to see if the Mount leans toward Saturn, whether the apex does likewise, and whether the finger of Apollo also leans toward Saturn. If so this will be the secondary type.

The Mount of Apollo will exert a favorable influence on the Saturnian child.

His ability to write well will be turned from gloomy stories to plays, in which calling he can be successful. He can essay the stage, and members of his type have recorded some outstanding successes. He can now turn to painting and produce some noteworthy examples of successful art. He can be most proficient in sculpture, especially if the tips of his fingers are square.

The Apollonian is far less deep than the Saturnian as a type; he is much more on the surface, so he does not add to the scientific ability of the Saturnian child, but he does add an ability to make scientific subjects more attractive, and so the Saturnian-Apollonian children can be successful in stores selling optical goods which the Saturnian child understands and which his secondary type enables him to explain and sell in a popular way. This child can be a successful optometrist. He can have success, owing to his technical talent, with a company making or selling heavy electric generators, coils, light plants, motors, or railway equipment, or for the same reason, in stores selling electrical appliances, washing machines, or he can succeed as an electro-therapist. The scientific ability of the Saturnian child adapts him especially to the scientific side in all these vocations, the Apollonian secondary type enabling him to meet, please the public and sell them.

MERCURY SECONDARY TYPE

The Mercurian is sometimes the secondary type to the Saturnian child and when he is, it will be shown by the absence of Jupiterian and Apollonian Mounts, with the Mount of Mercury high (Plate 50), and the apex leaning toward Saturn. The finger of Mercury will also be large and long. This formation, with the Saturnian development very strong, will show that Mercury is the secondary type.

As these two types are the bilious types, the combination of Saturn and Mercury produces some remarkable children and at the same time some very undesirable ones. The Mercurian is noted primarily for his shrewdness; he succeeds in business where other types fail. He has a sixth sense which tells him when to buy and when to sell. So when he is the secondary type, he will bring this faculty to the support of the Saturnian child who is made a better business man and can engage in more gainful employments. The strong inclination of the Saturnian child for agricultural employment can be turned to better account with the Mount of Mercury as the secondary Mount.

In Agriculture

Few realize the great number of first class opportunities that are to be found in what is known as agriculture. It does not mean what so many think, merely the tilling of soil and the raising of the ordinary crops, but agriculture has openings for men who have an aptitude for it, that are highly dignified and remunerative. The Saturnian child with his natural aptitude for agriculture, and his love of it, if he has Mercury for his secondary Mount, can take advantage of these opportunities. There is a large demand for educated agriculturists, for which vocation the Saturnian-Mercurian child has especial adaptability, and many of the colleges of agriculture cannot fill the requests that come to them for trained experts in a number of lines. These include animal husbandry, surveying, irrigation, drainage, milling, feeds, seeds, nursery stock, meat packing, stockyards, floriculture, farm machinery, publication of agricultural journals, advertising farm products, insecticides, farm colonization, fertilizers, dairy products, research experts, service men, and in all of these lines there are openings as executives at the head of companies engaged in these various lines of business. These openings are for the highly trained men and for those not so well educated there are innumerable positions of less importance in the same industries. Here you will be called upon to guide your child and place him in the grade to which he belongs and in a position according to his grade. It must not be thought that an education is not needed by those engaged in agriculture; it is absolutely necessary for those who are to be placed in the better positions.

In the Sciences

The Mercurian has a strong adaptability for scientific study, many of the best doctors belonging to this type. Here he can aid the Saturnian child materially, for he is primarily a scientist. So the combination of the two Mounts can produce the highest grade of work in analytical chemistry, biology, pathology, astronomy, geology, medicine, synthetic chemistry, metallurgical chemistry, food chemistry in the following fields, in which connections with large corporations are possible: Cellulose, dyes, fertilizers, gas and fuel, industrial and engineering chemistry, leather and gelatine, medicinal products, organic chemistry, paint and varnish, petroleum, physical and inorganic chemistry, in rubber, sugar, water, sewage, and sanitation.

As the Saturnian child has an inherent adaptability for work of this kind, and the Mercurian also has an ability in the same direction, this combination will enable a child who has it to achieve success in accordance with the degree of fineness he possesses and of the education which he acquires. When you find a Saturnian-Mercurian child, leave no stone unturned to give him the best preparation within your power by means of a thorough technical education under the best auspices. Another feature of the combination will be that the child will be able to turn his ability to better advantage from a financial standpoint.

The Saturnian child is not a money maker, and by himself he does not accumulate money. But with the Mercurian as his secondary type, he has the Mercurian shrewdness to aid him, and he secures more money for everything he does.

The Saturnian child does not often enter the world of business, except through scientific channels such as have been herein set out. He does not become a merchant, a manufacturer, or a distributor of similar commodities, but he has a much better chance of success in these lines of endeavor if he has Mercury as his secondary Mount. We need not feel so great a necessity to keep him away from the public as is necessary in the case of a pure specimen.

We must not forget that the combination of the Saturnian child with Mercury as the secondary Mount produces mean, undesirable people, and many criminals. These two types are primarily the criminal types, they are the bilious types and these are the criminals who practice every form of criminality from petty thieving to bank and mail robbery and murder. A low, coarse development of the two types will stop at nothing, and their pictures are in all the rogues' galleries. Between this low criminal and the high quality of the finely developed specimens are many grades all of which can be located properly by means of the tests.

MARS SECONDARY TYPE

When the Mounts of Mars, or either of them, are the secondary Mounts, it is shown by the large development of the upper or lower Mounts of Mars (Plates 52–54), which bulge into the palms of the hands and extend outwardly at the percussion. The Mount and finger of Saturn are high and large, and the finger is long. The apex of the Mount is centrally located and there is a well marked vertical line on the Mount. The other Mounts will be flat or poorly marked.

The combination of Saturn and Mars is not often seen, but must be considered as it sometimes occurs. If it is the upper Mount of Mars which is secondary, it will make the Saturnian child much more courageous and he will have the power of resistance. A pure Saturnian child may have a great deal of ability but lacks the courage to let it be known. In such a case, the secondary Mount of Mars will be a great help, for a child who has it will push himself forward; he will not hesitate to meet people, and has a much greater range of possibilities open to him than a pure specimen of the Saturnian type.

The occupations for which he is best fitted will take on a sturdy character and with his scientific aptitudes and the Martian backing, he can be highly successful as a mining engineer, a vocation which offers excellent remuneration. Mining is a hard business, and without the Martian secondary Mount the Saturnian cannot be highly successful in it. But no one has greater adaptability for mining than he, and with the Martian Mount to add to his physical strength and stamina, the Saturnian-Martian child can have a fine career as a mining engineer, for gold, silver, coal, iron, copper, zinc, manganese mines, or for asbestos, nitrates, potash or sulphur mines. This child can also be very successful as a professor of mining engineering in a college and he can write excellent articles for newspapers or magazines on the same subject. The Saturnian-Martian child of good grade can be assigned to the field of mining engineering in all its branches with full assurance that he will be successful, but he should be well prepared for same by a liberal education.

If the lower Mount of Mars is the secondary Mount (Plate 54), which will be shown by the bulging character of the

Mount, it will add aggression to the Saturnian child and this is a quality unknown to him. It will make him more likely to be a leader. While the combination with Jupiter as the secondary Mount would give the Saturnian child ambition, he might not work to further these ambitions. But with the lower Mount of Mars secondary, it will cause him to push his Saturnian ability to the utmost.

The Martian is always practical. He is not often a scholar, but would be most valuable as a second to the Saturnian child in a career in the various agricultural pursuits which have been mentioned earlier in this chapter. In every instance, the good grade Saturnian child will be more successful with a strong lower Mount of Mars behind him. Such a child can be successful in the sale of farm machinery, the installation of complete dairy systems, he could successfully run an ice cream plant, a cold storage warehouse, or a packing house. He could succeed as the representative of a meat packer, or have charge of the operation of his refrigerating cars; he could succeed as a special freight representative of a railroad running through farming communities. He could be a buyer of live stock, cattle, sheep, hogs, or horses and mules; he could conduct an inter-city trucking and express service, or be express agent in cities and towns.

This lower Martian Mount, however, will not be favorable as secondary Mount with a low or bad grade of Saturnian child. This child needs no added aggression to push his inherent bad qualities to greater extremes.

LUNARIAN SECONDARY TYPE

The Mount of the Moon is often the secondary type and it makes a great deal of difference whether the Saturnian child is of a fine or coarse grade as to whether it is a favorable indication.

The Lunarian at his best is a difficult person and while he has an admirable side, he has a very bad one too. When he is the secondary type to the Saturnian, the Mount of the Moon, (Plate 56), is bulging and extends not only outward on the percussion, but downward as well, so that it makes a prominent appearance on the hand, so much so that it is not difficult to tell that it is the secondary type. At the same time the

Saturnian development must be pronounced, and strong enough to show that it is the primary Mount.

The Lunarian as a type has a vivid imagination, and this sometimes goes to such extremes that he becomes a liar, but the best use he makes of this gift is to write well. This is the principal way in which he can be of use to the Saturnian child.

First of all, the Lunarian secondary type will enable the Saturnian child to write better technical books, and this will be true especially of books on chemistry and physics on which subjects he will be predisposed to write a great deal. It will enable him to write remarkable essays, lectures, or articles for newspapers or magazines on philosophy as relating to religion, and this child can have great success as a professor or teacher of this subject or as a lecturer on the same subject. He can be a most successful professor of psychology in a college, both the Saturnian and the Lunarian being mystics and having a talent for everything occult. Or he can be a metaphysician or hold a high place in theosophy, or practice mental hygiene or New Thought. He can also write very practical and impelling books and magazine articles or lectures on the subjects recommended for the Saturnian-Mercurian child in the paragraph dealing with the Mercurian as secondary Mount in this chapter. If he has a well developed Mount of the Moon as a secondary Mount, the imagination of the Lunarian will make him also an excellent writer of fiction, which he could not be without this assistance.

VENUS SECONDARY TYPE

The Venusian as a secondary type for the Saturnian is an unusual combination, for of all the types they are the most diametrically opposed. Still this combination is sometimes found.

It is shown by a highly developed Mount of Venus (Plate 58), and in order to be sure that Venus is the secondary type, it will be necessary that the other mounts shall be flat and Saturn strongly marked.

Venus as the secondary Mount will soften the Saturnian child in every way. He will be more agreeable, more sociable, will seek companionship, will strive to please, and so he will be better adapted to business pursuits. His writings will be more optimistic, his musical compositions in a lighter vein, and he will not withdraw himself and seek solitude. This combination will make it possible for the Saturnian child to be a salesman, and in agricultural lines of commodities, either wholesale or retail, he can be successful.

Thus he may be placed in positions in the retail merchandising business, such as piano and organ salesman, real estate salesman, and in sales positions in insurance, bond, stock, radio, electric equipment for the factory and the home, farm implements, feed, grain, or fertilizer. He will also be successful in the newspaper field, in positions such as reporter, editor, business manager, circulation manager, and in retail book stores.

For these positions, we are speaking of a fine grade of Saturnian child, but in the same lines of business there are many less important positions which can be filled by Saturnian children in the lower grades. This does not mean the coarse common grades, but those in the middle brackets. In all above lines of business there are many clerkships and similar grades of positions among the rank and file of those who make up these organizations, which are open to medium grade Saturnian children with Venus as the secondary Mount.

THE TEST FOR GRADE

Having now considered the Saturnian child as a primary type, and with the combinations which may occur as secondary types, we next begin a study of the tests to be made by which we seek to determine his grade.

FIRST TEST—TEXTURE OF THE SKIN

First we will examine the texture of his skin, to see whether it be fine or coarse. In the ordinary walks of life we will encounter far more of the better grade Saturnian children than of the coarse ones. So we will largely find skin of fine or medium texture (Plate 10).

These children should be assigned to the better grades of positions in the occupations which we have outlined in this chapter. There will be many different degrees of fineness found, in grades below the very fine skin, and as we reach these grades we should place the child in a position equal to the grade. From the president down, the scale runs through various department heads. Office managers, district managers, book-keepers, clerks, statisticians, analysts, laboratory chiefs, laboratory helpers, chemists, writers, reporters, editors, farmers, agronomists of all grades, and a vast number of minor positions in a large number of occupations and industries engaged in similar lines of endeavor which are recommended in other parts of this chapter.

And finally we come to the very coarse skin (Plate 11), telling of a very coarse grade of child who can only be the porter, night watchman, drayman, truck driver, cleaner, errand boy, and similar occupations. And in the list of those with very coarse skin, will be those who are criminals, and belong to the unassigned on whom we can make no impression.

Second Test—Color of the Hands

Yellow Color

Yellow is the color we expect on the Saturnian child. In the largest number of cases we will find it in some degree. This arises from the predisposition to biliousness which is inherent in the Saturnian type, and when very marked it will be a dampening influence. A severe shade of yellow color will affect an otherwise good grade of Saturnian child and make his character doubtful. Such a child cannot be placed where he must meet the public, so selling positions are out of the question for him. But he can, on account of his agrarian instincts, be a gardener and do the work himself if of a coarse grade, or he can succeed as gardener in charge of a public park, or amusement resort, or a private estate if of better grade, and could have a number of men under him. He can have charge of a laboratory building as superintendent of maintenance, or the same position with a college looking after a number of buildings and caring for the grounds. He can have charge of the shipping, the receiving department, or the wholesale or retail delivery, of a dairy products company, or for a meat packing company, or a commission merchant in fruits and vegetables.

White Color

White color is often found on the hands of the Saturnian child, and this adds to his coldness, his mysticism, his aversion to society, his desire for seclusion, and his dislike of mankind. When this is pronounced, it affects his ability to meet people and he should be placed in positions where he does not have to come in direct contact with the public.

He can be placed in an office, where he can do his work away from people. White color affects even the best grades of Saturnian children, and reduces the number of occupations open to them. This child should be prepared to use his ability as a writer. If he has the Lunarian Mount secondary, he can be especially successful in this direction. His best field would be in what has been denominated in newspapers and magazines as "muckraking." The coldness of white color, and the cynicism inherent in his type, fit him to be either a "muckraking" reporter who digs up all the scandals in a city government, or he can prepare scathing articles for magazines on the viciousness of trusts, or business alliances in restraint of trade. Or he can be a very critical foreign correspondent, and the qualities which enable him to do these things, will also, in coarser grades, make him succeed as investigator for corporations, or a secret service man in governmental departments, or an ordinary detective. Thus according to his grade he can be a successful reporter, editor, correspondent, investigator, secret service man, or detective.

Pink Color

Pink color is not often found, but it is sometimes seen, and when present it will make the Saturnian child less gloomy, less a pessimist, more approachable, and will open more occupations to him. Remember the various lines of endeavor in which the Saturnian child can engage with greatest success, his scientific ability, writing ability, musical ability, agricultural ability, teaching ability, and place him in some grade of these employments. Pink Color will enable him to enter more and better grades in all of these occupations.

Specifically, pink color will assist this child to succeed better in the occupations in which the secondary Mounts assist him. It will make him a more popular minister, or politician with Jupiter as the secondary Mount, or he can succeed better as a salesman, or organizer of a sales organization for agrarian merchandise, or on the stage, or as a painter or sculptor with Apollo secondary. He can be more successful in medicine or the law with Mercury. Or on his own account he can be more successful if he has pink color, in chemistry, mining engineering, biology, astronomy, or other scientific occupations for which he has talent, or as a writer on these subjects, or as a teacher or professor in all of them.

Red Color

Red color is very seldom seen, for the Saturnian child is not at best an ardent person. If it is encountered, he can be placed in positions requiring greater physical strength, and he will have more ability to dominate and direct any kind of operations. Thus he can be a superintendent of engineering parties doing prospecting or surveying both civil and in mines, or rights of way, or in road building gangs, or in railroad construction, or in building operations. He can be headmaster in a boys school, or conduct a touring party. He becomes less the shrinking timid person, and more the man of affairs.

THIRD TEST—FLEXIBILITY OF THE HANDS

The Flexible Hands

Flexible hands will often be found on a high grade Saturnian child for, in spite of his peculiarities, he has a keen elastic mind. This is proven by the fact that he has so many aptitudes. In the high grades this child can be a bacteriologist in charge of laboratories where great mental alertness is required, or a writer who needs imagination, a college professor in the subject of cosmography, or a composer for voice, orchestra, or instrumentalists who must have a highly endowed mentality. We are not therefore surprised to see the finer grade Saturnian children with hands bending back and forming an arch, which shows us the elasticity of their minds (Plates 14, 15).

Such a child can be fitted for the dean of a college, and in such a position he will supervise the work of all the departments, for which position he needs to know a great deal about all the subjects taught. Few are fitted for such an important position, which requires not only technical and academic qualifications, but executive as well. An ordinary mind could not grasp the whole range of the requirements, but a fine grade Saturnian child with flexible hands, such as are shown in the illustrations, could. With a strong thumb, a Saturnian child who has such hands should be given every advantage possible in education and training, with a view to having him begin in a teaching position, and advance as his qualifications become known, to the position of dean.

The Straight Hand

As the Saturnian child can also find a successful field of operation in agriculture, he needs a practical mind, and on one who makes this his life work, we wish to find the straight hand (Plate 13). This gives him a good balance of qualities, and when we find a Saturnian child with a straight hand, we should consider him qualified for some of the many positions in industries dealing with agronomy which have been listed in previous paragraphs of this chapter, or in the many side lines which a pursuit of that calling make necessary.

There is a wonderful field for him in the line of marketing dairy products, which a Saturnian child with a straight hand can make successful, either as an employee of a company engaged in this business, or in business for himself. If he is a nearly pure Saturnian he will have the shrinking qualities of the type, and to be in a business of this kind for himself, even if on a very small scale, will be agreeable and profitable to him. There are now so many ways in which dairy products can be disposed of through coöperative marketing, that a timid Saturnian child need not be a direct salesman, and as his straight hand and Saturnian qualities will enable him to produce the dairy products he needs to sell, he can be successful, for he will not be called upon to do the direct selling.

The Stiff Hand

As we go down the scale in the grade of children, we find hands grow stiffer even than the straight hand, and in these cases the mind is less elastic as the stiffness of the hand increases. This continues until we reach the lowest grade as shown by the elementary hand (Plate 12), where there is nothing but crass unintelligence, and a mind adapted to nothing but menial tasks. Children with such hands will be able to do only common labor.

Such a child can look after feeding or milking cows, or the machinery used in making butter or cheese. Or he could work in the killing pens of abattoirs, or do the feeding of cattle in stock yards and their loading for shipment. He could be a farm hand or janitor of a building, and if we find a child whose stiff hands and other tests show him only fitted for such inferior positions he will be better off in an industry for which his Saturnian type has qualifications.

Fourth Test—Consistency of the Hands

By means of consistency of the hands, we gauge the energy of the Saturnian child. Energy is not one of the strong qualities of the pure Saturnian, for his physical strength is not of the robust kind. Usually we find a consistency softer than the elastic, but not actually soft. This will indicate that the energy will be more mental than physical, and such a child will have all of the retiring, unsocial qualities of the type. He will do better as a laboratory man than as a salesman, and will have ability as a writer, but will lack the industry which is necessary in this calling.

Soft Consistency

If soft consistency is found, the child must be placed where he will not come in contact directly with the public. Here he will have to rely upon his mental qualifications and not upon physical energy.

If he has the musical talent usual to the Saturnian type, this child should have an education as a musician. He will do better as a composer than as an instrumentalist as he lacks the energy to do the necessary practicing. He could however be an excellent accompanist but not a soloist. Or he should be given a technical and academic education in preparation for teaching subjects for which his type is qualified, such as speculative philosophy which he will like very much, or religious history for which he has especial aptitude, or for psychometry. If he has spatulate tips he should be educated for a position in a research laboratory either chemical or mining. If this child is of fine quality he can be an excellent tutor.

Flabby Consistency

If flabby consistency is found, it will be a difficult situation. This child will be subject to the extremes of dejection, and his morbidness will be increased. He will sense his lack of physical vitality, and this will cause him to be exceedingly shy and reticent. As the Saturnian child has ability in mathematics, he should be placed in a statistical department for a life insurance company, or in an accounting office, or he may be in a company mining coal, a stenographer in an office which does typing work, but he will not have the creative faculty, nor the energy to take positions requiring him to take much responsibility. When his secondary type is either Jupiterian, Apollonian, or Martian it will help a flabby hand to be more independent, and to take some grades of positions in business organizations. But as far as possible he should be kept in occupations which are of a more routine nature. These may be in offices of corporations dealing in farm machinery, or as a clerk in wholesale packing houses, as stockkeeper, time keeper, filing clerk, record clerk in an automobile factory, or as a type setter in a printing office, a weaver, prescription clerk, or mechanical draftsman if the child be of good grade. If of lower grade he can occupy positions of less importance in these same lines of endeavor, such as messenger in an office, switch board operator, lunch clerk in a drug store, or making blueprints.

Elastic Consistency

When we find elastic consistency, where the hand will be resilient as you grasp it, the child will be full of energy and this will modify his backward tendency and make him more aggressive, less retiring, and able to take more prominent places in the professions for which the type has aptitude, and a greater range of positions in the business world. When we say business world, we mean business in lines in which the Saturnian has special aptitude. These will be in scientific studies, chemical companies, all companies dealing in products of or related to the agricultural or dairy business, book stores, many lines of newspaper work, companies engaged in all the applied sciences, and others which have been previously mentioned in this chapter.

This child has especial ability in adapting electricity to its many kinds of uses. The subtle and tremendous power of the unseen current appeals to the mystical side of the Saturnian child, who with the intelligent energy shown by his elastic hands and his natural scientific ability, can master the technical operations of electricity. Thus with proper training such a child can have great success in one of the big manufacturing plants either for radio, telephone, or general electric manufacture, in all of which they have complete research laboratories engaged in finding new uses for electricity and in inventing and perfecting new machines to improve its operation and usefulness. His success will be made more certain and easier for him if he has square or spatulate finger tips. It will be better if this child specialize in such plants as a radio or telephone engineer, in both of which he can be highly successful. Or he can specialize in companies manufacturing heavy machinery, such as turbine engines, large generators, or electrically driven engines for railroads. This child is presupposed to be of fine quality; others who are not can be placed in the same companies in positions in accordance with their grade but of a less degree of prominence. Saturnian children of all grades, but with elastic hands, can be successful in positions with electrical companies which are in accordance with their grade.

With any of the spontaneous types such as Jupiter, Apollo, Mars, Mercury, or Venus as the secondary type, elastic consistency will be a great asset, as it indicates intelligent energy in sufficient supply to make these strong types successful.

Hard Consistency

In the lower grades of Saturnian children we generally find hard consistency. Here is great energy, but it is too often blind energy. The child will do things unintelligently. He will be forceful, but the energy of hard consistency is not a mental quality. On seeing it we must at once go over all the tests to determine the grade of the child, for the harder the hand is, the lower the grade is. This child must be placed in the lower brackets of occupation in the various lines in which the Saturnian succeeds best. We constantly find the hard hand a reliable test in the lower grades.

FIFTH TEST—THE THREE WORLDS

We are much interested to know in which world the child will be strongest, and this information we get from the hand as a whole divided into three sections called the three worlds.

We also find the fingers divided into three worlds as shown by the first or nail phalanx which is the mental world, the second phalanx which is the practical or business world, and the third phalanx which is the lower or material world (Plate 1). By means of these three worlds, we find whether the child has most ability for mental pursuits, practical or business occupations, or in the lower world, and it will be found, that the fingers always corroborate the story told by the hand as a whole.

The Mental World

The Saturnian child can succeed in many lines which call for mental capacity, so if we are going to place him in any of these lines, we wish to see that the first phalanx of his fingers are the longest (Plate 17), and that the mental world of the hand as a whole dominates. It will be very necessary if the child is to be placed where he will use his scientific attainments that his mental world should be well developed. When this is the case, we may safely assign him to medicine, that is, if he is of superior grade, and in the mastery of medical subjects *per se*, and in their allied branches, he can be successful.

He may be a general practitioner, or a specialist in many subjects. Eye and ear, throat and nose, laboratory diagnosis, skin, pathology, microscopist, oral or rectal surgery, or he may go into a biological laboratory and be successful. Here he will do his work scientifically, but he will not aways get the most money for it.

The Saturnian child can be an excellent writer, and in this profession it will be very necessary that the mental world be well developed. He can write especially well on astronomy. If he is to be prepared as a teacher or a professor, in both of which callings he can be very proficient, he must have the mental world strong, and especially if he is to be a professor of mathematics. In all forms of employment, such as statistical, analytical, research, ad writing, office management, or similar occupations, he needs to have the mental world best developed.

The Middle World

If the middle or practical world is best developed (Plate 18), the child will find his best field of endeavor in the business world. While his personality does not fit him for contact with people, the development of the middle world will give him an urge which will overcome a good deal of his shyness, and he will be able to fill a position in the executive end, or in the manufacturing department of a railroad equipment company, an air reduction company, a powder plant, an asphalt plant, or in a hydro-electric company. He can be successful, as well, in the development of water power sites and the distribution of electric current in a chain of cities. These fields furnish an immense variety of positions where any grade of Saturnian child with the middle world developed can find an opportunity for future advancement. The telephone field will also be open to him, for here he can use scientific ability, and if this be linked to practical ability he will find a splendid field for his endeavors.

The Lower World

If the lower world be the strongest, which is shown by the large development of the lower portion of his hand and the third phalanx of his fingers (Plate 19), he will be able to do much in the same line of enterprises as are mentioned above, except that he will occupy a different stratum of their activities. He will do best in the building end of the companies mentioned, and can in some cases be the contractor who builds the plants, or installs the machinery if he be of high grade, and if lower in grade he can be the superintendent of workmen engaged on the enterprise. If of lower grade still, he can be the workman who performs the actual labor, or the day or night watchman, or the yard-keeper, or in similar positions.

Mental and Middle Worlds Developed

It is desirable to find the mental and the middle worlds equally developed, for here we have mental strength, supported by practical ability. The result is, that this child can be not only successful in his mental efforts, but he is able to turn them to practical account. Thus in all the enterprises mentioned above, he will be able to take part in their activities on both the mental and practical plane. This will give him a much larger choice of occupations in which he can be successful. In other words, he can either conceive, lay out, or plan the work of one of these companies, or he can build the plant, or execute any part of it.

SIXTH TEST—KNOTTY FINGERS

Knotty fingers (Plate 20) will often be found on the hands of the Saturnian child as his natural tendency is toward an analytical turn of mind, which is indicated by the presence of the knots.

Knot of Mental Order

We often see a hand with the first knot developed (Plate 21), and this aids the operation of the mental world materially, as the mental knot means a systematic and orderly mind. It is especially useful where the Saturnian child expects to engage in some of the scientific work for which he is so well fitted. In all steel and public service enterprises, the systematic mind shown by the first knot is of immense value. These professions call for an analytical mind, and a well ordered and systematized one at that, and here the first knot will help him, and make him more successful. As the Saturnian child is not an orderly person at best, and as he has so many characteristics which show a not too orderly state of his mental machinery, it will be a great advantage to find something like the first knot which is going to improve the order and system of his mental processes. Thus he can become a better writer on scientific subjects, not so predisposed to be erratic or flighty, and whether he be in a laboratory, or in the inventing end of a telephone company, in which enterprises he can be successful, or whether he occupy the lower grades of employment in these companies, a systematic mind will be a great help to him. The first knot will also be a help in the lower grades as well as in the higher ones, and will make them less liable to attain the ultimate in coarseness.

The Saturnian child, of all the other types, has the greatest adaptability for the study of philosophy. In no line of study does he reach such great depths as in this. And the fine grade Saturnian child with the knot of mental order is the greatest philosopher of all. As philosophy now embraces many subjects, the first thought that comes to mind on seeing a fine grade Saturnian child with square tips and the knot of mental order is, that this child should be devoted to studying, writing upon, and teaching philosophy in all its branches. Such a child when started on a study of this subject will withdraw himself from the ordinary contacts and absorptions of life, and will devote himself to his studies, and as he can succeed best of all in this direction, he should be given, as soon as his aptitudes have been recognized, as thorough an education as possible for a life work which will bring him the most happiness and success. As the study of philosophy is purely a mental exercise, the knot of mental order will help the child most.

Knot of Material Order

If the second knot be developed (Plate 22), it will make the child orderly in practical affairs. Thus in any business enterprise in which he is engaged, his office will be better arranged, there will be less lost motion in his daily routine, he will pay more attention to his personal appearance, and in any work which he has in his charge, it will be better systematized, and will proceed in a more orderly fashion.

If both the knots of mental and material order are found on the hands of a fine grade Saturnian child he will have both mental and material order and system. This is a good combination, especially if the finger tips be square. This child should be devoted to research work in the laboratory of one of the large drug manufacturing companies, who are constantly searching for new chemical combinations for drugs in the preparation of new remedies. Within the last few years some wonderful things have been done in this direction and there is no field where the Saturnian child with both knots can be so successful as in such work. The material order which the second knot will give him is quite necessary in such an occupation, for he must keep all his retorts and his workshop in order so that no fatal mixing of drugs, and no mistakes may be made.

If his second world be developed, and the second knot as well, he will be adapted to some form of business activity. There should be no hesitancy in placing him in some of the practical lines we have heretofore mentioned.

SEVENTH TEST—SMOOTH FINGERS

Smooth fingers (Plate 23), are not so often found, for the Saturnian child does not act upon impulse, and smooth fingers belong to the spontaneous types such as Jupiter, Apollo, Venus, and sometimes Mars. When found on a Saturnian child, they give him an intuitive faculty which will enable him to arrive at some of his conclusions more quickly and more easily than by the analytical processes which are more natural to him. This will give him confidence in himself, and he will not be so retiring or shy. But smooth fingers may lead him to rely upon impulse in his mental processes, and this is not so safe for a Saturnian child as to rely upon slower analytical methods which are more natural to him.

This child will not be able to write well on subjects requiring analysis or technical detail, nor will he be able to occupy positions requiring research, but he can be a successful composer of music for orchestras, trios, or of choruses in the lighter forms of composition, and he will do well as an actor, and, strange as it may seem, in comedy parts. There are many Saturnian actors who have taken the peculiarities of their type and successfully capitalized them into comedy. The smooth fingered Saturnian child can successfully conduct a school of music especially for beginners—all these, if his grade be fine.

EIGHTH TEST—LONG FINGERS

Long fingers (Plate 24), belong to the Saturnian type. There will be some difference in the degrees of length, but in all but a few cases the fingers will be long. This does not mean that the finger of Saturn alone will be long, but that all of the fingers will be of such a length that they must be classified as being distinctly long fingers.

The Saturnian child is naturally slow in his movements, and when he is long fingered, he is just that much slower. Such an one enters into all the details of everything he does, and in the scientific studies of the Saturnian this is a help to him, for here he needs exactitude and certainty, and these only come from going to the bottom of everything.

Long fingers will intensify Saturnian qualities and make the child retiring, and desirous of being away from the crowds and by himself. This comes from the fact that his mental faculties work slowly, and in order to accomplish, he must be free from excitement and confusion. Such a child should be placed in a laboratory making soil analysis, in a water company in charge of purification and purity maintenance, in the analytical department of a company making glass, or in a statistical department for the same company; in a company manufacturing coal tar products, either medical preparations or in relation to dyes or road building compounds. A high grade Saturnian child in such companies is likely to make discoveries of new products or to invent new processes.

It is not always easy to get started in these companies, as applicants are numerous, but the best prepared will win. Colleges and technical schools furnish by request lists of those who have shown the greatest proficiency, and upon discovering the hand formations which make such a career desirable, the Saturnian child should have studies chosen from the beginning which will lead up to good technical training in reliable schools as soon as he is old enough to begin them. A long fingered Saturnian child will advance rapidly in these schools and love his work.

In lower grades, the long fingered Saturnian child will do best in agricultural pursuits. He can be a farm laborer if of a very low grade and with no Jupiterian development to give him ambition, and from this point upward, he can occupy various positions in agricultural pursuits, all according to his grade. Such as: a breeder of cattle, hogs and horses, a poultry raiser, or buyer and shipper of grain. But he will not do so well in selling as in the actual farming end of agricultural enterprises, or in the manufacturing end of companies making products for farm consumption, such as farm machinery.

NINTH TEST—SHORT FINGERS

Short fingers (Plate 26), are very seldom found on the hands of Saturnian children. The qualities they indicate are the opposite of Saturnian qualities, and their absence on Saturnian hands is, to our mind, a further proof of a plan of creation by an intelligent Creator, for he has given long fingers to 98 per cent of Saturnians that we have examined, and we take it this ratio extends through them all.

When short fingers do occur, the child is not so profound, and does not analyze but relies on inspiration for his guidance. He will not have the certainty of correct first impressions as in the case of the spontaneous types to which short fingers belong, but will make mistakes. This will make him less accurate in scientific studies, and he should be placed in some of the occupations of a less technical character. If of fine grade, this child will do well as a lecturer, he will be quicker in speech than one with long fingers, or even than one whose fingers are of normal length. He will be inspirational in his style of delivery, and as in his case we must rely on the serious qualities of his type for the preparation of his lecture material, this quick delivery will be an advantage in making his points with an audience. He will be especially good in well prepared travel lectures, or lectures on English literature with dramatic illustrations, he can do well with lectures on the drama, or dramatic form, and can be successful as a dramatic or music critic.

TENTH TEST—THE FINGER TIPS

The Pointed Tip

Among the finger tips, two are often found on the Saturnian child, and two are seldom seen. The pointed tip (Plate 27) will not be found on two per cent of children, for while the Saturnian child is a moody person, introspective, and contemplative, his visions are of practical things.

Thus the pointed tip would in no sense be a help to him.

On the few cases where we do find it, the child will be idealistic, and dreamy but impractical.

He should not be placed in positions requiring original research, analysis, or scientific investigation of any kind. But he may be placed in a clerical position in a company manufacturing lenses for microscopes or telescopes, or in the filing room of a tire and rubber company, where he will deal only with routine in the tabulation of work done by others. On account of his pointed tips, he will have a more pleasing address than is usual with Saturnian children, and can do well with a manufacturer of perfumery in an office position.

The Conic Tip

Conic tips (Plate 28), are seen more often than pointed, and their owners are more practical. Saturnian children with conic tips will do best in the distributing end of the businesses for which Saturnians are best adapted, many of which have been mentioned in this chapter. They will not be so retiring and shy as those with square tips, and will meet the public better. Quite a field is open to them as a secretary, stenographer, typist, floor clerk, floor manager, salesman if they belong to a good grade, and in the lower grades as a stock clerk, file clerk, telephone operator, telegraph operator, switchman, glass blower, and in lower grades still, as helper in a cement mill, lime kiln, coal mine, or as a pressman, watchman, porter, and similar occupations in the industries in which Saturnian children do best. When conic tips are seen on a Saturnian child, if you will remember that this tip takes away much of the practical side of the type, you will be able to place him properly in one of the Saturnian occupations according to his grade.

The Square Tip

You will find more square tips (Plate 29), than any others on Saturnian children, for these are the tips indicating system, order, and regularity, they are always practical, and have good ability for analysis and research. This tip is found on the hands of many great scientists; they represent just the qualities which a Saturnian child needs. On a high grade child, they promise much in the scientific world. Here will be one who will be most proficient in all matters pertaining to physical science, who will be adapted to a thorough medical education, he can also be successful as a ceramic engineer, professor of mathematics or in mechanical engineering. As an archæologist, a palæontologist, automobile engineer, neurologist, orthopædist, plastic surgeon, pathologist, or a medical practitioner either in general medicine or in many medical specialties. In lower grades, the child can be an assistant in the above lines and many which are similar. He will have the same aptitudes for all these professions, but not as high a grade of ability, and he will not go as far in them as the Saturnian child of high grade.

In mechanics the Saturnian child with square tips has many fields open if he is of high grade. They are: heating and ventilating engineering, plumbing and sanitary engineering, sheet metal designing and drafting, boiler making laying out and inspection, steel ship laying out and plan reading, estimating for contracts, mathematics and slide rule reading, and in all of these vocations, there are positions open for Saturnian children of lower grades, all the way down to manual labor in the companies engaged in manufacturing commodities used in these different lines. In the highest grades, the Saturnian child may be placed at the head of these companies.

As a teacher, the square tipped Saturnian child can be successful in a number of subjects. There will be: algebra, biblical literature, economics, American history, philosophy, American literature, European history, American government, biology, applied grammar, child psychology, astronomy, English literature, and all mathematical subjects. And as a writer he can deal with all of these subjects in a satisfactory manner.

In all of the agrarian occupations he can be successful. Real estate in cities and farming lands, the laying out of additions urban and suburban, colonization plans; all of these if he be of high grade, and positions can be found in companies operating along these lines for Saturnian children of all the lower grades.

In agricultural pursuits, the square tipped Saturnian child can be successful. The high grade ones as owners, and the lower grades filling all the positions down to common labor according to their grades. In all the lines manufacturing commodities for the use of farms he can be successful, occupying positions according to his grade.

The Spatulate Tip

A good many Saturnian children will be found with spatulate tips (Plate 30), and these tips will exert a powerful influence. They will make him practical, more active than usual to the type, original, independent, and the love of nature of the spatulate tip will emphasize the Saturnian love of the country so strong in him.

The spatulate tip will make him much more skillful in games than is usual, and this skill will extend to all the activities in which he uses his hands. Thus he can be proficient in the mechanical arts, and can be successful in trades such as: manufacturing jeweler, diamond cutter, photo engraver, etcher, die cutter, silversmith, glass cutter, inlayer, watch repairer, watchmaker, shoemaker (hand), if he be of fine grade. Subordinate positions in all these trades as apprentice, journeyman and the like will be open to those of lower grades.

Spatulate tips (Plate 30), which indicate originality will, on high grade Saturnian children, show a talent for invention. Thus a child with this combination can have a successful future in the mechanical departments of many leading industries where new ideas are at a premium. The automobile industry offers splendid opportunities of this kind. Here they are constantly seeking improvements in their engineering problems or in methods of manufacture, in machines to increase production and cut down the number of operators, and improvements in any of the numerous things going to make up the total of factory operation.

As nearly all executives in the automobile organizations are chosen from those who show ability in the ranks, and mostly from factory operatives, there is a great opportunity here for a child so fortunate as to have a Saturnian type and spatulate tips. The same thing is true of the electrical industry, and the chemical industry, for here there are some rich prizes for those children who discover ways to produce synthetically some of the most needed articles. An enormous field is open in radio for inventors with mechanical ability who can solve some of the problems pressing for solution. In all of these fields, a high grade Saturnian child has more than an equal chance, if he has spatulate tips.

Eleventh Test—The Thumb

We have now reached the point in our study of the Saturnian child where we can visualize him, not only his personal appearance, but as a whole.

As he stands depicted in this chapter, he is a distinct personality, unlike any other human entity, his characteristics are very positive, and his possibilities clearly defined. But we know, that unless the child has the will to succeed, the most brilliant opportunities will come to nothing, and therefore at this time, we look to his thumb to tell us the amount of will he has, its strength and kind, for upon the answer to these questions depends his future success.

Thumb Curled Under Fingers

Our first observation of the thumb will be to see if it curls under the fingers, and to learn whether the child usually carries it in this manner. We have previously told you that the thumb so carried denotes a weak character, that will is in abeyance and that the child will not have this strong force to aid him. In such a case we cannot expect positive results in the development of his strong Saturnian qualities, and we must reduce the grade of employment to which he is assigned giving him less responsible positions.

Such a child should not be placed in a position above a clerk who carries out instructions, or he can be successful as a bookkeeper, a cashier, a waiter, a cook, a doorman, an elevator starter or operative, for in none of these positions will he have to exert strong will, and he will have no one under him.

Size of Thumb

The size of the thumb must next be examined, for from this we also determine strength of character.

Large Thumb

If we find a large thumb (Plate 31), we can expect much from the child, he can be placed in positions where he will have charge of others; for the large thumb indicates strong will power which enables him to control himself and dominate others. Thus in the various lines of endeavor in which the Saturnian child does best he can be given responsibility, and expected to develop competent organizations.

Such a child can be foreman or superintendent in a coal or lumber yard, an ice manufacturing plant, or he can occupy the same positions in a nitrate plant, in a copper, lead or zinc mine, and if his grade be fine he can be manager of a company selling farm machinery and appliances, or in a factory manufacturing the same. He can be secretary of a college.

Small Thumb

If we find that the child has a small thumb (Plate 32), it will negative many of the opportunities that would otherwise be available, and the small thumb will be a serious handicap. This child has a weak character, as weak as with the thumb curled under, and must be assigned entirely to subordinate positions, such as a machine operator in a shirt factory, or a board man in a broker's office, for with a small thumb he can neither control himself or others, and these positions require no exercise of will power.

High and Low Set Thumb

We next determine whether the thumb is set high or low. This will be very important when we come to assign a child to the mechanical arts or trades, and also among the ranks of skilled labor.

Low Set

With a low set thumb (Plate 34), he will be able to do work requiring skill with his hands. His thumb will be strong enough to oppose his fingers and form, mold, or fashion metal or other substances to required specifications or to express an artistic idea. The low set thumb will not only give him mechanical skill, but it will also indicate strength of character with a will sufficient to enable him to occupy positions of responsibility. Thus he may be put into a better employment than if his thumb be high set, and given more responsible positions in every line where Saturnians do best. The child with this thumb will make his way to the top if he is placed in the right vocation. With Mercury the secondary Mount he can be an excellent surgeon, with spatulate tips he can excel in golf and be a golf professional, with Apollo secondary, he can succeed as a painter, with Venus as a composer of spirited marches for bands, with square tips he can be most successful as a craftsman in metals, wood, or clay, and could make a name for himself as a sculptor, more certainly if Apollo be the secondary Mount.

High Set

If the thumb be high set (Plate 36), the child should not be put in positions requiring mechanical skill, or creative artistic ability in a manual way. Subordinate positions will be best for him. Nor should he be put in positions requiring the dominance of others, his shrinking Saturnian disposition with a lack of strength of will make such positions out of his range of possibilities.

Such a child can be a ticket taker for a movie house, a train caller, clerk in a concession in an amusement park, an extra on a movie lot, work in an auto checking garage, or in a green house, a nursery, or in a baseball park. None of these positions require skill, creative ability, or physical strength.

In judging all the thumbs so far mentioned, they must be applied to the grade to which the child belongs, and the various occupations chosen must be in his proper grade and of the kind his thumb entitles him to hold. The occupations possible to children of the lower grades are increased by the possession of a low set thumb.

Phalanges of Will and Reason

The two phalanges of the thumb will give us further confirmation of the facts we have just been considering, for from the first phalanx we determine accurately the strength of will possessed by the child.

Bulbous Will Phalanx

If we find the bulbous first phalanx (Plate 37), it will reduce the grade of a child even if other tests are favorable.

It is never quite safe to put this child in charge of others weaker than himself, for he may at any moment display the brutal character which the thumb indicates. He should be placed where he can be under someone of strong character, which may result in bringing out his better nature and developing the aptitudes which belong to his type.

A child with this thumb can succeed in the army where he will have the pugnacity and fighting spirit that goes well with his profession and does not fit into many other occupations; and he will at the same time be dealing with fighting men stronger than himself. If he be of fine grade he can be a commissioned officer. He can also succeed in expeditions which the Martian conducts in explorations for minerals and oils, and can be second in command of such expeditions if his grade be fine, for the fine grade will reduce the stubborn qualities of the bulbous phalanx of will. If he is of low grade, he can only be assigned to take care of the officers' horses, or look after the baggage on the Martian expeditions.

Long Will Phalanx

It is most desirable to find the first phalanx well shaped, long, and of fine quality (Plate 38), for here we have the operation of an intelligent will, sufficiently strong to give determination, but too intelligent to be stubborn or brutal. Such a phalanx will bring out all the best qualities of a Saturnian child, and will not emphasize those which are undesirable. If the child is of a fine grade, you may select a choice position for him in one of the industries in which Saturnian children do well, as listed heretofore in this chapter. Such a child also has talent in scientific directions; he may be placed in laboratories, observatories, in medical colleges, and given other scientific occupations already mentioned in this chapter.

As teacher or professor in schools and colleges he can also be successful. In fact this thumb will furnish the proper power to a good Saturnian child, which will enable him to operate at full strength in the direction of his best capabilities. It will also aid children of lower grades to occupy better positions. They may be foremen, superintendents, supervisors, inspectors, or occupy other positions to which some responsibility attaches.

This child with the long will phalanx has all the requirements for president of a college. As the Saturnian is primarily a student, the first choice of positions for him should be in mental occupations, and we have recommended various combinations for teaching and literary pursuits in former paragraphs. But the Saturnian child with this strong thumb can do more than write well or teach well, he is one of those who should head institutions of learning on account of his capability. In other words, children will be found who are superior to the ordinary run of children, and these must be placed in the highest positions in their vocation. Such an one is the Saturnian child with the fine thumb shown in Plate 38, and he should be started with the definite idea that he is going to the top and is preparing to be president of his college; and with this thumb he will stand a good chance.

Short Will Phalanx

If the first phalanx of the thumb be short (Plate 39), the child will not have will power sufficient to enable him to take any position where he will be called upon to have subordinates, he will not have command of himself, and can exert no influence on others. So he must be a clerk, or fill some other position where he is given orders. If his second phalanx be also short, his reasoning faculties will not enable him to take part in the many scientific occupations for which a Saturnian child has an aptitude, he will not be a good writer for he will not be a good reasoner, and in every line of endeavor where he might accomplish something with a large thumb, he must be content to occupy inferior positions.

Even though this child cannot fill any of the more responsible positions that his type is fitted for, he is still a Saturnian, and should be placed in some position in a vocation for which his type is adapted. If of fine grade he can be an orderly in a hospital, a filing clerk in a lawyer's office, a librarian in a college, or a proof reader in a print shop.

Second or Phalanx of Reason

The second phalanx is very important on the hand of a Saturnian child, for he so often chooses an occupation where the faculties of logic and reason are absolutely necessary. With a long phalanx of reason (Plate 38), the child will be able to be more successful in the medical profession and can be a clinical professor of the practice of medicine in a medical college. This covers a knowledge of all the diseases, and such a child can also be a very successful general practitioner, a branch of medicine now much needed. He can also be a professor of neurological surgery, for with his long phalanx of reason he will have mental preparation, and this will presuppose a strong thumb which is necessary to the practice of surgery. The long phalanx of reason makes the child able to excel in scientific studies, and he can be social hygienist for wholesale druggists which is much related to their business. He can also be an expert writer on zoögraphy, or director of research in a large corporation or foundation. He can be a professor of history and politics in a college or university, and in a technical school of radiography.

The Tip of the Thumb

The tip of the thumb will have one of the four formations, pointed, conic, square, or spatulate, which have already been described, and the qualities shown by these tips will apply to the qualities of the thumb in the same manner as they do to the fingers.

A pointed thumb (Plate 27), will reduce the strength of an otherwise good thumb. Such children must not be given positions of responsibility where they will be required to influence others, they belong to those who are led, rather than to those who lead.

The conic tip (Plate 28), will show greater strength of will and reasoning powers, but the child will be inspirational and rely upon intuition, and so will not be a deep student which the Saturnian child needs to be if he is to be a scientist, or engage in any of the more serious occupations of his type. If with the conic tip on the thumb, the tips of the fingers be also conic, the child may be placed in the distribution end of the companies producing products used by the agriculturists.

The square tip (Plate 29), found on the thumb, will assist with many of the occupations of a mechanical nature, all of the agricultural occupations according to the grade of the child, and he may be placed in scientific occupations, and as a teacher or professor in schools and colleges. The same line of occupations recommended for those with square tips in other portions of this chapter will be available, and the likelihood of success will be emphasized.

Spatulate tips (Plate 30), make any thumb much stronger. The will power is increased and the reasoning faculties function in many new ways. At another point in this chapter, the spatulate tip as relating to a Saturnian child is fully treated, and recommendations made as to occupations. If the thumb is spatulate in addition to the fingers, we would emphasize all of these recommendations.

CHART NOTE. The Saturnian type is not so hard to identify as some of the others. You will usually find the Mount not so high as the other Mounts, and your identification will likely depend on the apices and the leaning of the other fingers toward the Mount of Saturn together with a deep vertical line on the Mount. Other aids to identification will be found in the chapter on how to identify the Mounts.

TEST CHART

Types

Primary

Secondary

Others

Tests

1. Texture of skin
2. Color
3. Flexibility
4. Consistency
5. Three worlds
6. Knotty fingers
7. Smooth fingers
8. Long fingers
9. Short fingers
10. Finger tips

The Thumb

11. How carried.

How set.   High.   Low.   Medium.

Will Phalanx

Bulbous.   Short.   Very short.   Long.

Very long.

Phalanx of Logic

Long.   Very long.   Short.   Very short.

Will longer than logic.   Will shorter than logic.

Will and logic balanced.

Large thumb.   Small thumb.

Elementary.   Medium.   Fine.

Tip of thumb.   Pointed.   Conic.

Square.   Spatulate.

Age of Child.   *Sex.*   *Date.*

CHAPTER THREE

THE APOLLONIAN MOUNT TYPE

The Artist

All of the occupations recommended for children in this book are either in professions, or in branches of trade, manufacture, or service which are in successful operation at the present time. There are no obsolete or impractical vocations in the list. There is work that any grade of child can do, somewhere in the list if he is properly prepared for it. He will succeed better if he chooses the occupation for which he is best fitted.

CHAPTER THREE

THE third Mount type is the Apollonian, which is identified by the size of the Mount and finger, with the apex in the center of the Mount.

THE APOLLONIAN HAND

The Apollonian Mount is usually not so bulging as the Jupiterian, or Mercurian, but is generally indentified by the apex in the center, the other fingers leaning toward it, and by a strongly cut vertical line on the Mount, or a well marked star. Plate 48 is a hand marked in this way, and Plate 49 is an Apollonian hand marked by the bulging of the Mount together with other indications. These hands are those of men celebrated on the stage, one in heavy dramatic parts, and the other in comedy. Both have strong secondary Mounts which have aided them, but both are pure Apollonians.

DESCRIBING THE APOLLONIAN

From a composite description of the type prepared from pure specimens, the Apollonian is a handsome and manly type. He is of medium height, between the Jupiterian and Saturnian, is not fleshy like the Jupiterian, nor lean and lanky like the Saturnian, but is shapely, muscular, and athletic. The lines of his body run in graceful curves, and he is light and supple. His complexion is clear, his skin white, fine and firm in texture, and cheeks rosy. Pinkness of color gives the clue to a healthy condition and consequent attractiveness. The hair is thick, wavy, and black or auburn in color, fine and silky in quality, and when he has a beard it partakes of the same fineness and abundance growing over the chin, lip, and high on the cheeks.

His forehead is broad and full, but not high, the eyes are

large, almond shaped, brown or blue in color, with long lashes curling up at the ends. His cheeks are firm and rounded, showing no hollows. The nose is straight and finely shaped, the nostrils beautifully proportioned, and dilate under the play of emotions as is the case with all highly strung people.

The voice is musical and resonant. The lower limbs are graceful, muscular, finely proportioned, and never fat. The feet are of medium size, the insteps arching and high, which gives spring and elasticity to the walk. This is a particularly distinguishing feature of the Apollonian. In this type is presented a picture of healthy conditions, beautiful proportions, grace and symmetry of body, and to this must be linked a mind full of similar charms and attributes.

The Apollonian who is one of the spontaneous types does not present as many problems that must be worked out as does the Saturnian. His handsome appearance and the charm and graces of his manner open many doors to him, and occupations in many lines are not only open to him, but are thrust upon him.

The Apollonian Entity

The Apollonian is a distinct entity. He is a person. He has distinct characteristics, he is subject to certain diseases, he has his own idea of matrimony, and of religion. He has positive views on life in general. He has his own way of getting at things, and of getting others to do things for him, he knows how to get along without friction and at the same time to attain his ends. So it is valuable if we can know when we look at a very young child in its crib just what it is likely to look like and be like when it is grown up, and all the things it can do better than other people; for as we look at him we can plan his future if we have this knowledge, and mold him into it from the first days of his conscious life.

Conducting our study of the type in the same manner as we have done with the preceding types, we shall treat the Apollonian we describe as an adult male and a pure specimen of the type, and shall use the pronoun he, though there are just as many female Apollonians as there are males, all of whom follow in every way the characteristics as ascribed to the males. When we refer to the Apollonian child in reference to vocations, it will mean that he is fitted for them when he is grown.

Apollonian Characteristics

The Apollonian of fine grade is primarily *ARTISTIC*. He worships beauty in every aspect, in nature, dress, in pictures, sculpture, color, or form. He idealizes the spirit of beauty in every shape. He loves harmony in his surroundings, he is passionately fond of music generally of melodic character, and his very being radiates all these beauties which express themselves in his every gesture, in his smile, his very presence.

Thus the Apollonian child can be creative in the realm of art, in which he expresses himself by means of pictures, sculpture, musical composition, design, and in many processes of the manufacture of beautiful things.

We may place him safely as a painter, sculptor, architect, composer, landscape gardener, rug designer, or decorator, in all of which occupations he can find expression for his love of beauty, and his artistic sense.

The Apollonian of high grade has for his second strong characteristic *BRILLIANCY*, for his mind is exceedingly keen, and whether it be in talking about the things he loves or doing them, his mind fairly scintillates, and such a child is the welcomed one in any gathering.

He is in every sense a *DASHING* figure, confident of himself, filled with no gloomy thoughts and is healthy; he is of all the types one of the most *HAPPY*. And the combination of all these qualities make him *SUCCESSFUL*, which the Apollonian almost invariably is. We have in the Apollonian child one which has no very bad side. We find him of all grades, and the lower grades will not have as brilliant minds as the finer grades. As we descend the scale of grades we must not place a child of a lower grade in the creative artistic occupations which a high grade Apollonian can fill so well. In any grade, however, there will always be the love of beauty, he will aways be handsome, dashing in a degree, happy, and successful according to his grade. We will never find him mean, surly, vicious, criminal, or untrustworthy.

Thus we class the leading characteristics of the Apollonian as being:

Artistic sense
Brilliancy
A dashing figure
Always happy
Successful

THE APOLLONIAN AND MARRIAGE

In his marriage relations, the Apollonian is not uniformly successful. Having the beauty, the charm, and the social graces which belong to the type, he desires a mate of the same kind. For some reason he does not always succeed in securing such an one, and largely from the fact that he is the target for women who desire him, and who display their charms before him with many blandishments. He does not seem to be able to resist all of these advances and often chooses someone who, after he has been secured, does not keep up the effort to please or appear attractive, with the result that he finds himself tied to a wife who does not shine as he expected, and he is disappointed. He does not mate well with a Mercurian, a Saturnian, or a Lunarian.

APOLLONIAN HEALTH

The Apollonian is a healthy type, still there are several health defects peculiar to the type. He is first of all free from bile which is found so plentifully in the Saturnian and Mercurian. He is not a heavy eater as is the Jupiterian, consequently does not have the disturbances of his stomach which result from overloading it.

Nor is he a heavy drinker. He will not refuse to partake when it is offered, but he loves the social part of drinking more than the drink itself. His principal danger is from affections of the heart, which organ seems to be the weakest spot in his otherwise strong physique. This is a source of considerable danger, and any Apollonian child should be examined frequently so that the first sign of weakness of the heart may receive prompt medical attention. The Apollonian is subject to weak eyes, and is also susceptible to sunstroke and acute attacks of fever.

APOLLONIAN QUALITIES

The Apollonian is extremely versatile, his mind acts rapidly and he has the faculty of seeing a point so quickly that he astonishes those whose minds act more slowly. He is not a serious student, yet he seems well informed on any subject; in fact with a slight knowledge, and given a few facts, he will often confound those who have given years to a study, and his arguments will be sound.

There are few walks in life where the Apollonian cannot be successful. You observe we use the word cannot, for he will not always take the trouble to become profound in any subject and therefore he does the things that take the least exertion. If he can be aroused, he can become a scientist of attainments, or he can be brilliant in many different lines. There is not one of the types that can be successful in as many different occupations as the Apollonian.

THE SECONDARY TYPE

The first thing we wish to know, is which is the secondary type, and what it is going to do for the Apollonian child.

JUPITER SECONDARY TYPE

In many cases you will find that the Mount of Jupiter (Plate 8), is the secondary Mount. Thus the strong qualities of that type will be brought to the support of the child. In the first place he will have a large supply of ambition, and this will prove a great incentive to his best endeavors. The Apollonian child will not only have the fine qualities which belong to his own type, but he will have a great desire to take a leading position in society or business which he gets from the Jupiterian secondary type.

The Stage

This child can attain success on the stage, for from the ranks of Apollonian-Jupiterian children have and do come many of the leading exponents of dramatic art. The fine voice which both the Apollonian and the Jupiterian possess gives the necessary organ for a wonderful speaking voice, and the handsome appearance of the combined types give the child a commanding and attractive figure for the portrayal of heroic and dramatic rôles.

If you consult some of the leading authorities on the stage as a vocation, they will tell you that the great successes in this profession have all had a commanding ability to start with. Fine voice and fine physique, and that added to this they have a tremendous urge for the stage, and great industry. They will tell you that dramatic talent is inherent, and that by means of hard work it can be developed and perfected.

The stage presents a field for endeavor that is highly remunerative when successful, and a lure known to possibly no other occupation. A fine grade of Apollonian child possesses all of the qualities necessary to the greatest success on the stage. He has voice, physique, beauty, and if you will check up all his qualities, you will find that nothing is lacking to bring him to the highest pinnacle in the profession. If you will also check up all the qualities of the Jupiterian, which we are now considering as his secondary type, you will find that every one of them will be an aid to the success of the Apollonian child.

Good authorities say that to achieve success on the stage much study is necessary, much reading of the classics, the memorizing of rôles in all the leading plays old and new, voice training, the seeing of many plays, and the study of leading actors and their technique. Through the application of these methods, a fine grade Apollonian child with Jupiter as the secondary Mount can be made a distinguished actor.

In the lower grades, there are other branches of dramatic expression open to a child with this combination. Stock work, vaudeville, musical comedy, burlesque, farce, light and heavy character parts, utility, and later in life, old men and women parts, and positions as prompter, or assistant director. There is also open to those with dramatic talent a wonderful field as playwright and adapter. All of these are possible to an Apollonian child with Jupiter as the secondary Mount.

In Art

Next to the talent necessary for dramatic success shown by this combination, is its indication of talent in artistic directions. Such children can be successful artists, sculptors, mural decorators, designers, commercial illustrators, etchers, engravers and all those who transfer creative thought to canvas, or express it in other ways. The career of an artist cannot be said to offer inducement from a financial standpoint unless great celebrity is attained, but as the Apollonian-Jupiterian child has as one of his leading characteristics a large supply of artistic sense, we must not overlook an artistic calling as one best suited to many children. If they are so strongly marked in the development of their Mounts, and in the other tests which bear upon the Mounts, that it is plain that an artistic career presents great opportunity for them, then every effort should be made to give them the support which will develop their talents.

Moving Pictures

A new field has developed during the past few years, in which an Apollonian-Jupiterian child can meet with great success. This is in the moving picture industry. In every department of this, which is now the fourth largest industry, the Apollonian child with this combination has many positions open to him which he can fill better than is possible to any of the other types. In going over the different departments of this industry, it seems as if the Apollonian child had been created especially for the purpose of filling important positions in every one of them.

The three departments into which the work of the moving picture industry is divided are: the *production* of the *picture,* its distribution to the different places where it is shown, and the *exhibition* of the picture to the public.

In the first department, the Apollonian child's talent as an actor gives him a preëminent advantage in the filling of the parts necessary to the production of the picture. His artistic sense together with his fine appearance, his splendid physique and his beauty, make him an outstanding figure for photographic reproduction, and with the Jupiterian secondary Mount adding to all of these, he has an inherent advantage as a moving picture actor.

In the second department, which is the distributing of the picture to the houses where it will be shown, salesmanship is called into play. This is one of the Apollonian-Jupiterian child's most successful lines of endeavor. No one is his superior as a salesman. His manner, his appearance, his magnetic personality, all unite to make him supremely successful in salesmanship.

In the third department, which is the exhibition of the picture to the public, he brings into play all of his attractive qualities through the beautiful houses which his artistic sense enables him to imagine and build and the feeling of comfort with which he endows them, all of which bring many people to view his offerings and bring him success. There are thousands of positions of all degrees of importance in the dramatic field and in the moving pictures which are made to order for Apollonian children of all grades with the Mount of Jupiter as the secondary Mount. Of many of these we shall speak later when applying our tests.

Saturn Secondary Type

The Mount of Saturn (Plate 46), as the secondary Mount is not found in a large number of cases, as the qualities of the two Mounts are diametrically opposite. But in case the Apollonian development is very strong, Saturn can add some valuable qualities to the Apollonian child. He can be more of a student and he can be a better writer especially as an art and music critic. With this combination the Apollonian child is able to take some engineering positions, such as accoustic engineer or landscape engineer in which he will be successful on account of his pleasing personality and artistic qualities from his Apollonian side, and the studious habits he acquires from the Saturnian.

In Banking

The combination of Apollo and Saturn qualifies a child for success in the banking business, for from his Apollonian Mount type he has the address necessary for making friends which is needed by a modern banker, he is a good salesman which is also a requirement of a successful banker, and his intuitive faculties aid him in his judgment of men from whom he must select the customers of the bank.

In speaking of the banking business as an occupation please visualize just what that means, form an idea of what a big city bank is and what is done in it.

In the small banks of the villages and even of cities of small size, a position in a bank is a very personal one, the banker knows all his customers, and handles most of the business with them. In such a bank the child can start as bookkeeper, then cashier, and finally be president. Such an experience is excellent preparation for a position in one of the larger banks, and the ultimate in banking is to be connected with one of the big banks in the large cities.

Some of these banks comprise a small city in themselves. They are thoroughly departmentized and in every department are many positions of every grade up to the head of the department. The executive positions as heads of these banks, such as president, vice president, or chairman of the board, come after many years of experience in all branches of the banking business, but there are hundreds of positions as clerks of all kinds, runners, tellers, bookkeepers, auditors, foreign exchange experts, typists, stenographers, cashiers, bond salesmen, trust officers, credit men, insurance experts both life and fire, investigators and lawyers. Where the bank has a welfare department, there are many positions here, and as many banks have lunch and club facilities there are many positions in this department. In fact in some of the largest banks in the big cities, there are several thousand persons engaged in their daily operations, and in these banks Apollonian-Saturnian children of all grades can be placed according to their grades in positions in which they will be successful.

Every position in such a bank should be considered as training for the higher positions at the head of the bank. The more a man or woman learns in this way of the operations of the bank, the better chance for promotion. No position should be considered too unimportant by one deciding to make the banking business his career, as nearly all positions are filled from the bank's own personnel, certainly all that are possible to be are so filled. Banking offers a fine career, and a child who is an Apollonian with the Saturnian Mount secondary should be started along this line as soon as possible.

MERCURY SECONDARY TYPE

The Mount of Mercury (Plate 50), is often found as the secondary Mount in the hands of an Apollonian child. It will be recognized by the high Mount of Mercury, the apex leaning toward Apollo, and we also find bent or crooked fingers of Mercury on less desirable children, also leaning toward Apollo. These formations will be the means of identification of Mercury as the secondary Mount.

The Mount of Mercury is the business Mount, and its owner is always shrewd, calculating, and possesses an uncanny faculty of doing business at a profit. Fine specimens of the type number among them some of the most successful men in the business world. But as the grade becomes lower the Mercurian is tricky and resorts to sharp practice, until in the lowest grades he becomes a thief, and the very coarse ones petty thieves.

Salesmanship

The grade of the child will make a great difference in the class of employment in which he can be most successful with Mercury as the secondary Mount. In fine grades the Mercurian shrewdness, added to the super-ability of the Apollonian child as a salesman, fit him for the most important positions in the selling field.

Securities—Insurance

The ability to distribute merchandise and commodities is the most important part of business. No big business can exist unless there is first sold stocks and bonds to secure capital to finance the enterprise, and there is no one in the world who can be as successful in the sale and distribution of securities as the Apollonian-Mercurian child. There is no more important field than the sale of insurance as it is done today. In fact insurance of all the contingencies of life, fire, accidents of all sorts, health, old age, annuity, death, and the many forms of protection which can now be thrown around the family, the individual, or the business organization, offer to one who can sell policies for all these risks enormous returns, and of all the children of all the types, the Apollonian-Mercurian child can be the most successful in the insurance field. No large or small business enterprise can exist unless they can sell what they make, and world wide organizations are maintained by manufacturing companies in all of which this child can find a place, small stores need to sell, the farmer needs to sell, the minister has to sell, thus it is only a matter of choice which field the Apollonian-Mercurian child shall enter to successfully market his salesmanship.

Automobiles

We are of the opinion that there is no field which offers such wonderful opportunities to-day as the automobile industry. A fine grade Apollonian-Mercurian child whose parents select this as his life's work and prepare him for it, will be placing him in an occupation for which he is well fitted, for he is, on merit, entitled to have the best opportunity there is. No greater opportunity for success and profit can be found than as head of a big international sales department of a prominent automobile company, in which capacity a fine grade Apollonian-Mercurian child with fine skin, pink color, elastic consistency, and a strong thumb can have the ultimate in success.

MARTIAN SECONDARY TYPES

The Apollonian child will often have the Martian as the secondary Mounts (Plates 52-54), and here we must note whether the upper or the lower Mount is best developed as each will give a different kind of support. These Mounts are located by their bulging character, and the direction in which they lean.

The Upper Mount (Plate 52), which is located on the side of the hand, if it be full and bulging will add coolness, courage, calmness, and this particular Martian Mount will, if well developed, add a large measure of resistance. The addition of these qualities to the Apollonian child will make him more self confident, and such a thing as discouragement is unknown to him.

In Diplomatic Service

An Apollonian child with upper Mars secondary can be very successful in the diplomatic service, for he will have the fine address, the charming manner, the handsome appearance and magnetic personality of the Apollonian, and to these will be added the coolness, calmness, courage, and resistance of the upper Mount of Mars. Thus he will approach a diplomatic mission with tact, and yet with an unbeatable persistence.

In the regular diplomatic service of the Government, there are a very large number of positions in the various embassies and consular branches of the service. All of these positions can be filled with great success by Apollonian children of all grades. There are hosts of clerks, and many under secretaries; these positions can be filled by those of medium grade, and there are heads of departments for high grade children, who have under them a large force of employees all of whom can be Apollonian-Martian children of varying grades.

Foreign Trade

There is a division of business where the same qualities that bring success in the diplomatic field are needed, and we should start our child at a very early age to prepare for a career in this field. This is the business of foreign trade, which means the handling of our export and import business with all the foreign countries. It is a business in itself, and is capable of the highest specialization, in fact must have this kind of specialization upon the part of those who are to be successful in it.

There has never been a time when as many highly trained men and women were needed to handle this business as now. The war and economic conditions have changed the entire aspect of our relations with foreign countries, and it is not only desirable but necessary for us to distribute a large part of our manufactured goods abroad as well as our raw material and the product of our farms. To do this requires highly trained sales forces, who must speak the languages of the different countries, know their customs, and the manners of approach which will most appeal to them. These foreign trade organizations call for the highest type of talent in salesmanship and pay the largest price to get it.

Many large corporations send men to foreign countries whose business is to promote good will. They are in reality business ambassadors, and principally they get to know everybody worth while, they entertain, they make themselves liked, they know the most important people in the country and are on a social footing with them. These men keep their companies posted as to every phase of business, the kind of goods most desired, all changes in prices, and they become so situated that they can take up any matter with the heads of the government.

These positions require the highest grade of men, and the Apollonian child with upper Mars secondary is the combination most needed for success.

The business ambassador is the highest type of service in foreign trade, and from this, all the way down, there are positions of great importance. The big international banking corporations use a host of men for investigation, promotion, and sales. Manufacturing companies are building factories abroad, and every effort is being made to develop foreign trade. Great opportunities lie ahead for young men and women of the type combination we are considering, in the foreign trade field.

But they must be prepared for these opportunities, by reading and studying the right subjects, by becoming thoroughly familiar with the customs of all the foreign countries, and by learning at least two of the foreign languages. French and Spanish will give an entrée into a great many countries, and to know more languages in countries where trade opportunities exist is still better. There should be a thorough knowledge of economics, banking, commercial law, exchange of money, foreign investments, credit, transportation, and patent trade mark law.

These things can be taught a child in easy stages if one begins when they are young, and by the time they are old enough to accept a position it will only be necessary to apply to the foreign trade department office of any large corporation engaged in this business to be eagerly accepted.

If the Apollonian child has the *lower Mount* of Mars secondary, it will add aggression to his other qualities. Thus he will push to a conclusion everything he undertakes. He is admirably adapted to be the pioneer in the opening of new oil fields, and in their development. He can succeed in the real estate business in the development of new additions, in right of way work for railroads, and the lower grades make excellent superintendents, foremen, district managers, city managers, and they will be successful in all positions where they have the superintendence of men. They also make excellent army officers, commissioned and non-commissioned.

The Lunarian Secondary Type

We sometimes find the Mount of the Moon to be the secondary Mount for the Apollonian child, which is shown by the bulging of the Mount, and other indications already explained. The principal addition to the Apollonian child from this combination will be a supply of imagination and a large vocabulary.

The Lunar subject has a number of strong characteristics such as mysticism, coldness, and selfishness, but the Apollonian child is a stronger character than the Lunarian, and these qualities are minimized in transmission to him. The quality of imagination, however, which is strong in the Lunarian, has considerable effect on the Apollonian child which gives him the ability to express himself in well chosen language, for no one has a larger vocabulary than the Lunarian.

Through this combination, the Apollonian child can be a good writer with a large vocabulary and plenty of imagination, which he now gets from the Mount of the Moon. What he writes is logical and convincing. He is always a salesman, and now, with this combination, we have a salesman who writes convincingly and has the imagination to develop new ideas.

In Advertising

Thus he falls naturally into the advertising business. Here he finds an opportunity to coin new phrases, to say old things in a new way, to invent slogans, and to use his always masterful selling ability in the preparation of booklets, pamphlets, circulars, newspaper advertising, and all the countless inventions of the advertising mind.

The advertising field is one which offers as great opportunities to the right children as any which can be chosen. It is the field of large scale selling, a necessary part of the distribution plans of all large corporations. It is what has made possible the mass production in the automobile field, and all the other fields wherein production has reached such heights that better goods are now obtainable, at lower prices, than were possible during the era of small production. It creates new markets, and is in every way a benefit to those who have goods to sell or money to spend.

The amount of money spent for advertising every year is enormous, and a child who is found to be an Apollonian with the Mount of the Moon as the secondary Mount is especially fortunate, and peculiarly adapted for a successful career in the advertising field. When this combination is found, the child should be educated by having him acquire a knowledge of the things that will help him most in the advertising business, and the greater general knowledge he has, the better able he will be to prepare convincing advertising material.

By far the greatest amount of useful knowledge can be gained by reading which should cover all subjects relating to the manufacture and distribution of merchandise. He should learn to analyze, to plan selling campaigns, should practice writing, study illustrations which he must understand thoroughly, and learn type setting, engraving, and printing. The best preparation is to start at the bottom in a good advertising agency, where he can learn every branch of advertising.

The agency is both the buyer and seller of advertising space, prepares the copy, plans the campaign, studies the possible field for every product, and becomes the intermediary between the producer and consumer. A complete education can be obtained in an agency which will be much more valuable than that to be had in any other way. Fine openings are available to all young men and women who have a thorough knowledge of advertising, in department stores, on newspapers, in large corporations, and with the railroads and public utility corporations. In fact no large enterprise can succeed today without a large expenditure for advertising which opens a vast field of operation for the Apollonian child with the Mount of the Moon as the secondary Mount. For this calling he can be prepared from the beginning.

Venus the Secondary Type

When we find the Mount of Venus as the secondary Mount, it does not add much strength to the Apollonian child as these two Mounts are so much alike that it simply amounts to making the Apollonian qualities more intense. Both are handsome, attractive, spontaneous, and fond of beauty. They are artistic, cheerful, graceful, and in every way delightful in personality. The Venusian secondary Mount will bring to the combination no new strengthening qualities, nor any new qualities, but it will insure a more intense operation of the good qualities of the Apollonian child. So it may be taken, when present, as an earnest of the fact that he will more surely be able to do successfully all of the things which we have outlined for him.

THE TEST FOR GRADE

By this time we have a very clear idea of the Apollonian child, and of many things he can do better than other people, in fact he now stands before us as a definite personality, a more complete picture of a human being than can be obtained in any other manner than by the examination of his hands. We are now going to apply to this entity a number of tests to see what further information we can obtain from them.

FIRST TEST—TEXTURE OF THE SKIN

First there is the texture of the skin on the hands, which gives us information as to the grade of the child. As has been stated, we do not expect to find a criminal tendency, even in the lowest grades of Apollonian children, and beyond the fact that his instincts are not the most refined, the lower grades do not present serious problems. We find, most often, skin on the hands of Apollonian children of the softest velvety texture (Plate 10), even on the hands of adults, and the hands of very young children are always of soft fine texture. If the child is inherently of a coarse grade, the skin will coarsen as he grows older until it reaches the grade to which he belongs, where it remains stationary. By the time he is twelve years old, his skin will accurately indicate his grade. From very fine skin, the texture gradually coarsens as the grade of the child becomes lower, until, in some cases, it becomes as coarse as the skin shown in Plate 11, though this grade is not common with the Apollonian child.

We have outlined in this chapter a number of lines of business in which very great opportunities are open to the Apollonian child. We cannot too strongly recommend those in which he comes in direct contact with the public, where his fine appearance, charming manner, and magnetic personality give him a preëminent advantage. Those children with fine texture of skin can be the ones who will occupy the best positions in all of the sales organizations and wherever we have suggested that they be placed. Those of lower grades can find in these same organizations innumerable positions of lesser responsibility which they can fill.

SECOND TEST—COLOR OF THE HANDS

The color of the hands should next be considered, as this will give an idea of the amount and character of the physical strength present, and this will exert a considerable influence on the career of the child.

With a very young child, the thing that is supremely important, is to locate his primary and secondary types and choose the occupation best suited to him. Preparation for this chosen occupation can begin at once by directing his play so that he will become interested in the things which are at a future day to become the tools of his vocation, and by the time he has arrived at an age where it is possible, the color of his hands will help you to know him better and thus be able to help him more.

White Color

White color is not the normal color for an Apollonian child. He is full blooded, and pink or red are his natural colors. When white is present, he should at once be given a medical examination. A weak anæmic condition will, if not corrected, have a strong influence on his whole career. There will not be the virility in this case that is needed to bring the splendid qualities of the Apollonian child to their best development. He will be listless, he will lack energy, he will put things off, his type qualities will not develop to the fullest extent, and he will not achieve the possibilities which are inherent in him. Many times white color accounts for unexplainable indifference on the part of talented children and their failure to become what we know they are capable of being.

This child, in spite of his white color, still has the Apollonian type advantages, and while he cannot engage in occupations requiring great energy he can do those things which do not tax his strength. So when we see white color on a fine grade child, we should prepare him for a critic of music or of art. He will have natural talent for both, but it will be better to have him specialize in one or the other. If music is chosen he need not try to be a concert performer, but he can master harmony, theory, composition, and study all the best composers and their compositions. In other words he can learn what is needed to enable him to judge of the performances of others. In this field he can be successful. If art is chosen, he need not try to be a painter or sculptor, but he can learn how to judge the work of others and thus have success in this direction too.

Pink Color

Pink color shows the full operation of a healthy blood supply which is nourishing and enriching the brain activities, is feeding the nervous system with the elements it needs, is supplying all the organs with new matter, and carrying off that which has been used up and needs to be eliminated. So we find that when pink color is present, the child will be active, interested, virile, and will develop his type qualities to the fullest extent.

Such an one, if he be of fine quality, can attain the highest positions in any of the occupations for which we have recommended him, and the lower grades can find occupation in the less responsible positions.

This child should be prepared for an important position in foreign trade, he can even be a business ambassador if he is given the proper training and handled right. He should be started as suggested in a former paragraph in this chapter, and should have the opportunity to master the subjects as outlined in this same paragraph. He should learn the political situation in all the foreign countries, their language and customs, then he should select some prominent house engaged in foreign trade and associate himself with them in a minor position from which he can rise, and where he can learn all about the business. In this way he can get his start and, so prepared, this child can achieve a fine success and secure a large income in foreign trade.

Red Color

Red color shows that there is still more force, with the result that the child becomes very intense in everything he does, he pushes his projects with great vigor, he is less tactful, he forces things instead of having people do things because they like him, he needs restraint so that he does not go too fast.

With this color it is well to examine closely and identify the secondary type. If the Martian Mounts are secondary this child should be fitted for a building contractor. He will be even more successful than the Martian, for the red color will give him the virility he needs, and the Apollonian type will make him able to get the contracts. If Saturn is secondary he should, if of fine grade, choose the mining profession. Such a child can be, if of fine grade, not only a mining engineer but he can be at the head of a mining company mining for coal, iron, gold, silver, copper, or other metals.

Yellow Color

The Apollonian child seldom has yellow color. When it is present it is an abnormal condition, and a medical examination should be given. It shows the presence of bile in the system in sufficient quantity to tinge the skin. We know from this that some organ is not functioning in a manner natural to the Apollonian type.

Yellow color, which produces irritability, deprives the Apollonian child of his ability to come in direct contact with the public which is one of his greatest assets. So we can only place this child in a position where his Apollonian talents can be used, but where he will not have to make direct sales. This can be done by training him for commercial illustrating for which he has talent on account of his type qualities. It will not be difficult, by sending him to good art schools, and giving him private instruction in addition, to prepare him for a successful career as an illustrator.

THIRD TEST—FLEXIBILITY OF THE HAND

Flexibility of the hands will tell us much about the elasticity of mind possessed by the Apollonian child. Even in very young children we may get an idea of this quality of mind, and as the child grows older we find his hands giving us more and more information on this subject.

The Stiff Hand

In young children we will not find the extreme stiffness of hand that is shown in Plate 12; such a case as this develops later in life, if at all, but we will find that as the child grows older his hand takes on stiffness if that quality is inherent in him.

An Apollonian child with such a hand will still have his type qualities but in a crude form, he cannot occupy the high positions which others of his type can who are of fine grade, but he can fill some position in occupations in which Apollonian children are successful. In every advertising agency one of the prominent forms of advertising is that of outdoor signs which often take the form of huge affairs covering a large space. The painting and hanging of these signs is an important matter, and while the stiff handed Apollonian child cannot excel in the higher forms of art he can be taught to be an excellent painter of outdoor advertising signs which is important to his company and for which he will be well paid. Thus he will be successful in one of the Apollonian occupations, that of advertising, though not in the highest position.

The Flexible Hand

The flexible hand shown in Plate 14, and extreme flexibility shown in Plate 15, belong with the finest grade of Apollonian development. Here we have a mind that can adapt itself to any situation; which is clever, versatile, keen, and such a mind will bring out the strongest side of Apollonian development in any child. He will be able to fill the highest positions in all the occupations for which the Apollonian child is best fitted.

In the banking business, more certainly with Saturn as secondary type, he will be one who can master the details of the business, and with his numerous advantages he can advance to the highest executive positions. As a salesman, he can, whether in foreign trade or in the organization of large corporations, occupy one of the best positions, and as an advertising man he will have an advantage owing to his mental elasticity, so that he can adjust himself to any situation. His mind is keen enough to see through any proposition which is brought to him and discover all of its points of appeal which must be stressed. In fact, flexible hands are the indication of an extremely high grade organism which applied to the Apollonian indicates that he can achieve the highest forms of success.

An Apollonian child with flexible hands is a fine combination, and this child should be placed where he can take full advantage of his opportunities and his natural advantages; such as an important art gallery in one of the large cities, where the best in painting and sculpture, including the work of modern artists and the old masters, are brought together; and where in widely advertised sales there are gathered the most important collectors of art from this and foreign counties. In these sales the *objets d'art* are sold both at auction and by private sale at high prices. These art galleries gather collections of antique furniture, glass, china, silver, books, tapestries, and other rare and costly merchandise. In such a gallery, either at the head of it, or connected with it, there is the greatest opportunity, for the Apollonian child with flexible hands, for contacts with those who value and buy high priced art. In such a place, this Apollonian child, if of fine grade, could, owing to his charming personality and sales ability, find a great opportunity and establish a clientèle that would bring him a large income and permanent success.

Flexible hands will also materially aid an Apollonian child of the lower grades, and with these hands he can fill more responsible positions in all of the fields in which his type is most successful. Flexible hands will not be found on the lowest grades of children.

The Straight Hand

The straight hand (Plate 13), will often be found on Apollonian children and this will mean that the child is well balanced, and occupies a medium position when it comes to elasticity of the mind. He will not be nearly so brilliant as his brother with the flexible hands, his mind will not be adaptable to as many different things, but he will be steady and reliable, and while he will be more of a plodder, he will retain what he learns.

The Apollonian child with straight hands will be practical, and while he will have all the qualities belonging to his type, he will not have the high artistic sense which would make him a great artist or sculptor, but he is an artist, as every member of the type is, so we must use this talent in a practical way and prepare this child for a career as a scene painter in which vocation he can have great success. He can have a studio, and if he receives good training and proper advantages, he can become famous in the theatrical world and be called on for work in all the prominent theatres. He can make more money than the painter of pictures, and such a child should be started early to understand what he is going to do and his training should begin as soon as he is able to hold a brush.

Fourth Test—Consistency of the Hands

Consistency of the hands is an important test, for no matter how brilliant one may be, if laziness be present little will come of it. We will not be able to use this test with very young children, as their hands are uniformly soft, but a hand that is soft on a very young child will grow to be elastic or hard as the child grows older. At the age of twelve, the hand takes on the consistency that belongs to it, and from that time on we know how much help energy will give in shaping his future.

Flabby Hands

If the hands remain flabby when the child grows older, he will have little energy, he will have all the strong qualities that belong to the type, but he will always be putting things off with the result that he makes no particular headway even if he is given the best of opportunities.

Manifestly it will not do to put this child into a business position, for there competition is keen and one must be up and doing to keep up with the procession. Such a child would only invite failure in attempting to enter any big sales organization, an advertising agency or foreign trade, but he has all the artistic ability of the Apollonian type and he can succeed as an artist, and even though he is lazy, he can paint pictures which will command attention. Therefore we advise that this child should be given thorough instruction in art and as soon as possible placed under a competent teacher, so that instead of merely drifting through life he may make a name for himself.

Soft Hands

If the hands of the child are soft, he will not be quite so hopelessly lazy as if they are flabby, yet he will not be full of energy, he will need someone to keep him at work. Such a child seldom reaches the highest positions in any organization.

He should be given as much work as possible in a gymnasium, where he will be made to go through vigorous exercise. He should be given a camp life out of doors where he will have to cook and do other things before he can eat and have a place to sleep, and in every way he should be kept busy doing things which require work that he is *forced* to do. In this way work may become a habit and a measure of energy may be built up.

In placing this child in the occupation for which he is best fitted we must remember that he has the Apollonian talents, the principal one of which is salesmanship. We must not depend upon his using this talent however to its fullest extent if he has soft hands. We cannot place him in high pressure sales organizations, but we must find a place where he can make use of his salesmanship with the least amount of exertion. As we know, he can be a writer, we can therefore place him with safety in a position as a writer of sales literature. This may be either in an advertising agency, or it may be in the advertising department of a department store, or a manufacturing company which does a large amount of advertising and distribution of mail matter. In such a position the Apollonian child with soft hands can be successful.

Elastic Hands

The elastic hand is what we wish to find on an Apollonian child, for the elastic hand means not only energy, but intelligent energy; it means that the child will do all the work necessary to bring him the largest measure of success. His type gives him the mental qualities and the characteristics which produce success, and the elastic hand supplies the energy to bring them to fruition. No matter what the grade of the Apollonian child, elastic consistency gives him a better chance for success.

There is no place where energy is so much needed as in positions where sales are solicited and made by direct calls upon prospects. Many miles a day are traveled by a salesman in calling on those he expects to sell, and as the Apollonian child's greatest talent is in selling, he will find the intelligent energy of the elastic hand a big asset, and we must take advantage of it in placing him in the occupation where he can have the most success. Among the recommendations for an Apollonian child is the insurance business, either as a representative or manager of a general insurance agency. In either case the sales ability of this child and the energy of the elastic hand will enable him to have great success in the insurance business and to make a large profit from it. We should therefore prepare this child for this business and secure him a connection with a good company.

Hard Hands

Hard hands show an excess of energy but not such intelligent energy, and this consistency is not often found on hands of the highest grades of Apollonian children. It is preferable to soft or flabby hands, however, even on a high grade Apollonian child, but its presence shows that the child is not of the finest quality.

The newspaper field has openings for Apollonian children and there is an attraction about it which appeals to the type. In this case however as in all others we must fit the child into a position according to his grade. We find, therefore, when we discover a child with hard hands, that we should not place him in the editorial chair, but there is a place where he can be successful and that is as an advertising solicitor. The great energy he gets from his hard hands will enable him to do the real hard work necessary in such a position, and the type love for newspaper work will give him the proper approach and the salesmanship necessary to success.

Fifth Test—The Three Worlds

The three worlds of the hand are very important tests. The Apollonian child is so versatile that he may enter many parts of a number of different kinds of organizations. They may relate to art, the theater, to advertising, to writing, selling, to diplomacy, to banking, to foreign trade, to scientific study and occupations, and to innumerable positions in the business world. It will be better for a child to be placed in the branch of all these lines of endeavor where he has the most aptitude, and from the three worlds we learn whether he is stronger in the mental world, the practical or business world, or in the lower or material world.

First we examine the hand as a whole, on which the divisions of the three worlds are shown as in Plate 16. We also find that the fingers by means of the phalanges, likewise show the three worlds (Plate 1). We always find that the worlds as shown by the hand as a whole, and by the phalanges of the fingers, corroborate each other.

The Mental World

When we find the mental world dominant (Plate 17), the child will be best fitted for occupations where his mental powers can be brought into play. Thus in the advertising business he can succeed in the copy writing department where all advertisements are written, and with his artistic taste he can do well in the art and illustrating departments if properly prepared. He can also do well in the public accounting business where a trained mind is necessary, especially in the collection departments, and in planning sales campaigns which are recommended to clients. As in the big accounting companies the distribution of products is a part of their service, he can do well here. He can also do well as a teacher or professor of art in schools and colleges, and can succeed in the newspaper business, especially in the editorial end.

In all of the sales organizations of large corporations there are many positions where literary ability is of great assistance, and in these portions of a sales organization an Apollonian child with the mental world best developed will be most successful. He is always a salesman, and where he can best express himself he will be most successful.

In the insurance business where fine fields exist, the mental world will fit him for the preparation of most effective sales literature, and in the field of the stage, one of his strongest aptitudes, the mental world will enable him to see and appreciate the higher values of his art.

It is in this latter field that a well developed Apollonian child with the mental world best developed will do best, and, if he is prepared for it, he can make a success as a producer. So many poor plays are produced today which could be avoided if producers had the talent for the stage inherent in the Apollonian child, and with this, had mental and literary ability to see the faults of the plays presented to them. It requires more than business sense to be a successful producer, it requires the artistic instinct even more. Financial backing can be furnished, or business management, but unless the producer has a sense of dramatic value, he will produce poor plays. An Apollonian child has this necessary ingredient if his mental world dominates, and for this reason he should be prepared by early study of the fundamentals as laid down in an earlier paragraph in this chapter, and his vocation should be that of a theatrical producer.

The Middle World

The middle world if best developed (Plate 18), will give the Apollonian child a practical turn, and if he selects art as a career, he will not be carried away by fads in painting or sculpture. He will not be a cubist but a realist, and his work will show things as they really are, consequently he will be a greater financial success and will sell more pictures.

He will have great ability for interior decoration and mural painting. In these occupations there are positions ranging from those of fine grade who do the most important work, to those of lower grade who fill in backgrounds and work of a supplementary character.

In the banking business the middle world will be of great assistance. It will take away every thought that the child is a dreamer, and will show that he can be eminently practical in all things and as a consequence safe and conservative—two qualities most necessary in the banking business.

It will be of great help in the world of salesmanship, for here all things are practical. It will enable him to realize the advantage he possesses in his fine appearance, his rich mellow voice, and his magnetic personality, and he will lay plans to use all these advantages. Such children, if of fine grade, are fitted for the more important positions in sales organizations, and plans can be made even while the child is quite young, looking toward his filling places at the head of such organizations. It is even possible to select the identical company in which you intend to place him.

The Apollonian child with the middle world well developed will find his greatest opportunity in foreign trade which is really a refinement of salesmanship. The opportunities are so great at this time that no better choice of a vocation could be made. As there are a number of different departments in foreign trade the child should select some particular department and specialize in it. He can become an international lawyer as law is one department, and he will be more successful in the law if Mercury be his secondary Mount. Or he can specialize in foreign banking, for many of our larger banks have foreign branches, in which he will be much helped if Saturn be secondary. There is transportation which is a huge field covering rail and shipping by air and water. In this department the child will be much assisted if the Martian Mounts be secondary. Then there are the sales departments of which there are all kinds, and in these the child can be most successful and if of fine grade he can rise to high positions. In these Jupiter can be of help if secondary. There is both importing and exporting, and there are many kinds of merchandise to be manufactured and sold. Each one of these is a specialized part of foreign trade, and the parent should choose in which the child is to operate and prepare him for the work he is to do. If thought is given to it by the parent, an Apollonian child of fine grade with the middle phalanx well developed can have a successful career in foreign trade.

The Lower World

With the lower or material world best developed (Plate 19), the child will still be practical but his efforts will not be effective on such a high plane as is the case when the other two worlds are best developed. He will have more of the sensual about him, and his thoughts will be of coarser things. He will be fitted for the less important parts of the work in all the occupations for which an Apollonian child has been recommended. He will have the Apollonian advantages, but they will not lead him to the most responsible positions.

This child will not be fitted for occupations which require mental effort in literary directions, nor will he be successful as an actor or artist, but he can be successful as a salesman, which is an Apollonian qualification, and it should not be in stores handling fine merchandise. He can be successful as a hardware merchant, and could run such a store for himself or be a salesman in one, he could sell heavy machinery, or tractors, plumbing supplies, laundry machines, or printing presses and supplies. Or be a stage manager in a theater.

The Middle World in Combination

The middle world makes a good combination with either of the other two, for with the mental world the intellectual qualities of the Apollonian child will have a practical side, and he will not be a theorist; his mental ability will be devoted to practical ends.

If he writes, it will be on practical subjects, and his efforts will be to secure practical results. So in sales literature he will first desire to induce sales rather than to produce literature, and in every effort which he makes in the mental world, he will always have in mind the results he is going to achieve in whatever field his operations may lie.

There is a field in which this Apollonian child can be especially successful, and this is in the diplomatic service. His brilliant qualities, his charming manner, his fine appearance all fit him to make friends, and he can capitalize all of these qualities as a diplomat. With the mental world developed he will add the attraction of a proper understanding of the correct way to appear in society, it will give him poise, and in dealing with other diplomats he will be keen enough to hold his own. If the middle world is also developed he will in addition have the benefit of business ability. Thus he will be a good business man and in everything he does as a diplomat he will see that it is done in a businesslike manner. The result of the combination of his Apollonian talents with the mental alertness of the mental world and business ability of the middle world make him fit to hold a position as ambassador or consul in the diplomatic service for which he should be prepared.

If the middle and the lower worlds are the two best developed, he will be best fitted for very practical positions. He will not do well as a teacher, professor, or writer, but he will be a good contractor, superintendent, foreman, salesman of farm implements, tractors, trucks, and in similar capacities.

Sixth Test—Knotty Fingers

Knotty fingers (Plate 20), are not common on the hands of the Apollonian child. His best results are not brought about by analysis. But there are cases where this combination is found, and our first consideration will be to see whether the first or second knot is developed, or only one of them.

Knot of Mental Order

If the first or knot of mental order (Plate 21), is alone developed, we have mental system, and order in thinking. This will indicate that the child will not depend upon inspiration, but will have all his facts well arranged, and there will be no possibility of a confusion of ideas.

He can make a good writer often on technical subjects, he can organize well thought out sales campaigns, he will plan all of his work, he will demand order and system from those about him, and he will be extremely well fitted for the mental side of a number of Apollonian occupations.

This child can be successful as a newspaper reporter or editor. If his grade be fine he can hold the higher positions, but he will not be able to get into an editorial chair in the beginning; he will probably, until he has demonstrated his ability, have to take a much lower position from which he will advance. But the Apollonian qualities will make themselves felt, and the mental organization shown by the knot of mental order will enable him to do such a superior class of work that if he is well prepared with a good general education and wide reading, he will rise to the top. In other of the Apollonian occupations the knot of mental order will be a help, but in none of them as much help as in the newspaper or magazine field in editorial positions. This will prove the best field for an Apollonian child with knots of mental order.

Second or Knot of Material Order

If the second knot is best developed (Plate 22), he will have system in material things, his dress will be immaculate, and everything he plans will be laid out and thoroughly considered. He can be an exceptionally good organizer which can make him a leader in many of the Apollonian fields.

Order and system are prime requisites for success in the organization of a sales department for a large corporation, especially if the business of the company extends over a wide territory. Unless there is the most perfect system in such an organization there will be no reports, no careful checking of expense accounts, and none of the other innumerable, invisible, but most essential details of organization which spell either success or failure in such an enterprise. And while we know that an Apollonian child of fine grade will have the highest type of ability as a salesman, and while he has all the qualifications necessary for success as an individual salesman, if he has not the ability to systematize, he cannot be successful as the leader of a widespread sales effort which is the purpose of a large sales organization. When we find on the hands of a high grade Apollonian child, however, the knot of material order, we know that this child has not only individual sales ability, but he has sales organization ability. Such a child should makes sales organization his life work.

Both Knots Developed

If both knots be developed (Plate 20), the child will have greater qualities of analysis than is usual with the Apollonian. Here he will be able to enter several of the engineering fields. He is, so far as an Apollonian can be, a scientist, and he can find success in psychology, ceramic engineering, automobile engineering if he is of a fine grade, and if of a lower grade, he will do well as a superintendent, sanitary engineer, or building inspector in these same industries.

In the fine grades he can also do well as an architect, a surveyor, a telephone or telegraph engineer, or a civil engineer. He can also be the ultra-conservative banker.

SEVENTH TEST—SMOOTH FINGERS

Smooth fingers (Plate 23), are natural to the Apollonian child. He being one of the spontaneous types relies on intuition and inspiration rather than analysis. And as we have all along been considering a pure specimen of the Apollonian type, it has included the fact that he has smooth fingers which we expect. Such recommendations as have been made are predicated upon the fact that the child has smooth fingers. These children should not be placed in the engineering professions, but in the large list of theatrical or artistic occupations which are open to the Apollonian child many of which have been enumerated in this chapter.

Eighth Test—Long Fingers

Long fingers (Plate 24), with their love of detail, make the Apollonian child slow, and in only a few cases are they a benefit. In some of the engineering occupations where mathematics are needed they will be helpful, such as mechanical engineering, and in astronomy. A child with good Apollonian hands and long fingers may be placed in either of these branches of engineering, and as teachers of these subjects they can be successful. They are also adapted for, and are excellent as, accountants and auditors, bookkeepers, certified public accountants, and in telegraphy.

In a research department for a medical college, in statistical work, in analytical work in the engineering department of an automobile manufacturer they can succeed, and as there are so many of these kinds of departments, it opens the way for good positions with many of the larger corporations. Also with brokerage houses, steel companies, or with railroads. A good many sales organizations have departments which gather various kinds of sales information, showing the number of possible customers in a given territory, their purchasing power, their location locally, and a large number of facts which will help a sales manager plan a sales campaign. In such a department, the Apollonian child with long fingers can be successful on account of his natural sales ability and the detail of the long fingers. Such a child can go to the head of such a department. He should be started at the bottom and will naturally rise to the top. But he should be prepared for the work beginning at an early age.

If the child is of fine grade there is a department of the art of portrait painting in which he will have great success. This is the painting of miniatures. This is a specialty and few artists attempt it. The drawing and brush work is so small, and in order to be a success must be so fine, that no one who is not a master of detail would dare to essay the task. But to an Apollonian child with long fingers and fine grade, miniature painting presents no difficulties; but to do it, the child must have thorough training in color mixing and blending, drawing, and brush work. With such training the child can make a name for himself and as this form of painting commands a good price he can also make it very profitable.

Ninth Test—Short Fingers

Short fingers (Plate 26), are found on the hands of Apollonian children in a large number of cases. They are especially favorable when the indications point to the stage. The natural talent of the Apollonian child for dramatic work needs a quick way of thinking, for often emergencies arise where the whole performance depends upon a quick answer, and the short fingered Apollonian child will never be at a loss. In addition to this he must have intuition in order to get the dramatic spirit of many rôles, and inspiration, a quality of short fingers, is one of the chief requisites of an actor. The same is true of children for whom the movies offer the best opportunity as shown by the proper markings in their hands, and for all of these, short fingers will be favorable.

They are not always favorable for Apollonian children in the business world and the sciences, for here a slower method of thought is needed in order not to make mistakes. They will not be so favorable in the banking business where quick decisions are not desirable.

In the field of salesmanship short fingers will make the child mentally alert and he will be able to take advantage of every opening for the purpose of making a good impression, he will be intuitive in judging the best method of approach to a customer, and quick to seize every opening given for the use of his favorable personality in the making of a sale.

There is a branch of selling where the Apollonian child with short fingers will be most successful and this is in the conduct of an auction house. The Apollonian sales ability will furnish salesmanship, and the short fingers the quick wit and repartee which an auctioneer needs to be the most successful. This is a business which has great possibilities. A number of men have become wealthy as auctioneers of real estate in large cities, selling large buildings and ranking among the leading citizens. Auction houses for art collections are very successful, and altogether this is a vocation worthy of a high grade Apollonian child. The one with short fingers should be started in a good auction house at an early age so that he may learn the best methods; afterwards he can engage in business for himself with profit.

TENTH TEST—THE FINGER TIPS

The tips of the fingers will have a great deal to do with determining the best place to use the Apollonian talents, for the qualities indicated by the tips are fundamental.

The Pointed Tip

In the first place the pointed tip (Plate 27), will make the child too impractical to enable him to fill a place in the business world; this much we determine at the start. But if he is hyper-artistic, he can be devoted to creative art, and the pointed tip will be of great assistance.

The pointed tip indicates that the child has artistic sense which we know as soon as we identify his type, and with both vision and artistic sense, he can be dedicated to art with the expectation of success. In fact the surest indication that art is his best occupation is to be found in the pointed tip.

This art may take the form of portrait painting, landscape, still life, cattle, horses, street scenes, or water pictures; these are specializations in which children with this combination can do well, and as an artist must have something from which he can earn his daily bread, this child can use the imagination of pointed tips in commercial art.

The pointed tip will also be helpful in a dramatic career. There must be vision in the creation of a rôle, and this the pointed tip will give, but the owner of this tip will be most temperamental, and seldom has the capacity for hard work necessary for success on the stage. Children with this tip who have succeeded on the stage and in literature have been natural geniuses filled with type talent and the imagination and vision of the pointed tip.

This tip also gives ability in the field of literature, especially in fiction writing and in poetry. When this combination is seen on a child, it will be a mistake to try and force him into a career in business, it will only cause unhappiness and failure.

The Conic Tip

The conic tip (Plate 28), is found very often on the hands of Apollonian children, for the conic tip is known as the artistic tip. But the child with this tip will be able to fill many positions in the business world too, in fact the world is now full of those who are doing so.

The conic tip will be a help in foreign trade, especially in Latin countries, for here so much depends on personality. It is those who have the ability to charm who succeed in the introduction of new lines of goods in foreign countries, and who increase the sales of the established products of a corporation.

There are splendid openings for Apollonian children with conic tips, as export managers, import managers, foreign sales executives, agents abroad for American manufacturers, managers abroad of American wholesale houses, banks, mills, and factories, electrical companies, telephone companies, assembling plants, automobile manufacturers, textile mills, bond and stock houses, engineering companies, agricultural companies, and companies engaged in mining, motor transportation, advertising, oil exploitation, and resident buyers abroad of raw materials in metals, foodstuffs, chemicals, coal, potash, and innumerable articles necessary for manufacture and trade. All of these departments of American companies doing business abroad also maintain legal departments specializing in patent and trade mark law, maritime, international, and commercial law.

In every one of these vast international organizations for the promotion of trade in foreign countries, the Apollonian child with conic tips has a place waiting for him which is in accordance with his grade. The fine specimens of the type must be placed in the more important positions, and those of lower grade must fill the clerkships and other subordinate positions. As stenographer and typist, there are many positions which children with this combination can fill better than anyone else, and in these positions they will, on account of their personality and versatility, receive a higher salary than others doing the same work in the same place.

The Square Tip

The square tip (Plate 29), on the Apollonian child of fine grade, indicates ability in all of the engineering professions, in medicine, in chemistry, physics, photography, surgery, as a trained nurse, manufacturing chemist, and he will be very successful as manager of a sanitarium. Also as an osteopath and chiropractor, Roentgen operator, dentist, pathologist; and in the medium and lower grades; as telephone operator, drug clerk, jewelry repair man, clothing cutter, linotype operator, electrician, switchboard operator, wireless operator, locomotive engineer, plumber, steam fitter, printer, carpet weaver, lace curtain weaver, silk or cotton weaver, or roofer.

There are peculiar qualifications necessary in each of these trades and professions which are more plentifully supplied by an Apollonian child with square tips than by other type formations. Each of them present opportunities with adequate pay, but the child should have his preparation begin at an early age for the vocation selected, with a definite idea that this is to be his life work.

The square tips will give the Apollonian child ability in mathematics, and he will be able to teach all of the branches successfully. He will also have ability in mechanical engineering, statistical work, bookkeeping, accounting, auditing, and actuarial work for life and fire insurance companies.

In the realm of art, the Apollonian with square tips will be a good sculptor but an indifferent painter.

In the business world he will be successful in the production end of large corporations. In the automobile business he will have exceptional opportunities for a brilliant future in the manufacturing departments where they are constantly seeking young men of ability.

Here brains count for as much or more than in any other field of effort, for here is where savings in production methods are made, new engineering ideas originate, and from which men are chosen for the most important executive positions. In fact, in most of the larger automobile companies, the best opportunities for executive advancement are from manufacturing and production departments and many of the best salesmen and sales executives are chosen from these departments. For all such choice positions, a high grade Apollonian child with square tips will advance over the heads of people of any other type formation.

In banking, the square tip will be of great help, for here we need system and order in all the daily operations, and a well ordered and systematic mind, and of these things an Apollonian child with square tips has a full supply. Consequently we may safely choose the banking business for a child with such a combination, especially with Saturn secondary type, but we should at the same time begin his preparation for it at an early age.

In addition to learning every department of a bank, he should be well informed in economics, commercial law, English, composition, at least one foreign language, mathematics, the history of money, and by all means shorthand and typing.

A position as secretary of some of the officials which the last two will assure, will give him great opportunities to learn many of the inside workings of the bank. A child who is an Apollonian with square tips, after such a preparation as this, need have no fear that promotions will not come in the banking business.

The important positions in a bank are for high grade children, but there are large numbers of less important ones that can be filled by those of a lower grade. Such children may be started in the banking business with the same assurance of success that we feel concerning those of higher grades, and while they may not attain the more important positions, they will easily secure the best ones according to their grade and preparation.

The Spatulate Tip

The spatulate tip, (Plate 30), will give the Apollonian child originality, which will enable him to do old things in a new way; thus in laboratory experiments, he can discover new compounds, and separate new elements from old bases. He can invent new processes, and so, when we find a child who has this combination, we can with safety place him in various positions in chemical companies and research laboratories. In the most important positions if he be of fine grade, and in the subordinate positions in accordance with his grade.

Such a child will only need a start with a good company when the Apollonian qualities together with those of the spatulate tips will soon be noticed and he will be promoted to more important assignments. Such a combination will ultimately take him to the best positions in his department and higher. Spatulate tips also give the Apollonian child inventive genius in mechanics, and he can be placed in the mechanical departments of electric, automobile, telephone, telegraph, mining, radio, or airplane companies, where he will be sure to discover something which will add to the efficiency of their operations.

The Apollonian child with spatulate tips can succeed in the advertising business on account of the originality given him by the spatulate tips. He will write well and be original in his form of expression which is a great advantage in this business.

He will also be a good writer of fiction, and many places will be open to him in the newspaper field in the editorial departments. There has never been a time when original ideas have been at such a premium, and you will find, if you have a child with this combination, that he will be showing this originality at home even when quite young, and will be devising all manner of odd things which are unlike other things. You should then make up your mind in which of the industries we have named you will place him.

Even before he is old enough to show signs of the spatulate originality, you can decide this question and devote every energy toward preparing him for it.

ELEVENTH TEST—THE THUMB

Having examined the various formations of hands beginning with the identification of the type of the child, through all of the tests that have followed, we now come to the thumb, which is all-important. From it we shall discover whether he has sufficient will power to force the development of his talents.

Thumb Curled Under Fingers

First we note whether the thumb is curled under the fingers, for if it is, the child is weak in character, and we must not place him where he will be required to display leadership over others. This indication is seen in the hands of very young children, and we can know this fact from the very beginning, so the preparation of this child must be for subordinate positions but not the leading ones in the organizations which have been recommended for Apollonian children. He will have adaptability for these various lines, but not for leadership in them.

The Thumb Erect

If we find the thumb standing erect at the side of the hand, independent and free in appearance (Plate 33), we may place the child in the most responsible positions in accordance with his grade, for he will have will power and reason to aid him, and he can dominate himself and others. In all the Apollonian occupations he can be a leader.

Such a child can fill positions such as president, vice-president, or the assistants to each, or cashier, auditor, trust officer, personnel or credit manager of a bank if of fine grade, or positions as teller or loan clerk if of medium grade. He can be at the head of an advertising agency, and can be an artist whose paintings will be bold and full of vigor.

Size of Thumb

We must note the size of the thumb, for in a general way a large thumb will indicate strong character and abundant will power. The child with a large thumb (Plate 31), may be trained for positions of responsibility in Apollonian occupations, such as those mentioned above, and the one with a small thumb (Plate 32), for subordinate positions such as clerks, bookkeepers, or in the safe deposit department of a bank.

High and Low Set Thumb

We must carefully note whether the thumb is high, medium, or low set.

High Set

If it is high set (Plate 36), the child must not be prepared for positions requiring manual skill, for the thumb high set has not the power to oppose the fingers which is necessary for those who are to do work requiring skill with their hands. The high set thumb will show an inferior will power, and this child must be placed in subordinate positions in the Apollonian occupations.

This child will have the Apollonian qualities in spite of his high set thumb, which means that he is still a good individual salesman. He cannot head a sales organization, but he can sell himself. If he is of fine grade he can succeed in a bond or stock house of issue, and can build a clientèle for himself. He will not be known as strong, but he will have a pleasing personality and can make people like him. When a thumb with this setting is found, the child can be prepared for a successful career as above indicated.

Medium Set

If the thumb has a medium setting (Plate 35), the child will be well balanced, he has good will power, and can be placed in all the Apollonian business occupations, such as foreign trade, salesmanship, banking, insurance, and advertising.

Such a child should sell group insurance. This is a day of specialization, and in each line of business there are special departments. Thus in the insurance business there has grown up a department which is writing an enormous lot of business and this department offers large remuneration and requires a business viewpoint to succeed best in it. This is the department of group insurance, where hundreds, sometimes thousands of employees are insured under one policy, and this form of insurance has grown to be a specialty in itself. For the child who has the thumb with a medium setting, it offers a great opportunity to be successful in an important line of business which is growing constantly. The medium setting gives him the business viewpoint necessary to present the matter properly to a client, and the Apollonian salesmanship will do the rest.

Low Set

If the thumb is low set (Plate 34), the child will have strong will, and adaptability for all manual occupations. He will have a higher grade of intelligence than with the high set thumb, and may be placed in Apollonian business occupations and in many of the mechanical arts, and any skilled labor. There is one line of endeavor in the mechanical arts for which this child is especially fitted, and that is as an etcher and engraver. This is a form of art expression that will give the Apollonian talent for artistic things full sway, in fact it is just another way to record creative thought. The low set thumb will make the child who has it peculiarly well fitted to be successful as an etcher and engraver. He will have to have good preparation which can begin quite early once you have identified his type and made the tests. Children of fine grade can do the fine steel engraving, those of lower grades the more ordinary work, such as zinc etching or photo-engraving.

Phalanges of Will and Reason

The first and second phalanges of the thumb considered separately, must be applied to the type qualities of the child, to determine the amount of will and reason which are present.

Will and Reason Balanced

What we desire to find, is that the two phalanges balance each other, that is, that they are of equal length and size. If this is the case, the child will have an abundance of will power, and good reasoning faculties. If his grade is fine, he can occupy the higher positions in the Apollonian occupations. A balanced thumb is shown in Plate 38.

Balanced will and reason are the expression of a balanced temperament which will enable the child who has it to command a large number of people. He will have poise and will command respect. Such a thumb on a Apollonian child of fine grade will fit him for a producer of moving or talking pictures. It is necessary in such a position to have a high degree of artistic sense, for some of the pictures are examples of real art in photography and could not be produced unless one had this sense, so with a combination of artistic sense from the type, with good reasoning powers to guide the judgment from the second phalanx, and strong will from the first phalanx, with both of these qualities balanced, the child can be prepared as a director in moving pictures, one of the Apol-

lonian occupations, with the assurance that he can be successful.

Shape of Will Phalanx

Considering the first phalanx separately, if we find a bulbous first phalanx such as is shown in Plate 37, it will indicate
a stubborn child whose will is of a common variety, and this
thumb will be found most often on the hands of children of
lower grade. But if found on the hand of a high grade child,
it will show an excess of will operating in an unintelligent
manner which will make him domineering, and he will lose
much of his Apollonian attractiveness and charm, and consequently much of his ability to be successful. Such a child will
find it hard to keep his place in an organization regardless of
his inherent ability.

This thumb, with its stubborn will, puts this child in a class
which cannot take a place in the organizations where the fine
grade Apollonian child finds his best expression; but he still
has the Apollonian talents though they must operate in a
coarse way. He should not be put in any of the better positions
in the occupations which have been recommended for Apollonian children. But he can operate a linotype machine in a
newspaper office, which is as near as he can get to the newspaper business, an occupation of his type; and as near as he
can come to art, is as a lithographer. In such positions he
can do very well, and no better occupations can be chosen
for him.

Short Will Phalanx

The opposite of this thumb is the one with a short first
phalanx (Plate 39), which shows deficiency of will and this
means a weak character. This child will never be able to reach
high positions, and must at once be prepared for those of a
subordinate nature in the Apollonian occupations.

Such a child can take minor parts in a dramatic performance, or he can have unimportant parts in a moving picture.
He will, in spite of his weak thumb, have an ability for the
stage, the difference being that an absence of will makes a
listless child, who will never take a commanding position no

matter what his talents. He can succeed as clerk in a department store, in the better ones if his grade be fine, or he can
clerk in a haberdashery, and in such a position will attract
customers, but he cannot manage the store.

Long Will Phalanx

A fine looking first phalanx, balanced with the second, not
bulbous, and not short or flat, but broad, and with a fine
texture of nail, will be the one we expect and wish to find on
the hands of a fine grade Apollonian child (Plate 38). This
will mean an intelligent, evenly balanced will, which makes
him able to take responsibility and influence others, and this
child will go to the top in any of the Apollonian occupations.

There is a field in which a fine grade Apollonian child with
this strong thumb can have great success, and this is in the
hotel business. As the manager or as the head of a chain of
hotels he could bring into play his charming personality, and
his genial disposition, which would attract customers to the
hotel who would even go out of their way to stop with him.
The fine thumb shown in Plate 38 is only a part of the fine
Apollonian child who owns it; if he has such a thumb he will
be fine all the way through, and this means that he can be
the genial host par excellence, and can sell himself and his
hotel to the general public. Parents can well afford to devote
a child with such a type and thumb combination to the hotel
business, which when successful is very profitable.

Phalanx of Reason

The second phalanx will, by its length, show the reasoning
and logical qualities possessed by the child. If this phalanx
be long (Plate 38), the child will have good reasoning faculties, will think out his problems, and will not take chances,
consequently he is the one who can fill important positions, and
is the best counselor and adviser.

The long second phalanx showing good reasoning powers
will fit this child for a successful career as a teacher. He has
all the versatility of the Apollonian type and with this thumb
he will have in addition the power to reason out all questions
with which he comes in contact. His talent for art can make it

easy for him to teach this subject, or he can be successful as a teacher of advertising. If of fine quality he should prepare to be a professor in a technical college, but if of a lower grade as a teacher in a high school.

If the second phalanx is longer than the first (Plate 39), he will be a better adviser than executor, and he should be placed in the departments where the planning is done and let others execute them.

If the second phalanx be very short (Plate 40), the child will plunge into things, he will be determined, but not always right. He should be placed in departments where the planning is done for him, and he is given the carrying out of these plans. He will do things but not know the reason why, whereas with the second phalanx longest he will know the reason why, but will not do them.

In the examination which we have been making of a child, we wish to find a first phalanx of thumb which shows a strong *intelligent* will, for from such a one we know that the necessary and right kind of power is going to be furnished the child-engine, he will have the steam to make him go. At the same time, we want to find good reasoning powers, for it is best that a child should *know why* he is doing a thing. These two desirable conditions we find when the first and second phalanges balance each other.

CHART NOTE: It will be found that the Mount of Apollo will most often be identified by the size and length of the finger, the central location of the apex of the Mount, and the fact that the fingers of Saturn and Mercury lean toward it. When there is a strong development of the Mount type, the Mount will be high and full, and very often a clear single line, deep and well cut, runs from the bottom to the top of the Mount. When you have formed your conclusion, note it on the chart under the proper heading.

TEST CHART

Types

    Primary.

    Secondary.

    Others.

Tests

    1. Texture of skin

    2. Color

    3. Flexibility

    4. Consistency

    5. Three worlds

    6. Knotty fingers

    7. Smooth fingers

    8. Long fingers

    9. Short fingers

    10. Finger tips

The Thumb

    11. How carried

        How set.   High.   Low.   Medium.

Will Phalanx

    Bulbous.   Short.   Very short.   Long.
        Very long.

Phalanx of Logic

    Long.   Very long.   Short.   Very short.
    Will longer than logic.   Will shorter than logic.
    Will and logic balanced.
    Large thumb.   Small thumb.
    Elementary.   Medium.   Fine.
    Tip of thumb.   Pointed.   Conic.
        Square.   Spatulate.

Age of Child.   *Sex.*   *Date.*

CHAPTER FOUR

THE MERCURIAN MOUNT TYPE

The Business Man

A type is a type—a child is a child. His race, nationality, or the language he speaks do not matter. Whether his skin be white, black, or yellow, he will belong to one or the other of the types, and type qualities will guide him. In either case, he can do some things better than others, there is an occupation for which he is best fitted. In all races, nationalities, and colors, there are children of fine, medium, or coarse grades. Fine grades should have fine positions, medium grades medium positions, and coarse grades must do the manual labor in industries for which their type is best adapted. Their hands show each his proper place.

CHAPTER FOUR

THE fourth of the Mount types is the Mercurian, whose Mount and finger are the fourth on the hand, forming a part of the percussion. A high bulging Mount, with apex in the center, and a large and long finger of Mercury with the other fingers leaning toward it, identify the Mount of Mercury as the primary Mount.

THE MERCURIAN HAND

In order that you may have an idea of a Mercurian hand, we insert at this point Plate 50, which will show you the bulging Mount and the large long finger of Mercury. The hand from which this plate was made is that of a leading surgeon of New York City, a man of national note, and is quite typical of the development which has produced success for him in one of the Mercurian's leading directions, medicine.

We are able to show you in addition to this strongly marked hand, one on which the Mount of Mercury is entirely absent (Plate 51), and the subject from whom this plate was made is as lacking in Mercurian qualities as the hand is deficient in Mercurian Mount and finger. Between these two hands, there are many degrees of type development, which it is our mission to locate and estimate, but with the two hands here shown, it should not be a difficult task.

It is, however, an important one, for the Mercurian presents a side which is extremely good, and one which is extremely bad, and from these extremes we must estimate the child. This will not be hard to do if you will follow closely the directions given in this Chapter.

DESCRIBING THE MERCURIAN

From a composite description prepared from actual specimens of the pure Mercurian type, he is small in stature, averaging about five feet seven inches, he is compactly built, trim in appearance, tidy looking, and with a strong forceful expression of countenance. His face is oval in shape, features inclining to be regular, with the expression changing rapidly, showing the quick play of his mind. The skin is smooth, fine, and transparent, tending to be olive in color, and showing the passing of the blood current underneath by alternately turning red or white when excited, embarrassed or in fear.

The forehead is high and bulging, the hair is chestnut or black and inclined to be curly on the ends. The eyebrows are not thick but are regular in outline, running to fine points on the ends, and sometimes meeting over the nose. The eyes are dark or quite black, restless, and sharp in expression.

The nose is thin and straight, somewhat fleshy, the lips are thin, evenly set and often a trifle pale or bluish in color. The neck is strong and muscular, connecting the head with shapely shoulders, lithe, sinewy, and graceful in outline. The chest is large for the stature, well muscled and containing big lungs.

In our treatment of the Mercurian type, we will follow the same method as with former Mount types, by considering him as a pure specimen of the type, and an adult male, though the female members of this type are plentiful and in appearance and characteristics closely follow the male. When we speak of the Mercurian child in relation to his vocation, it will mean that he is fitted for it when he is grown.

Mercurian Characteristics

Of all the types, none of them equal the Mercurian for *SHREWDNESS*, which is the leading characteristic of the type, and to make his shrewdness effective, he has a formidable array of qualities, some of which are good, and some are bad. It is this mixture of good and bad qualities which makes the Mercurian a many-sided person. He is adroit in all the grades from the finest to the lowest, he is crafty, and it is seldom that any of the other types gain an advantage over him. He is inherently a schemer, and is constantly laying plans whereby he gains an advantage over some other person. If he is of fine grade these qualities do not take the form of dishonesty, or an unfair advantage, but in the lower grades he stops at nothing, until in the lowest he becomes a common thief, a liar, a swindler, and of all the types his shrewdness is the most acute and the most successful.

In the finer grades, he plays a prominent part in the world of medicine, science, law, and business. Some of the leaders of the world in all these vocations are high grade Mercurians, and in the underworld he is supreme, for his tremendous shrewdness enables him to devise new schemes for swindling, to lay the plans for burglary, to engineer bank robberies, and the lowest specimens of the type are pickpockets, and petty thieves of all sorts.

The second characteristic of the Mercurian is *INDUSTRY*. This is one quality which makes him formidable, for whether he be engaged in the most beneficial of occupations, or in the lowest form of criminal practice, he will work hard, and will spare no effort to produce a successful outcome of the venture in hand. It is this tireless industry which keeps him constantly on the go, and as most of the types move more slowly than he does, he often accomplishes what he starts out to before his slower moving brethren become aware of the fact that he is "putting something over on them."

His next characteristic is *QUICKNESS*, and none of the other types can keep pace with him, for before they know what he is thinking about, he has laid his plans, executed them, and is on his way to some other field of operation. Not only are his physical movements extremely quick, but his mental operations are just as rapid, and in this respect, it does not matter to what grade he belongs, he is in every case the embodiment of quickness, both physical and mental.

These are some of the reasons for his supremacy in *BUSINESS*, which is his next marked characteristic. If we comb the world for distinguished examples of success in business, we will find that by far the largest number are Mercurians. There is an inherent ability for business possessed by those of this type which makes them almost invincible. It is the instinct of trade and barter, it is the uncanny knowledge of supply and demand, it is the willingness to do almost anything to secure trade, even to accept humiliation to make a sale. It is the get-the-money spirit, backed by judgment of human nature, intuition, shrewdness, industry, mental and physical quickness, adroitness, craft if necessary, scheming if it will bring the results; all of these qualities; with a pleasing manner of approach and a likable personality.

The Mercurian has also much talent in scientific directions, which is most often expressed in the medical profession, which brings us to the next strong characteristic of the type, *SCIENTIFIC* attainment.

The Mercurian doctor is not only proficient in the practice of his profession, but he makes it pay as well. He is possessed of an intuitive faculty of diagnosis, skill with his hands which makes him a good surgeon, and a scientific turn of mind which causes him to realize the benefit of laboratory assistance, so he is a safe doctor to employ, and he brings to each case an inherent ability in the diagnosis and cure of disease. His quick mind helps him here as everywhere else, and his judgment of human nature and intuition are powerful accessories. He also has a great deal of occult power which assists these latter qualities to function.

It is not alone in medicine that the Mercurian shows scientific ability, but he has a scientific mind, which enables him to take in many branches, and as he is a good writer, he can be the author of scientific books, and the editor of scientific publications. He is talented in mathematics.

This enables him to be successful in some of the engineering professions. He can also make an excellent lawyer, in fact he is as able in this direction as he is in medicine. He is primarily an orator, and this ability to speak well helps him to be a good trial lawyer. One able to speak well usually writes well, so the oratorical ability can again help him in editorial work.

We have been considering so far the good qualities of the Mercurian as we have spoken of his successes in business, medicine, law, editorial and scientific work, but we must remember that there is a very undesirable fellow, who has all the same characteristics as the fine grades, which he does not put to good uses. Rather he prostitutes these talents, and uses them for criminal practices. These lower grade Mercurians stand always as a menace, and we must seek them as we go along, so that we may, if we discover these tendencies when they are very young, endeavor to start them on a road which, through being interested, may *lead* them *away* from evil into a measure of good.

We must also remember that in using the pronoun *he* we are doing it as a matter of convenience, for there are innumerable examples of success which come to Mercurian women through possession of the Mercurian characteristics, and there are many low and vicious creatures as well. We now enumerate the leading characteristics of the type, which we have just considered. They are:

> Shrewdness
> Industry
> Quickness
> Business Ability
> Scientific Attainment

which as we have seen, make the Mercurian an important figure in the operation of the universe.

THE MERCURIAN AND MARRIAGE

The Mercurian is predisposed to marriage. In fact it is most unusual to find either a male or female Mercurian who remains single after the attainment of their majority, and in many cases they enter matrimony while yet in their teens. This does not arise from the fact that they are passionate, but it is because they are home lovers and desire a home of their own as soon as possible. They are even so much in favor of marriage that they make matches among their friends, and in crowded cities it is not unusual to find small communities of young Mercurian friends, and all married.

The Mercurian is very particular in his choice of a mate, he is small in stature, and wants a wife who is the right height and in proper proportion. So he most often chooses his mate from one of his own type, for women of this type are neat and trim in appearance, and when young are quite handsome. They have delicate skin, olive complexion, black eyes, which are bright and flashing, soft black hair, and red lips, making an attractive person of whom one could be proud in any company, and to be proud of his wife is one of the necessary things to a Mercurian.

He is liberal in the expenditure of money for her clothing and other wants, and furnishes his house generally in good taste. He has children, and sometimes a large family, to whom

he is kind, and of whom he is very proud. He educates them
and is an excellent provider.

The Mercurian woman, unless she is exceedingly careful,
becomes stout at an early age, but this does not affect the
male, for we see many happy marriages where this condition
exists.

In the lowest grades of Mercurians, we find the mating to
be that of the "Apache," which represents a most elemental
display of the forces of nature as applied to the marriage
relation.

MERCURIAN HEALTH

While the Mercurian is a healthy type, he still has health
defects. He is first of all intensely nervous. This is the principal cause of most of the Mercurian's health difficulties. Sometimes it is not severe enough to make him actually ill, in which
case it expends itself by making him very restless and desirous
of change. This gives him a great flair for travel, and in this
manner he uses a good deal of his energy. Very often the
nervousness disarranges his digestive functions, and results in
an excess of bile which makes him irritable and results in giving him his olive complexion if the case is not severe. In some
cases he has a decidedly yellow complexion. This is particularly true with the lower grades, and in the extremely coarse
grades yellow color is marked.

The Mercurian nervousness in some cases results in a para-
lytic condition when very severe, and when this is the case it
is almost always the arms and upper part of the body which
are affected.

MERCURIAN QUALITIES

The Mercurian child is admirably adapted to the rôle
he is to play in the drama of life. It is his province to come
in direct contact with people in all of the various callings in
which he is most proficient, so he has a winning smile, and an
air of frankness which gains him confidence, but back of all
this he is planning the method by which he is to attain his
end.

As a judge of value, the Mercurian has no equal. It makes

little difference what the object is, he can with a glance estimate its worth, and this makes him a shrewd trader who never
comes out second best.

In the manufacturing business the Mercurian child can
play a conspicuous part as a maker of many kinds of wear-
ing apparel, and here he shines, as he not only knows the value
of what goes into his merchandise, but of the labor that turns
it into a finished product. He is masterful in securing help, and
as well in selling his goods after he has made them.

He can be successful in the loan business owing to his judgment of values. In the lower grades you will find him everywhere with things to sell which he carries from door to door
or sells from the street in crowded cities. He has the trading
instinct, and nothing is too large for him to attempt, nor too
small if he can make a profit.

He is the inhabitant of cities, and will never be seen as a
farmer, seldom as a common laborer, never as an explorer,
but always where many people are gathered together with
whom he can trade and to whom he can sell.

Even in the professions Mercurian children will exhibit
their mercantile ability, and locate where they can reach many
people upon whom they use good selling methods and from
whom they gain many clients.

The Mercurian child can be conspicuous as a banker. Some
of the largest banking houses in the world are owned and
operated by Mercurians of high grade. These banking houses
they have built up themselves, or they have been founded by
their ancestors and have been handed down from generation
to generation. They are very clannish, and in their establishments are found a majority of Mercurian employees. This
applies to whatever kind of business they are engaged in. They
seem to sense the business instinct of their own type and to
surround themselves with Mercurians.

THE SECONDARY TYPE

The secondary type will play a prominent part with the
Mercurian child, for with his own characteristics always pronounced and of a fundamental character, the secondary Mount
will often determine which direction they shall take.

When we find the Mount of Jupiter as the secondary Mount, we have added to the Mercurian type qualities a very strong set of forces. There will be ambition, desire for leadership, religion, love of nature, honor, pride, and dignity, and some of these can be of immense assistance to the child.

In the Law

The ability of the Mercurian child can expend itself in several directions among the professions and in business, and Jupiter as the secondary Mount adds great strength to all of them. One division of the professions in which the Mercurian child can be most successful is the law, for the things needed by a successful lawyer are just the things which the Mercurian child has in abundant supply, and many of the things which he has not, and which are needed, are supplied by the Jupiterian secondary Mount.

The modern lawyer is not only versed in the law but the most successful lawyers of the present day are good business men. Those who have risen to the point where they command large fees and are employed by the big corporations, are men of vision, with a liberal education on all subjects as well as a thorough knowledge of the law and an immense amount of common sense. To all of these must be added a business mind, and inherent business instincts, all qualities which belong to the Mercurian child.

He has in addition great shrewdness, quick thinking and acting, he is naturally adroit and crafty, which qualities all help a lawyer. So it is plain to be seen that the Mercurian child is equipped by nature with those elemental qualities which preëminently fit him for success in the law. And it is also plain that a secondary Jupiterian Mount adds to the strength of the combination.

There are many kinds of lawyers. Some specialize in real estate law, others in business law, some in criminal law, many in corporation law, which is probably the highest paid of all the specialties, and lawyers practice in all the courts from the Supreme Court of the United States to the police court.

In the offices of the legal departments of large corporations, and in the offices of real estate corporations and of lawyers with a large private practice, there are openings for young men and women of marked ability; innumerable positions in the collecting, filing, research, and other departments, and no child with talent for the law can fail to find an opening waiting for him after due preparation. The more preparation he has, the higher place he will find in the profession at the beginning, and the higher place he will have at the end.

In Medicine

The Mercurian child with Jupiter as the secondary Mount can be successful in the medical profession, and many of the leaders of this profession have this combination. There has never, heretofore, been any way in which those best fitted for the medical profession could be culled from the mass of young men and women who annually make this their choice as a calling in life. With the placing of the Mount types before the parents of the world as we are now doing, this can no longer be said, for here, in the Mercurian type, with Jupiter secondary, is the child who is preëminently fitted to become a doctor. He should be started on his career of preparation as soon as the identification of his types have taken place.

Many branches of medicine, one of which is surgery, require great manual dexterity, and this is a leading qualification of the Mercurian child. As we scan other characteristics needed for success in the medical profession, we find that the Mercurian child with Jupiter secondary has all of them.

There are great opportunities today for research work in all the hospitals, where new remedies for special diseases are being sought; in the offices of physicians with a large practice who need assistants, in biological work, in chemistry, physics, in private practice, in the medical departments of large corporations, and an enormous field in all the specialties which medicine has developed in the past few years.

It is confidently stated that the general practitioner even in large cities is coming back. He now exists as an important part of every rural community, and competent judges state that his place has never been filled in the matter of real service to his patients and that a need now exists for many well trained general practitioners.

These are some of the opportunities in the medical profession open to Mercurian children, and it may be stated that those belonging to the type combination we are now considering will far outdistance those of any other types in the race for success.

SATURN SECONDARY TYPE

In considering the Mount of Saturn as the secondary type, a combination which sometimes occurs, we have brought together the two bilious types, and the two who number in their ranks most of the real criminals. It is therefore apparent that if we find this combination on the hands of very *low grade* children they will have none of the splendid qualities which each of the types possesses.

But if we find the child to be of fine grade, we shall have the benefit of the fine qualities of a high grade Saturnian to aid those of the Mercurian child.

This child should never be placed in any of the agrarian occupations, for he is never a farmer but is a city dweller. He can be successful in sales departments which sell to farmers, he can travel successfully through rural communities for companies selling fertilizer, farm implements, or any product distributed among farmers, but he will not live in the country.

A Writer

The ability of the Saturnian as a writer will add much to the Mercurian child who can also be a writer, and it will enable him to deal with technical and scientific subjects. This will open a field for the Mercurian child in newspaper work in the editorial departments. He can be successful as a reporter, columnist, dramatic critic, and as editor, for in each of these departments his business instinct will be aided by his shrewdness, and with the serious turn his Saturnian secondary Mount gives him, he will write well on a wide range of subjects.

A Teacher

The Saturnian secondary Mount will give the Mercurian child ability as a teacher, especially of mathematics. His Mercurian ability in mathematics, to which is added that of the

Saturnian secondary Mount, will make him especially brilliant in this subject.

Engineering

He can also enter the engineering field, gaining his strength in this direction from his secondary Mount. Thus with this combination he can be successful as a mechanical engineer, a chemical, electrical, ceramic, civil, radio, and automobile engineer, and in chemical laboratory work. These fields are opened to him by the secondary Mount, but unless Saturn is secondary, the Mercurian child should not attempt engineering. In all of the engineering fields mentioned above, there are very large companies doing extensive work in various lines, and these companies need an army of employees to carry on this work.

There are positions in such companies, ranging from night watchmen up, through all grades of employment, to the executive at the head of the corporation. These opportunities are open to Mercurian children with Saturn secondary. Those of the lower grades will not find their way to the head of the companies, but somewhere along the line there is a place where they can be successful.

APOLLO SECONDARY TYPE

The Mount of Apollo (Plate 49), when found as the secondary Mount, will prove a fine combination, and will aid the Mercurian child to achieve distinguished success in the business world. Far more Mercurians are found in business than in the professions or in scientific occupations, and in this field they occupy every position from the most humble to the most exalted. The Mercurian is a natural trader, and as the Apollonian is a master salesman, he brings to the combination such force in this direction that the Mercurian-Apollonian child can be highly successful in business.

The Department Store

One important field in the business world, in which large numbers of Mercurian children can be extremely successful, is in merchandising, commonly called storekeeping, and in this direction a great advance has been made in the past twenty-five years, almost entirely due to Mercurian mercantile ability.

The evolution of the country general store into the modern department store is the most conspicuous example of what is meant, and the department store is a fertile field in which to start a Mercurian child.

If we find the Mercurian primary type strong, with a well developed Apollonian secondary Mount, there is almost no limit to what the child can achieve in the department store business. The large department stores in the big cities call for an army of people, both men and women, to carry on their business. They are highly organized into departments, each of which is a large business enterprise in itself in which there must be the department head or executive, with a complete corps of assistants and a large force of salespeople. As the variety of merchandise which they handle is so great, this means many departments, and in a store with a hundred or more departments we can imagine the great number of openings that exist for those who can properly fill them.

Among the many important positions which can be filled by Mercurian children are merchandise managers who must have a broad knowledge of merchandise, of values, of the tastes of the public, who must know where the right goods may be obtained at the right prices, and have an organization of buyers who can instantly secure these goods when wanted.

Under the merchandise manager will be a large force, including buyers in many cities and many countries, assistant buyers, stock clerks, office clerks, salesmen, and a large number of those who do the little things, run the errands and other seemingly unimportant but always necessary parts of the daily routine. All of these positions can be successfully filled by Mercurian-Apollonian children.

In the financial departments there are controllers who have charge of financial operations, prepare balance sheets, figure inventories, and determine profits. These have assistants, credit managers, accountants, analysts, statisticians, and other helpers, all positions which Mercurian-Apollonian children can fill.

Then there are those who design and dictate styles, who have a large force of helpers ; and the advertising departments which have writers, illustrators, copy men, which in the large stores means practically an advertising agency. All of the positions we have mentioned are but a *part* of those who make up the personnel of a large department store. We have not even mentioned the army of salespeople who far outnumber all the rest, and the delivery departments, the postal, and other service rendering departments. In the department store field alone, there are positions waiting for all competent Mercurian-Apollonian children of the proper grade. If space would permit the enumeration of all the qualities needed to win success in each of the departments of any department store, we would find that as we check them off, the Mercurian-Apollonian child has them. It is as if this combination was built especially for the department store business. A roll of honor of all the great department store heads would disclose that the Mercurian type could claim nearly all of them.

All Mercurian-Apollonian children cannot be among the great department store heads, or even engage in the department store business, but they can be successful in every kind of a store, selling every kind of merchandise. They can be in business for themselves in many instances, employees in others, and in the great throng of all kinds of merchants it will be found that a majority of them are Mercurians. We find a vast number as itinerant vendors, selling from door to door, some pushing carts, others standing in a market. These represent the lower grades. Grade will determine which stratum your child can occupy. The tests which we apply to him will tell you his grade.

You can safely place any Mercurian child who has Apollo as the secondary Mount in the merchandising business, with full confidence that he will win success in the positions suited to his grade. But make your decision as soon as you have determined his types, and prepare him for his future work. Then start him in the lowest position, so that by going through every part of the organization he will know the requirements of each, and have no fear but that he will be singled out and put into his proper place.

The Clothing Business

The predominant qualifications of a Mercurian child for a business career, to which so much is added by having the

Mount of Apollo as the secondary Mount, open to him great opportunities in the manufacture and wholesale distribution of men's clothing, also in their retail distribution and in the manufacture and wholesale and retail distribution of women's dresses, coats, and suits. Very large corporations with an immense number of employees exist for the purpose of carrying on the above activities, and in all of these the majority of the personnel are Mercurians.

Great business acumen is needed for the successful conduct of these enterprises, and the Mercurian child of all the types is most richly endowed with the necessary qualities. In fact the Mercurian type dominates these trades almost to the exclusion of all others.

Unless we stop to think, we do not realize how large a percentage of all the people who wear clothes buy them already made, and we must also realize the great improvements which have been made in the character and quality of ready made clothing in the past fifteen years. First in the cloth which is used, which must now follow the advanced styles in colors and pattern. This has necessitated the development of extremely skillful merchandise men who buy millions of dollars worth of material of all kinds, long in advance of their use, and these men must be able to judge what the public taste will approve and buy sometimes a year in advance. For these positions the highest grade Mercurian children are fitted, and they need the good taste of the Apollonian secondary Mount to aid them.

Then there must be those who can judge what the styles will be, often a year in advance, and these stylists and designers must come from the same grade of Mercurian-Apollonian children. These two important departments offer great opportunities for positions which pay large salaries, and these men and women have many assistants of all kinds in which positions young Mercurian-Apollonian men and women can train for the leading places.

These clothing manufacturers have a large personnel. There are executives, who generally come from the ranks of those who have begun at the bottom and learned all the departments, having been promoted step by step until they reach the top. There are also immense office departments, credit departments, hosts of buyers and their assistants, an army of machine operatives, cutters, and literally thousands of salespeople, both wholesale and retail. In all of these departments, the Mercurian child with Apollo as the secondary Mount will outstrip all the other types.

We have just been considering the possibilities of a connection with the large manufacturing companies, and the taking of an important position in the trade, but there are innumerable small factories making cheap and some of them fine goods, all operated by Mercurians of the medium and lower grades, and all of these factories together employ a vast number of people. Many low and medium grade Mercurians own their own shops, and cater to a neighborhood trade, but all of these employ almost none but Mercurians.

In a retail way, there are hundreds of small shops in large cities, and many in cities of smaller size, who sell clothing of every description, much of it cheap in quality and cheap in price. These are nearly all owned by low and medium grade Mercurians and manned with Mercurian help. These people are all successful according to their grades. So we may set it down as a fixed fact that a Mercurian child who is a combination of the Mercurian-Apollonian type can achieve success in the clothing industries, either in a large or small way according to his grade.

Banking

Another field in which the Mercurian-Apollonian child can be extremely successful is that of banking. Here his shrewdness comes into play, as well as his affability and good business common sense. Many large and internationally famous banking houses owned and operated by Mercurians have existed for a great many years, and have played a conspicuous part in world finance. No more successful career can be chosen for a high grade Mercurian-Apollonian child than that of banking. The banking business has become so highly specialized that it is not necessary that one should be the president or chairman of the board to occupy a position of importance and distinction in the banking world: the organization of a large bank numbers so many positions of importance that to fill any one of a large number will be to achieve success. Besides the conspicuous positions there are many which may be filled by Mercurian-Apollonian children who are not of the finest grades, but the lowest grades should not hope to be countenanced in the banking business, and such are not found in it.

Brokerage

The brokerage business is another in which the Mercurian-Apollonian child of high grade can be successful. This may be the brokerage of stocks, bonds, cotton, corn, wheat or other grains, or of insurance, metals, chemicals, sugar, or other raw materials, real estate or other commodities or articles of value. These various brokerages require salesmanship, business judgment, a good address, industry, shrewdness, a knowledge of values, and all of these the Mercurian-Apollonian child has. A child with this combination can be started in the brokerage business with full confidence, but whichever line you decide to have him follow, he should have an early and thorough preparation. He should learn all there is to know about the article he is to handle, its methods of production, growth, or mining, he should know all of its past history, markets, and values over a period of many years, all of which he can study without great difficulty, and all of which is necessary to his success.

The brokerage business is an exceedingly profitable one, and one in which a Mercurian-Apollonian child can be successful. Many find it difficult to get a start in this business owing to lack of preparation. This should be the parent's concern, but it is neglected in too many instances to the great detriment of the child. The average broker is forced to select young men and women at random, and wait to see if they develop into anything worth while. He would warmly welcome a well prepared young man or woman of good address, and would give them every opportunity. This is all a Mercurian-Apollonian child would need; given the opportunity, his type qualities would insure his success.

MARTIAN SECONDARY TYPE

The Martian is often found as the secondary type on the hands of Mercurian children, sometimes one of the Mounts and sometimes both. The *Upper Mount* (Plate 52), is a good ally for it brings with it physical strength, courage, calmness, and a tremendous power of resistance. These qualities can be a great help to the Mercurian child in whatever occupation he chooses, for they will back his natural talents with the courage and strength to develop them. The quality of resistance is especially helpful, and if the Upper Mount of Mars be well developed the Mercurian-Martian child will know no such thing as defeat in any of his undertakings, for the Martian never knows when he is beaten.

There can be no greater help to a Mercurian child who is to make his way in the world than to have aggression, as this is, next to will power, the strongest driving force. If the *Lower Mount* of Mars (Plate 54), be large, he will have aggression, which will drive him hard at whatever he undertakes. If *in addition* he has the *Upper Mount* of Mars strongly developed, he will *also* have *resistance* which will prevent him from becoming discouraged, and with the two qualities of aggression and resistance, we may be certain that whatever the Mercurian child determines to do, he will go through with it to the end.

The Mercurian child has a much keener mind than the Martian child, he is more shrewd, a better judge of human nature, and infinitely superior as a business man. The Martian does not bring him any addition to his talents in this direction, but he *does* bring him *aggression* and *resistance*, and these he needs, for to place aggression and resistance as supporting forces behind him will make the Mercurian child infinitely stronger in every direction, and in placing this child in any one of the occupations for which he is fitted, we may feel more certain of his success with the Martian Mounts to support him.

With the Martian Mounts secondary, the Mercurian child will have a fondness for the army and navy which will even tinge his mercantile efforts. Thus he can be successful as a manufacturer and retailer of officers' uniforms for the army and navy, of flags, banners, and insignia, and of uniforms for uniformed fraternal organizations, which will lead quite naturally to costumes for degrees in the same organizations, in which lines there are a number of very large corporations engaged where the child can find congenial employment, and, if of fine grade, hold important positions. In these same companies there are positions such as cutters, designers, and machine operators in which children of lower grades can be placed with an expectation of success.

As the Martian succeeds as a building contractor and a prospector for oil and mineral companies, the secondary Martian Mounts will enable the Mercurian child, on account of his inherent mercantile ability, to be successful in the builders' supply business, selling lime, cement, lumber, hardware, and paint, and a large number of new inventions in building specialties, and also pipe, joints, drills, derricks, and other oil well supplies.

The Martian secondary Mounts will enable the Mercurian child to have great success in the sale of guns, pistols, and firearms of all kinds. With this combination of Mercury and Mars, no better selection can be made for the child than to place him in a store dealing in such goods or in a factory making them. The Mercurian shrewdness will assist this child in finance and the business end of factory operations, and also in the retail end, where his knowledge of storekeeping will enable him to build up a successful business.

THE LUNARIAN SECONDARY TYPE

The Mount of the Moon (Plate 56), does not add to the strength of the Mercurian child who has few of the qualities which belong to the Mount of the Moon, and that Mount has little to offer which will help him. There is only one direction in which the Mount of the Moon will help the Mercurian child, and that is in the supply of a great amount of imagination. This will aid the Mercurian child in case he is to engage in writing, for it will enlarge his vision and increase his vocabulary.

It has been stated that the Mercurian child has great talent for medicine and the law. We cannot recommend that a child with the Lunarian type secondary be placed in either, but we find that such a child can write valuable treatises on medical or legal subjects; if he is of fine grade, he can also write excellent selling literature, or conduct schools of business, which with this combination will be his best vocation.

In the law there is needed in every large office a man who can prepare briefs, pleadings, and other law papers requiring research and a shaping of the English language so that it may not say what it does say, and no one can be found who could do this better than a Mercurian child with the Lunarian secondary Mount. While the child with this combination cannot successfully practice law, he can be of exceptional value to a law firm to prepare the papers they often need. Many large firms are willing to pay good salaries for such service.

Venus Secondary Type

With the Mount of Venus (Plate 58), as the secondary type, the Mercurian child will be more fond of the ladies than is his natural wont, he will have added to his already pleasant manner an increased supply, he will be fond of society and pleasures of every sort, and in general will not take life so seriously. While the Venusian type when secondary cannot give the Mercurian child robust qualities, it can and does give him charming ones. Its influence is not so much in specific lines as in making the good qualities of the Mercurian child more effective. It does help the child to engage in a finer line of merchandising. Such a child can be exceptionally successful, if of fine grade, in a business of his own, or as an employee in a high grade men's tailoring establishment where he caters to fine trade. This is an excellent business and affords an opportunity for building up a large clientèle of people of wealth and influence, especially in a large city; and as a career offers the Mercurian-Venusian child a successful future.

This child can also be successful in a store selling fine jewelry, furs, or luxury lines, but owing to the Mercurian's inherent talent in the clothing business, his greatest opportunity will be in a high grade tailoring establishment such as is described above.

The Mercurian and Chain Stores

The Mercurian is the only one of the types who has been able to conduct his little store and not be put out of business by a chain store in the same line of business, in the same vicinity. If you will go along any business street in which chain stores congregate, which is largely in marketing localities, you will find other little stores thriving and doing a good business. And if you will examine the people who are running these stores, you will find that they are Mercurians. If you will inquire, you will find that a large number of small stores which were formerly in the locality have gone out of business, and if you could examine the owners of these stores, you would find that they were not Mercurians. It has been the survival of the fittest as applied to business, and the Mercurian type has been the fittest.

There is no question but that the chain store idea of a large buying power which enable them to sell for less money, a centralized management with reduced overhead, and the application of a large number of fundamental ideas all of which reduce expenses and costs, is the correct and best method of distribution.

Men who are well informed believe that distribution in the future will be increasingly through chain stores, and it follows that the Mercurian child who has successfully held his own *against* the chain stores can be tremendously successful *in* the chain store business.

The inherent business ability which he possesses in large quantity, gives him a splendid opportunity to achieve success with the correct distribution idea of the chain stores to work with. The very qualities which enabled him to *compete* with chain stores will make him more successful in working *with* them. So among the army of employees of every grade who are operating the chain stores, and the larger number who will follow as the stores increase you may with safety prepare for, and place a Mercurian child in a career in the chain store business feeling confident of success.

In choosing which chain store field the child shall enter, we should select one in which his type has ability. For a fine grade child he can succeed best in a chain of stores selling women's suits, cloaks, hosiery, or in men's wear, ready made suits, overcoats, hats and shoes. There are many such chains operating successfully in which a child can be placed to learn the business, and if he has Jupiter as the secondary type he will not stop until he is at the head of the business. Children of lower grades can be placed in chains selling groceries, meat, fruits, and vegetables, in positions as managers, and if of still lower grade as clerks.

MERCURIAN SUCCESS IN LUXURY LINES

The Mercurian child of fine grade can be exceptionally successful as a dealer in jewelry and precious stones, in laces, lace curtains, and draperies, in oriental rugs, in paintings, etchings, engravings, wood cuts, all objects of art, and in antiques. Some of the finest grades of Mercurian merchants in the mercantile world are engaged in these lines, doing a business with intelligent and wealthy patrons, and themselves wealthy as the result of their merchandising efforts.

It will be noted that in every case mentioned the merchandise is such that its value is not easily determined by a layman, who must therefore rely to a great extent upon the word and judgment of the dealer from whom he buys. Sugar is so much a pound everywhere, the layman knows the price and the quality. This is not true of a diamond, a piece of lace, an oriental rug, a picture, or an antique. Intangible values enter into the price of all of these, and no greater judge of values, intangible or real, exists, than a high grade Mercurian child. For this reason he is the master buyer, and the master salesman of all these commodities whose real value he alone knows, and for these reasons he is immensely successful and deliberately chooses these lines of business.

In the best grades of stores, he is careful not to have his prices too high, and he takes pains to see that no misrepresentations are made as to the quality or authenticity of his merchandise. He gains a reputation for reliability. But it is plain that his Mercurian shrewdness has engaged him in a business where he has every advantage over his customer whether he takes advantage of it or not.

There are splendid opportunities in all of the lines just enumerated for high grade Mercurian children, whose preparation should begin early. They should have a liberal education, be taught the history of whichever line they are to engage in, travel extensively, and in every way gain a cultural background for their business activities. With such preparation, a fine grade Mercurian child, especially with a secondary Mount of Apollo, can achieve the utmost in success.

THE TESTS FOR GRADE

FIRST TEST—TEXTURE OF THE SKIN

It will be apparent from our study of the Mercurian child up to the present time that a great deal will depend upon his grade in our selection of an occupation for him. No type has more possibilities for good and evil than he. It behooves us therefore to very definitely judge the grade of a child so that we may know where his place is going to be in the scale of human endeavor. If he has the grade to justify it, we want to assign him to the highest positions, and as his grade decreases, we want to find a place for him among those of his own class.

In order to arrive at the proper conclusions as to grade, we must apply the various tests to him of which we have so often spoken, the first of which is the skin on his hands, whose texture will determine whether he is of a fine or coarse grade. Plate 11 shows the coarsest texture of skin that we have ever seen, and this may be taken as a basis from which to judge the texture of the skin in an ascending scale. You will never find any coarser, and you could not find any human being coarser, than the man whose hand we photographed to make this plate.

Coarseness means more on the hand of a Mercurian child than on any of the other types except the Saturnian, for with these two types who produce criminals, the criminality increases as the skin and other of the tests coarsen.

If the skin be very fine, soft and velvety (Plate 10), like the skin on a baby's hand, that fact must be recorded on the chart which will be the child's first passport looking toward a location in the higher grades of occupation in which Mercurian children can be successful. As the texture of this skin becomes coarser, positions of less importance are open to them in the same lines of business in which the fine grade Mercurian child is likely to be the head. Finally we come to the very coarse texture shown in Plate 11, which tells us that he is to occupy only the lowest positions, and which at the same time raises the question of possible criminal tendencies. All children will grade somewhere between the fine skin of a baby's hand, and Plate 11, and they will all do best in Mercurian occupations which correspond in importance to the texture of their skin.

SECOND TEST—COLOR OF THE HANDS

The color of the hands will be the next test which we will apply which should be determined by the color in the palm of the hand and under the nails.

White Color

White color is not often found on the hands of Mercurian children, especially the backs of the hands, but it is sometimes seen in the palm which in this instance has a bloodless look. This will indicate that the child is cold and liable to be cruel, and in the lower grades will cause them to have little feeling for their fellows. The Mercurian child of any grade with white palms will be very calculating, which added to his natural shrewdness and craftiness will make him uncompromising in a business transaction, and while he may keep this tendency covered up, he will always be on the edge of taking advantage of someone.

Such a child will not do well in the occupations which call for great vitality, and should not be placed at the head of a business. They have all the keenness of the Mercurian type, however, and such a child can make a success as a buyer for a cloak and suit manufacturer, as his coldness will not be overcome by the zealous salesmen who come to sell him goods. He will also be successful in the credit department of the same factory, and in the collection department. Such a child can be successful in the loan business, in what is called industrial banking, where small loans are made on personal security, and the lower grades can succeed as pawnbrokers.

Pink Color

Pink color is often seen, as the Mercurian child is a healthy person, and in his case the palm of the hand, and under the nail will be best to use when examining for color. If pink color is found, it will make the Mercurian child much better morally, much more jovial, and it will largely increase his chances of success. His mind will be keen and alert, his viewpoint on life will be pleasant, and he will more easily win success in whatever occupation he may be engaged. This color is most often found on the hands of high grade children.

Pink is the color we wish to find on the hands of children we expect to assign to the high grade stores selling fine jewelry, precious stones, silverware, fine rugs, curtains, and draperies, and it will add very much to the chance of success of the child we recommended for the fine grade men's tailoring business who had Venus as the secondary type. Pink color will be a great help to the child we place in the department store. Such a child should not go into this business simply for a job. He should be given to understand that merchandising in a large way is to be his future vocation, and that the department store is its fullest expression. There are plenty of children with less desirable color qualities than those with pink, who can do the ordinary things in a department store, but when a child is fortunate enough to have pink color, he should make the most of it by preparing himself for success.

Red Color

Red color is more often found on the hands of Mercurian children of the lower grades, and very seldom on those of the finer grades. The intensity which red color indicates is not typical of the Mercurian child. He does not achieve his success through physical strength and ardor but through his quick mental processes, so red color is an abnormal indication.

It will usually be accompanied by hard consistency and such a child should be placed in a grade of merchandising such as keeper of a market for fish and sea food, or a second hand book store, a second hand clothing store, or furniture store. He can succeed in one of the little stores on side streets which sell imitation jewelry, and he can succeed as a small manufacturer, or in the conduct of a store selling furs made to imitate finer skins. He can conduct an employment agency, or conduct a store selling musical instruments popular songs, radios, or victrolas. In all of these he will be very energetic and some of these stores make a good deal of money. Generally the wife and children help in the store.

Yellow Color

Yellow color is natural to the Mercurian child and is found on many Mercurian hands. It will often be seen on the back of the hand and in the palm as well. Many times the palm will show a yellow which is faded and almost shades into white. These children have a cold, cynical viewpoint toward their fellows, in proportion to the depth of color, and while they do not show these things outwardly, they harbor the inward thought and are constantly tempted to use their shrewdness to take an undue advantage. From pale yellow, we find yellow color deeper in shade until it becomes quite pronounced.

While yellow color shows some disagreeable qualities ethically, still the child with this color can be, and they almost always are, successful. We find them in the various Mercurian trades and stores, and of all grades, and they present one of the real problems in assigning children to their proper vocation. There is one place above all others where this child can be successful, and that is in the law. If he be of fine grade, he will be one of those lawyers you read a good deal about in the papers; they get into big cases and some of them are most successful criminal lawyers. Properly trained, such a child can have a large income from the practice of criminal law, and be most successful in winning cases. No mistake will be made in assigning him to the law as a vocation.

THIRD TEST—FLEXIBILITY OF THE HANDS

Flexibility of the hands is useful in enabling us to determine the grade of the child, for the greater the flexibility the finer the grade and the more elastic the mind. As the Mercurian child can engage in so many forms of business activity as well as the professions, we may get a very clear idea of where to place him from the flexibility of his hands.

The Stiff Hand

We very seldom find a stiff hand as pronounced as shown in Plate 12, and such stiffness would not show in the hand of a very young child; but we do find it in the hands of children as early as the age of twelve. These children will have such inelastic minds that they cannot successfully engage in the most important forms of business and professionl activity which are inherent in the Mercurian type, but must be placed in lower brackets.

They have a low form of cunning, extreme shrewdness, and can be successful as push cart peddlers who sell their wares for all they can get, short-change you if possible, and are extremely sharp in trading. This low grade of child is not often found in the legal and medical professions, but they are found among the low Mercurian criminals often operating as a "fence" from which source they derive most of their merchandise. Many such are engaged as truck drivers for importers and wholesale houses, and much merchandise disappears from the trucks they arive.

The Straight Hand

Passing to a better grade we come to the straight hand, shown in Plate 13. Here is a well poised mind, not the dullness of the stiff hand and not the elasticity of the flexible, but a mind well adapted to business of a practical nature, a common sense balanced person. This Mercurian child will have all the shrewdness of the type, will be an excellent trader, a good judge of human nature, and will have inherent business instincts. He cannot be successful in the most important positions in merchandising, banking, the law, and medicine, but in planning his future, a medium position in one of the lines in which Mercurians succeed should be chosen.

This child can be a treasurer, secretary, or manager of small or medium sized companies, he can be successful as manager of one of the stores of a chain store group, such as groceries, hats, or drugs. Lower grades can make good operators of soda fountains and lunch counters, and better grades can succeed in a restaurant as owner or proprietor.

In the banks, he can be placed in the collection department, in foreign exchange, as a teller, but does not often reach the higher offices. In the wholesale and retail merchandising business, these Mercurian children can be successful in an office as office manager if the rest of the grade be good, or in the stock department as a stockkeeper, or as an assistant buyer, but they do not reach high executive positions. The reason for this is, that the Mercurian children with flexible and extremely flexible hands who generally occupy these positions have such brilliant minds, and are so quick in thought and action and so shrewd, that they outclass the children with straight hands.

The Mercurian child with straight hands will however be steady and persistent, and will often pass those of other types, even if he does not attain to the heights reached by his flexible handed Mercurian brothers. The straight hand should be identified by the time the child is eight to ten, and this may be said about him, if he is well prepared for his future occupation, he will attain greater heights than if he is started through life unprepared. Thus if you begin at an early age and get him ready, you can advance him several degrees in the positions he will ultimately reach, over those he would otherwise have attained.

The Flexible Hand

Fine specimens of the flexible and extremely flexible hand are shown in Plates 14 and 15. They indicate extremely flexible minds, sharp and keen, versatile and adaptable to any situation. Consequently, children with these hands can grasp any subject, they think like a flash, their intuitions are remarkable, and the flexible hand brings out to its fullest extent the shrewdness, adroitness, skill, and inherent ability of the Mercurian child in the professions of law, medicine, or the world of business.

A child well identified as a Mercurian, with a strong secondary Mount of Jupiter or Saturn, and flexible hands, can be most successful in the law. His mind will be so quick that he will never be surprised in the trial of a case, and he will perpetrate many surprises on his opponent. His natural skill in oratory will make him a good trial lawyer, which not all well informed lawyers are. No mistakes can be made with a child who has such hands, in planning a career as a lawyer for him. These indications can be identified on the hands of a very young child, and his whole training can be such as to fit him in the best possible manner for a successful outcome in the law.

In medicine his scientific aptitudes may be brought to the highest point by flexible hands. His skill with his hands will enable him to be a successful surgeon, and his naturally keen mind reinforced by the flexible hands will make him a fine diagnostician. For a fine grade child with flexible hands medicine may be chosen, especially if on the Mount of Mercury there are a number of fine vertical lines, which we call the "medical stigmata."

A high grade Mercurian child with flexible hands has a great advantage in the business world. No other type can compete with him. Here we have one who possesses so many qualities that aid in barter and trade or business that he outmatches any of the other types.

He can occupy the highest places in Mercurian occupations such as merchandising, banking, manufacturing, and wholesale and retail distribution of clothing, brokerage, the jewelry trade, oriental rugs, laces, paintings, art objects, antiques, and in the chain store business, as well as importing and exporting furs, silks, and perfumes.

We have noted before that a Mercurian child with Saturn as the secondary Mount can make a success in engineering, and if he has flexible hands, this success will be much greater.

Flexible hands improve the possibilities of every grade of child. If we find one who has flexible hands whose grade is not the finest, we can, by identifying these facts early in life, and preparing him for a definite position in a definite business in which a Mercurian can be successful, advance him several degrees in his ultimate success beyond the point to which his grade usually attains.

Fourth Test—Consistency of the Hands

Consistency of the hands is very important to the Mercurian child, for he is naturally energetic and industrious. A great deal that he accomplishes is due to energy. With the natural keenness of his mind, if he has industry, this child can reach high in the business or professional world.

Flabby Hands

If we find flabby hands, it will be unfavorable, for here is indicated a lack of energy which will seriously interfere with his success. You will find hands which are flabby, where the rest of the hand shows great ability, but you can never plan that this child will attain to the positions to which his talents entitle him. His mind will be keen, he will make a good impression, he will have many opportunities, but others will pass him in the race; he is very bright but he is lazy, and the world of affairs does not count laziness as one of its assets.

It will not do to place this child where he has much responsibility, he cannot be successful at the head of a business. We must find him a position in which he can use his talents where energy is not required. Even flexible hands will not justify us in placing him in too important positions. He can be a cashier in a retail store, he can clerk in a cigar store, he can conduct a rental library, he can run a billiard hall, he can clerk in a stationery store, he can conduct a shop selling rubber stamps, dies, and checks, he can run a shop collecting and selling postage stamps. In none of these will great energy be required, and in all of them he can, by reason of his type qualities, make himself so useful that it will mean a good position for him.

Soft Hands

Soft hands will not indicate the degree of laziness shown by the flabby, but there will still be lacking the energy which belongs to the Mercurian child. What he accomplishes will be largely a matter of his secondary Mounts, for he will have to gain assistance from some source to counteract the softness of his hands. You should, upon discovering softness, give careful attention to the secondary Mounts, and your final estimate must largely be based upon what you find there.

Softness indicates a lack of energy, and when you take from the Mercurian his energy or any part of it, you have lessened his chances of success. The final reading of his chart will show a much reduced estimate of his possibilities which will affect the entire outcome. When we find soft hands on a Mercurian child we will have to bring to his assistance as many qualities as possible which will tend to compensate for the softness of his hands. The Mercurian's natural love of *money* and *profit* will be one set of forces which will help him, pride of success will be another, made more potent if Jupiter be the secondary Mount. Other auxiliary forces may be sought for and applied to the reading of his chart. You may recognize as fundamental, however, that he will have all the talents and possibilities of the Mercurian type, only diminished energy is going to handicap him.

You may remove some of this handicap by beginning early to develop forces which will minimize his lack of energy. A conscientious parent can do much to help in such a situation. With Jupiter as secondary type he can be secretary of a political club, with Saturn, assistant in a chemical laboratory, with Apollo or Venus, salesman in a jewelry or music store, with the Martian Mounts, office manager for a building contractor, and with the Lunarian type, secretary of a small newspaper or magazine.

This child cannot be placed in the professions of law and medicine, for it takes hard work these days to be successful in either, but he can be quite successful in the conduct of a dancing academy. This is a large field in which there are many opportunities for profit, especially in the large cities. The Mercurian is pleasing in manner and easily makes a good impression and gains friends, he is good looking and graceful and well fitted to be a teacher of dancing, or a dancing partner. His natural business ability will enable him to make dancing profitable, and such a business is well suited to a Mercurian child with soft hands. He can be successful in running a check room for coats and hats, or if of fine grade he can be secretary of a club, run a magazine subscription agency, a novelty gift shop, or custom made shirt shop.

Elastic Hands

Elastic consistency is what we hope to find on the hand of a high grade Mercurian child, for here is intelligent energy which will bring out the strong qualities of the type. This kind of energy will be a constant stimulus to effort and such a Mercurian child is tireless. This means that he is constantly on the alert, his quick mental faculties are at work, he is planning his next move and is energized to execute it; thus no opportunity for profit or advancement is overlooked or neglected. This elastic energy is like a coiled spring, constantly forcing its mechanism into action.

A fine grade Mercurian child with elastic consistency must be placed where he can use the business ability of the type and take advantage of the energy shown by elastic consistency. The manufacturing business can make full use of these advantages if the child is placed in the right company. As a manufacturing furrier this child can have great success. This is a good business and a profitable one when properly conducted. It requires that the child be familiar with all the markets for skins, he must be a stylist to know which fur is to be the popular one each season and the cut of the garments to be worn. He must know how to buy the skins at the right prices, and how to sell them after they are manufactured. Every one of these things is second nature to the Mercurian child with elastic hands, but he needs good preparation and study of the fundamentals of the business, which can begin at an early age. If he is placed with a good company until he thoroughly learns the business he can safely go into business for himself.

Such a child can be successful in the wholesale distribution of women's wear, such as cloaks, suits, gloves, hosiery, or in men's ready to wear suits and overcoats. With these lines he is inherently familiar, and he can safely be placed with a good company doing a wholesale business in these lines, or he can be successful in the distribution of similar lines at retail.

Hard Hands

Hard consistency belongs to the lower grades. These have Mercurian industry, and hard consistency forces it to operate but with less intelligence. They do not approach a question softly, but with full force, and for lower grades a less tactful method of operation is sometimes necessary. The lower grade Mercurian child deals with a less refined set of people, their trade is among a lower strata, and among the lowest grades (not criminal) strenuous methods are required in making sales or doing any kind of business. It requires great energy to conduct trade as these low grade Mercurians do it, and hard hands are a benefit for they indicate physical energy which to them is a prime requisite. Hard hands do not indicate mental energy so much as physical. Elastic hands indicate both.

The hard handed Mercurian child can be most successful in a small shop of his own in a location that does not attract the finest trade. In this shop he can handle a variety of merchandise, but he will incline to clothing, imitation jewelry, shoes, hats, or he can be successful in the loan business. A child with hard hands can be successful in the building business, or the real estate business, he can run a coal or lumber yard, or a trucking and express company. There is money to be made in the handling of scrap iron, old automobiles which are broken up into scrap, old pipe, rags, or paper, if the business is conducted in the Mercurian manner. This child, of all the types, is the one who can make such a business pay, and there are conspicuous examples of Mercurians who have accumulated a fortune from such a business. In the lowest grade of Mercurian children with hard hands, they can succeed as peddlers, in running market stands, fish stands, and especially in the delicatessen business in second rate locations.

FIFTH TEST—THE THREE WORLDS

In applying the three worlds to the Mercurian child, we desire to know whether his best success lies in the mental, the practical, or the lower world, and this we learn from the hand as a whole divided into the three worlds (Plate 16), and from the individual phalanges of the fingers which have been explained fully in other chapters.

The Mental World

Considering first the application of the three worlds to the mental occupations for which the Mercurian child is well fitted, we find that if the first phalanges of his fingers be long (Plate 17), it will greatly increase his ability as a lawyer and a doctor. In fact one of the most certain indications on which we rely in a judgment that either of these professions are the ones best suited to the child under consideration, is the fact that we find the first or mental phalanx on the finger of Mercury long.

Such a child will have the gift of oratory which is one of the determining factors in deciding upon the law as the occupation for him. We also find that in the profession of medicine, a long first phalanx of the finger of Mercury, with the medical stigmata well marked on the Mount, indicates a decided talent for medicine; and as the Mercurian child has great talent as a writer, and has been recommended for editorial work, the development of the mental world will mark him as well fitted for this kind of work. It will also be necessary if he enters the profession of teaching, and whenever he adopts any of the engineering professions.

Such a child can have great success as the editor of a business magazine. He is especially well adapted for editor of a trade magazine specializing in the garment trades. His natural Mercurian ability for business in general, together with his inherent instinct in the clothing line and with the mental world developed, particularly well fit him to write the kind of articles, and give the kind of information, which the garment trade wants. There is a big field in this direction which will pay a child well for choosing it as his vocation. He can be more successful than any of the other types who may attempt the same kind of work. If Jupiter is his secondary type he will not stop until he reaches the top, though he will have to start at the bottom to get a start.

He can also be successful in conducting a business college, where he can either teach himself, or manage the school. He will be well adapted for business law, and can do well as the publicity man for a college or law school, or for an actor or as a political writer.

The Middle World

The middle world (Plate 18), is particularly the world of business, and when found on the hands of a Mercurian child emphasizes the business side of his qualities. He will do better in the world of business than in the professions and it is only when we find the mental or both the mental and the middle world developed that we can recommend the law and medicine. On the hands of a fine grade child the middle world fits him to be successful as a banker, much more certainly if Apollo or Saturn be the secondary types. In a bank such a child will be more successful as a trust officer where he must meet customers and care for their trust matters. This is a growing business in banking, especially in large cities, and the trust business has devised many ways to benefit those who are not experienced in the handling of securities and money, especially widows and dependents not old enough to look after their affairs. Insurance companies have devised trust policies payable to the trust department of a bank, and this money can be much better cared for in this way than if left to those who may dissipate it. In a capacity such as a trust officer, a Mercurian child with the middle world developed can find a vocation for which he is well fitted.

The middle world will fit the child to be successful in all the business occupations which have been recommended for Mercurian children. According to his grade he can succeed in manufacturing and selling clothing and furs. In the retail stores in selling hats, shoes, or clothing, jewelry, rugs, furniture and household equipment, and in any of these lines the child can be placed, and will make a success.

He can specialize with success in a trunk store selling various kinds of luggage, or in a fine store specializing in tapestries and upholstery goods for interior decorators. He can specialize in silverware both as a manufacturer and in retail stores, he can specialize as an importer of Chinese and Japanese goods, both cloth and art objects. He can be very successful as a manufacturer of lingerie and corsets.

The Lower World

We seldom find the lower world (Plate 19), best developed on the hands of fine grade Mercurian children. When we do find it, the child cannot be placed in as high grade positions. On a fine grade child we find the lower world when best developed, longer than the mental or middle, but we seldom find it puffy, bulging, or thick. The lower world shows that a coarser set of qualities will dominate this child, consequently he cannot be placed in the best positions in the Mercurian occupations. But he can operate successfully as the owner or as an employee in a coffee house, a sandwich shop, a low price clothing store, as a rental agent in a low priced locality, in an employment agency, an auto tire repair shop, a chattel mortgage or salary loan office, a low priced furniture store, or as a bailiff or process server in a magistrate's office.

Sixth Test—Knotty Fingers

Knotty fingers (Plate 20), are not usual with the Mercurian child. His mind is not analytical and works too rapidly for the slow processes of knotty fingers. We do find them, however, and they have a profound effect on the operation of the child. These fingers have either the knot of mental order, or that of material order, and sometimes both plainly marked.

Knot of Mental Order

When we find the knot of mental order developed (Plate 21), it will be so prominent that it attracts attention and forms a distinct knot. This child will have system and order in all his mental operations. He will gather facts, and they will be so systematized that he can give them to you on a moment's notice. There will be no confusion in his ideas, and everything that he does will be well thought out. These fingers indicate that the child should be examined from every standpoint for the engineering professions.

We have already indicated that with certain combinations these professions should be chosen for him, and the development of the knot of mental order will be strong evidence in this direction. The study and preparation necessary for entering engineering professions is considerable, and the average Mercurian child will prefer to enter business for which he has inherent talent, unless he has the mental knot. This gives him the power of analysis and turns his thought toward the professions.

The mental knot is often found on the hands of successful Mercurian doctors, and these knots have added a great deal to the scientific attainments of their owners. Their presence on hands of fine grade Mercurian children should at once direct your attention toward the medical profession, and finding other evidence from the three worlds and the medical stigmata, you are safe in concluding that a career in medicine would be successful.

The Mercurian child being a born mathematician, one with the mental knot can find a successful occupation as a teacher or professor of mathematics. Such a child will have ability as an astronomer, and with Saturn secondary he can be a biological analyst, and can make quantitative analysis of chemical compounds, he can specialize in analytical and microscopic examinations for poisons, he can be a Bertillon and fingerprint specialist, and a writer on medical subjects for newspapers or magazines.

Second or Knot of Material Order

The second knot (Plate 22), when developed will be distinctly bulging and plainly show a knot. This is the knot of material order and the child who has it will be exacting about his surroundings, he will be neat in appearance and will insist that those with whom he comes in contact shall be the same.

His office will be clean and he will suffer no disorder, his home will be the same, he will have a place for everything. The material order with which this child surrounds himself makes him exceedingly valuable in any position where orderly procedure is required. He can be placed in a position as a statistician in a stock broker's office, he can be a cost accountant in a mill or factory, an auditor, bookkeeper, secretary, an office manager, in the latter of which positions he will find his greatest opportunity. His order and system will make him capable of conducting an office of any size if he be of fine grade and in the selection of his assistants his Mercurian shrewdness will be a great help.

There are a large number of positions in offices of the large steel companies and with accounting firms in the tax departments where a Mercurian child with the knot of material order can be placed; in the more important positions if of fine grade, and there are a very large number of less important positions in these same offices in which those of lower grade can find successful employment. Their natural business ability will enable them to surpass those of other types in the same office and secure the preferred positions.

Mercurian children with both knots developed (Plate 20), make good historians, and professors of philosophy, and as this type has an ability for writing, the teaching of history or the writing of books or articles on historical subjects and philosophy opens a wide field for successful endeavor. They also make expert chess players.

SEVENTH TEST—SMOOTH FINGERS

Smooth fingers (Plate 23), are expected on the hands of Mercurian children whose minds are quick and active, and the intuitive faculty of smooth fingers is a great aid in the judgment of human nature which helps in their ascendency in the business world. We do not find that Mercurian children with smooth fingers excel in technical occupations, we should not place them in engineering positions, theirs is the realm of business.

A fine grade Mercurian child with smooth fingers can be most valuable as the assistant to the president of a bank. In this position he will perform many of the duties of the president and will see many callers before they get to the president. His shrewd judgment of human nature will enable him to dispose of many cases and relieve his chief of a great deal in the course of a day's business. This child can fill similar positions in other large corporations, and while this cannot be called strictly a secretarial position, for he will not do stenography and typing, he is in fact the personal representative of the president and in the past many who have held such positions have succeeded to the presidency at a future date. This is a specialized position and well worthy the preparation necessary before the child attempts to fill it.

EIGHTH TEST—LONG FINGERS

Long fingers (Plate 24), need careful attention when found on the hands of a Mercurian child. Their effect is to slow down both his mental action as well as his physical, and as quickness in both is one of the leading assets of the Mercurian child, the effect of long fingers is to make him deliberate, and give him a desire to go into the detail and minutiæ of everything with which he comes in contact. This is not the usual mental operation of the Mercurian child, consequently we must consider the child with long fingers as out of the ordinary, and we must analyze him most carefully in order to find out what effect this slower mental and physical action is going to have upon him.

In the first place, it will make him more of a student, he will not take as much for granted, he will go into the detail of things, and this will make him preëminently fitted for the scientific professions such as chemistry or physics, and as a neurologist, plastic surgeon, osteopath, chiropractor, pharmacist, or roentgen operator. Long fingers indicate an analytical mind which enables the Mercurian child to be successful as an engineer in mining, mechanical, chemical, electrical, ceramic, radio, or automobile engineering, especially with Saturn as secondary type.

It must be understood that it is only when knotty or long fingers are found, or with Saturn as the secondary type, that we can place a Mercurian child in these engineering professions, as normally they are not suited to him without the long or knotty fingers, or the secondary type, but we may be sure that with his keen mind, the addition of deliberation, and the analytical qualities of long fingers, adapt him for a successful career in some of the engineering professions.

Long fingers will enable a Mercurian child to do work requiring great detail. If he has a low set thumb he can make a success as a diamond cutter, or a steel engraver. He can have great success as the head of a statistical bureau, especially in financial matters. There are a number of such bureaus, some of them very large, which gather statistics on every kind of business and all the large companies. These bureaus furnish their service to the most important banks, brokerage houses, international banks, underwriting houses, foreign governments, manufacturing corporations, newspapers, and wherever the actual facts are wanted about any industry, or the supply and demand of any commodity. Many important houses never act on any question until they have these reports before them. In such a reporting bureau a long fingered Mercurian child will find a great opportunity for a career.

Ninth Test—Short Fingers

Short fingers (Plate 26), are found on many Mercurian children. They help the child to be quick and active, they help his intuition, they help him to make up his mind quickly, and a quality peculiar to short fingers is that their first impressions are their best; second thought in their case causes them to make mistakes. Much of the success of the Mercurian in business may be attributed to his quickness in seizing an opportunity; this faculty comes from short fingers.

Such children when of fine grade can plan and execute the largest enterprises. The short fingered child will never go into the detail of anything. He sees everything as a whole. He has the ability to visualize a completed building of the largest size, and a public service enterprise. Consequently he can make a great success as promoter of a building company, a real estate development in any part of the world, a water works company, a hydro-electric company, a storage dam, and no enterprise can be brought to him too large for him to undertake. He can finance companies to build all of these promotions, for he can sell the securities of such companies. His enthusiasm will secure underwriting. He can impress the best character of contractors so that they will take contracts to build his promotions, so when we find a Mercurian child of fine grade with short fingers, we can safely assign him to the business of promotion as a worth-while career.

The finger tips, which are four in number, all different in shape, are one of the most important indications on the hands. They are especially important on the hands of a Mercurian child, as the different tips indicate in a large measure the vocation best for him, and as this child has several directions in which his talents lead him, the tips will be of great assistance to us.

The Pointed Tip

This tip has been fully described in former chapters and is well illustrated in Plate 27. It is quite distinctive in appearance, and we find them in many cases on the hands of both men and women. The Mercurian child is psychic, and pointed tips show that he is extremely so. Thus we find that a child with such finger tips can succeed as a psychiatrist if he be of fine grade, also as a psychoanalyst. There is a good deal of interest in these studies at the present time, and some very prominent scientists are devoting much time to specializing in them. A fine grade Mercurian child with pointed tips has the talent and natural aptitudes for success in psychiatry and psychoanalysis. This child can have success in psychotherapy, and owing to the increasing number who believe in the treatment of disease by mental suggestion he will have a large field in which to operate. It is quite worth while to give a fine grade Mercurian child a thorough preparation in these subjects, one which will fit him to teach them and write upon them, and a child so prepared will undoubtedly achieve success in two fields where he will not have much competition and where his type qualities and pointed tips will aid him.

The Conic Tip

We find the largest number of Mercurian children with conic tips (Plate 28). These are called the artistic tip, which

in the case of the Mercurian type expresses itself in their universally neat appearance and tasty way of dressing if they
be of fine grade. They are well groomed and this helps them
in the better and best stores in which they succeed so well.
The child with the conic tip does not do well in occupations,
which require studious preparation, his forte is in capitalizing
his good appearance and taking advantage of his natural
shrewdness in the avenues of business. We must not, therefore,
assign him to engineering professions, or to positions requiring analytical and statistical qualities of mind. He can succeed
best in positions where he comes in contact with people, and
thus in the luxury stores selling fine jewelry, rugs, laces,
precious stones, and antiques of every sort, he can have great
success if of fine grade, or he can succeed in retail stores selling women's wear of all kinds, dresses, hosiery, suits, gloves,
beauty preparations, millinery, or he can be very successful
in selling men's wear, custom or ready made tailoring, hats,
shoes, or in a haberdashery where they sell shirts, custom and
ready to wear, neckties, handkerchiefs, or he can be successful
in the wholesale end of all these different lines of trade.

If such a child is properly prepared for it, he can have
great success in the antique business. Conspicuous examples
exist of members of this type with conic tips who have grown
rich by the collection of rare pictures, old silver, much of
it from ancient estates in foreign countries, old and rare
jewelry, with precious and semi-precious stones, furniture of
various periods, tapestries, and an enormous variety of articles
which have a value to collectors. The value of all these when
they are purchased will be an easy matter to the Mercurian
child with conic tips, and he will also know what to ask for
them when he comes to sell them. This may well be chosen as
the vocation for a fine grade child. A position should be
obtained in one of the prominent stores, where he can learn
all he needs to know to make him successful.

The Square Tip

Square tips (Plate 29), are not plentiful on the hands of
Mercurian children, but when found they make them very
systematic. Such a child is not quick and active, nor is he as
rapid in his movements, but he is reliable, and from such chil-

dren should be chosen all those who are to be in, or have charge of, the accounting end of Mercurian enterprises. If his grade be fine, this child can take an advanced position in the accounting world, he can head a large accounting firm, his inherent business ability makes him exceptionally valuable in the advisory capacity which is such a large part of the business of public accounting at the present time. The square tips will indicate his accuracy in all matters, and the business ability of the type will make a combination which will insure success in the business of public accounting which may well be chosen as the vocation for a Mercurian child with square tips.

The successful public accountant of today needs to be much more than a mechanical handler of figures, he needs to be a business doctor, as he is largely employed to discover what is the matter with a business enterprise.

He is expected to audit the books of a company, to verify their records, to compile this information in such a way that it will show just what the cost of operation is, whether the business is solvent, what the income is, and the profit derived from operations. The modern accountant must in addition to all this, make recommendations whereby the sales may be increased without undue cost, where the cost of operations may be reduced without interfering with production, how the profit and loss account may show a larger balance on the right side with the same capital, and it is his business to devise a system by which all these may be done, and complete and accurate accounts be kept, which will tell at any moment just how things stand.

To accomplish all this, the public accountant of today must have a thorough knowledge of analysis, selling, collection, accounting theory, economics, finance, business organization, business law, statistics, and bookkeeping, and in addition to all this, if he is to achieve great success in his vocation, he must have inherent business sense, that intangible thing which will lead him to correct business conclusions. The Mercurian child has this business sense; square tips indicate the systematic mind which will enable him to do the mechanical part of the work.

There is a large field in accounting for the tax accountant. Many large corporations have departments which do nothing but look after the tax accounting of the company. Taxing has become very complex and it requires an expert to prevent large losses in this direction. A Mercurian child with square tips can specialize in tax accounting alone with great success. Another large field is bank accounting and audits, and still another is hotel accounting, for both of which the Mercurian child with square tips is well fitted. He may successfully specialize in any of these directions.

The Spatulate Tip

Spatulate tips (Plate 30), on a Mercurian child reinforce some of his existing qualities, and give him new ones which are influential in his vocational possibilities.

The Mercurian child with this combination can be very successful as a railroad promoter, a railroad contractor, a steamship captain if of fine grade, and a junior officer or sailor if of lower grades. He can be exceptionally successful in foreign trade. Here his business ability will be linked with a love of travel inherent with spatulate tips, and as he is naturally a salesman, he can, if of fine grade, occupy lucrative and to him pleasant positions, promoting trade for American corporations in foreign countries.

He can also be successful in governmental positions in the diplomatic corps, as his shrewdness and tact and his love of travel fit him exceptionally well to represent his government abroad.

The great originality of spatulate tips, added to the keen mind of the Mercurian child, will make him a searcher for new ideas. Thus in the medical professions he can be one who makes discoveries of new methods of treatment, new remedies, new ways of applying existing knowledge in the treatment of disease, and consequently spatulate tips give a Mercurian child an especial fitness for the medical profession.

With their constant desire to try new things, and to do old things in new ways, spatulate tips give the Mercurian child an especial fitness as an inventor or a patent attorney. At the present moment, he has great opportunities in the field of aviation. In this newest method of transportation, there are so many problems yet to be solved that it affords a wide field for original investigation for which the Mercurian child with spatulate tips is so well fitted. His inventive genius can find in this field an outlet for his best endeavors.

The thumb on the hands of a Mercurian child will inform us as to his strength of will, and his reasoning powers, and whether he is likely to take advantage of his type qualities and their combinations, or whether they are to remain dormant. When we have identified the type of a child and applied various combinations and tests to him, it is then a matter of will power as to whether he uses his talents in the development of his possibilities, for only through strength of will and logic can he enjoy the fullest measure of success.

Thumb Curled Under Fingers

We sometimes find the thumb curling under the fingers, and if we watch the child when he does not know that he is being watched we will find out whether this is accidental or his habitual way of carrying the thumb. If we find him carrying it in this way a great deal of the time, we may decide that he has a weak character, that his will is weak, and we must not place this child in responsible positions. In spite of his weak character, however, he has the Mercurian qualities, and we can place him in the Mercurian stores as cashier, window dresser, assistant to a buyer, clerk in a piece goods department, superintendent of a beauty parlor, in a theater ticket office, clerk in a telegraph office, or file clerk in a bank or broker's office.

Size of Thumb

If we find the thumb of the child small as in Plate 32, this child has also a weak character and will, and his chances of success are diminished. It does not make any difference how brilliant such a child may be, he will not have the ability to assert himself, and often such children are passed on the road by those of less ability who have large thumbs. With his Mercurian ability, however, this child with a small thumb may be successful if he is not given too great responsibility and required to have charge of a large number of people. With his inherent good taste this child can make a success of a ladies' tailoring shop. If his grade be fine he can cater to an exclusive trade and have a good location, but if it is medium or still lower he must choose a less prominent location and sell to a medium class trade. Such a child can succeed in one of the many small stores seen in large cities where they sell newspapers, magazines, candy, pencils, books, fountain pens, and a large number of novelties. Some of these stores enjoy a good trade and in some cases the owners have amassed a considerable fortune. This is an especially good business for a Mercurian child of medium grade.

The Large Thumb

We find many Mercurian children with large thumbs one of which is shown in Plate 31. This thumb, standing straight and independent and free from the hand, shows a strong character and a strong will. This child has command of himself, and he can command others. He may be placed in positions of responsibility, and can hold the best positions in his organization if he be of fine grade. With a thumb such as this, both the first and second phalanges are long and evenly balanced, consequently this child is guided by both a strong will and powerful reasoning faculties. He can be prepared for the banking business, for he has the strength to say *no* when it is necessary, and he can occupy prominent positions in the bank. One of the best positions for this child and one he can fill with great credit is the department in charge of opening new accounts. Here his intuitive faculties will aid him and his judgment of human nature will be a big asset.

He can also be successful in foreign trade. In charge of an agency for one of the prominent automobile manufacturers, he could make friends, especially in the Latin countries, and he would be successful in developing trade and building up the business. Such an occupation could well be chosen as the vocation for such a child, and proper preparation be given at an early age.

High and Low Set Thumb

We find on the hands of Mercurian children, thumbs that set high, that is they rise from the side of the hand at the top of the Mount of Venus. Such a setting is shown in Plate 36. This is the least favorable setting for the thumb, as it denotes a reduced grade of intelligence, its owner is less human, and while he may be firm, even stubborn, his is not the operation of an intelligent will. On the hand of a Mercurian child it shows that he must not be placed in the best positions, he will not do at all in the finer grade of stores, he must not be placed in engineering positions, and he will seldom be a writer. In the law and medicine he will be out of place, but we must find a place for him for he still has Mercurian qualities. Such a child can run a luncheonette and be very successful. He is shrewd and has a talent for business, consequently he will conduct his place so as to attract trade, and will learn the wishes of his customers and cater to them. He can make such a shop pay a good profit. If he cannot have a shop of his own, he can work at one of the numerous soda fountains and serve customers satisfactorily.

He can work in a cleaning and dyeing establishment where they do pressing while you wait, clean hats, and he can have a shoe repairing outfit in connection with it. Many such are doing a good business.

He can run a laundry office even though he does not do laundry work himself, for he can be an agent for a laundry which does the work, while he solicits and builds up the trade. In this way it appears as if he owned a laundry while he has nothing more invested than the fixtures and rent. The Mercurian child is quite smart enough for this, and there are many operating in this way.

Medium Set Thumb

The medium set thumb (Plate 35), rises in the center of the Mount of Venus and this child will have a goodly quantity of will power and will be very practical and have common sense. He can occupy positions requiring responsibility, but should not be placed in the highest places. With Jupiter as the secondary Mount he can do well in the ministry, or make a good captain in a political organization. With Saturn secondary he will make a good teacher in a secretarial school, with Apollo he can be successful with a moving picture theater, with Mars he could do especially well in the building and operating of an apartment house, with the Lunarian Mount he can be most successful in an advertising agency as a writer of business literature.

Low Set Thumb

The low set thumb (Plate 34), is the best of all, for it shows a stronger character and a firm but intelligent operation of the will. This thumb also opens a large field for the Mercurian child for it enables him to work with his hands. The low set thumb rises low at the base of the Mount of Venus, is generally a large thumb, and stands away from the hand in a bold and independent manner. When the thumb is capable of opposing the fingers it enables the child to be an artisan. Unless his thumb is set so that it strongly opposes the fingers he cannot be, and the low set thumb from its position gives the child a hand that enables him to firmly grasp an object, hold a tool, and thus he can be a craftsman. There are exclusive shops which do fine work in gold, silver, copper, brass, aluminum, and other metals, and in these shops the Mercurian child with this thumb can make a great success. If he have spatulate tips he will be original and will design bowls, plates, cups, jewelry, candelabra, picture frames, and many odd and unusual things which appeal to a fine trade. In such a shop this child can be successful and after he learns the business he can have a shop of his own if he is of fine grade. This child can be a watchmaker and do watch repairing. To specialize in watches is a good business, and the Mercurian child can do this well especially with the low set thumb. He can be a wood craftsman and engage in woodcarving, in which some shops specialize with success. This child can run such a shop. He can specialize in steel engraving and have a shop which makes plates for invitations to weddings and other occasions. These are all vocations in which the Mercurian child with a low set thumb can be successful.

Phalanges of Will and Reason

Bulbous Will Phalanx

The first phalanx of the thumb, called the will phalanx, by its shape and length, tells us the *amount* of will power the Mercurian child has. The larger the phalanx, the stronger the will. This is not always favorable, for we sometimes find a will phalanx shaped like Plate 37. This bulbous phalanx is the ultimate in stubbornness and unintelligence in will power, and its owner cannot be placed in any position requiring the finer qualities of the type, but must be placed in coarser occupations. He can be a machine operator in a cloak or suit factory, or a men's clothing factory, he can be a cutter in the same factory, a stock keeper or a time keeper. He can be foreman in a fertilizer factory with Saturn as the secondary Mount, or accompany the Martian on his prospecting expeditions if Mars be secondary. He can have a yard selling scrap iron and junk, but he must not work in a fine jewelry store, or haberdashery, or any of the stores selling women's wear. This thumb shows the coarsest kind of will power.

Strong Will Phalanx

There is a phalanx of will which is more often seen on the hands of Mercurian children which is broad, well formed, with a fine smooth nail, and the phalanx is long (Plate 38). This thumb denotes physical energy and strong will whose strength is used to forward the efforts of its owner in an intelligent manner, but is not brutal as is the one just described. Such a phalanx will enable a child to be successful in the Mercurian occupations, and is strong enough to force success through effort. This thumb will be a great help to a Mercurian lawyer or doctor, it will enhance the chances of a banker to win success, and it is a big asset on the hands of a manufacturer of the many lines made by Mercurians. A child with such a thumb can specialize in medical and surgical supplies. His natural taste for medicine will help him, and his business sense will enable him to assemble the proper articles and work up a trade. He can specialize in mortgage loans where his ability in financial directions will teach him where to place the loans and get the money, and to find the people to borrow it. He can specialize as a jobber, and as a manufacturer of millinery where his taste in dress and business ability will combine to manufacture a salable stock and sell it. A Mercurian child with this phalanx of will can succeed in any of the above mentioned directions.

Fine Will Phalanx

There is another will phalanx, equally long and well shaped (Plate 41), with a fine textured nail which is smooth and fine, and this phalanx indicates a will power that is very strong yet refined, one that gets what he goes after yet without offense, and the fortunate child who has this phalanx can have success in the finest grade of Mercurian occupations which have been mentioned in this chapter.

The second, or phalanx of reason, should be of the same length as this will phalanx. It should also be the same thickness. This will show a well balanced thumb, for will and reason are equal. The reasoning faculties are very necessary as a support to the will, and when the second phalanx is long we have this condition. With such a combination the Mercurian child has the forces that will support his talents and enable him to achieve the utmost in success.

Such a child can be successful in some of the more profound studies if he has Saturn as the secondary type. In this case he will have a philosophic turn of mind and can take up such subjects as mental hygienics, and can work in a psychological laboratory. With his ability in the direction of medicine he can specialize in the psychology of digestion which is attracting considerable attention at this time. Dietitians are trying to improve digestion by selected food, and psychologists are trying to do likewise by mental processes. The Mercurian child with this balanced thumb is shrewd enough to make a good deal of such an occupation.

Short Will Phalanx

A short phalanx of will seriously handicaps a Mercurian child. Such an one is shown in Plate 39. In this case the child has the same weak character as he has when the thumb curls under the fingers, or when he has the small thumb. This child must not be placed in important positions nor have the direction of others. He can, however, be successful as a stenographer. If he has the Lunarian type secondary, he will have a good command of language, and his natural quickness will enable him to be a court and law stenographer, which is a highly paid occupation. He will not need great strength of

will in this sort of a vocation and he has all the other necessary requirements.

The Thumb Tip

The tips of the thumb follow those of the fingers. We find
the pointed tip (Plate 27), which indicates the artistic viewpoint, and this child can be placed in the buying department
of a clothing manufacturer where his inherent good taste and
the artistic qualities of the pointed tip will guide him in his
selection of materials, or he can be in the designing department of such a factory where the same qualities will assist him
in choosing the styles in which garments shall be cut.

The conic tip (Plate 45), fits the child for sales positions
in various stores selling merchandise such as has been already
recommended for Mercurian children.

The square tip (Plate 44), and the spatulate tip (Plate
43), qualify the child for positions in finance, and in the offices
of Mercurian manufacturers and storekeepers in lines such
as banking, brokerage, production, and distribution of merchandise.

CHART NOTE:

When Mercury is the primary Mount, the finger will be
conspicuously larger and longer than the others. When such
is seen to be the case, have the child extend his hand, palm upward, toward you, and it will be seen that this finger is held
independently and that the other fingers lean toward it. It will
also be seen that the apices on the other Mounts lean toward
Mercury and the Mount is high and full.

When the apices of all the other Mounts lean toward Mercury, it should at once call your attention to the Mount, and
closer examination will in most cases identify this as the
primary Mount. When identified, note on the chart, with
any remarks that will enable the chart reader to judge the case
more clearly.

TEST CHART

Types
>   Primary.
>   Secondary.
>   Others.

Tests
>   1. Texture of skin
>   2. Color
>   3. Flexibility
>   4. Consistency
>   5. Three worlds
>   6. Knotty fingers
>   7. Smooth fingers
>   8. Long fingers
>   9. Short fingers
>   10. Finger tips

The Thumb
>   11. How carried
>   How set.   High.   Low.   Medium.

Will Phalanx
>   Bulbous.   Short.   Very short.   Long.
>   Very long.

Phalanx of Logic
>   Long.   Very long.   Short.   Very short.
>   Will longer than logic.   Will shorter than logic.
>   Will and logic balanced.
>   Large thumb.   Small thumb.
>   Elementary.   Medium.   Fine.
>   Tip of thumb.   Pointed.   Conic.
>   Square.   Spatulate.

Age of Child.   *Sex.*   *Date.*

CHAPTER FIVE

THE MARTIAN MOUNT TYPE

The Fighter

From the occupations listed in this book and adapted to various formations of the hand, a vocation in one of the main branches of industry, or of the sciences or professions, can be selected for children. For those whose hands show unusual combinations, there is a supplementary list which contains unusual vocations, and no child lives whose hands will not show that he is fitted for some one of these vocations. There is work for everyone. There can be no such thing as failure to find the position for which the unusual child is best fitted, from his hands, nor doubt of the ability to select the best occupation for him from this list.

CHAPTER FIVE

THE Martian Mount type is identified by the *two* Mounts of Mars, the positions in the hand which these Mounts occupy being well illustrated in Plate 1.

Knowing the location of these two Mounts, it is not difficult to identify a Martian child, and as these Mounts show quite plainly at the earliest age, we are in a position to begin with the preparation of the child even when he is still an infant.

These Mounts are the first we have encountered which do not have a finger to help in the identification, and we will be forced to rely upon the extent to which they extend at the side of the hand and into the palm in the case of the upper Mount, and the extent to which it bulges into the palm in the case of the lower Mount.

THE MARTIAN HAND

In order that you may have a correct idea of the appearance of well developed Mounts of Mars, we here refer to Plate 52 from which you will see the strong upper Mount bulging out at the side of the hand and into the palm as well, and also Plate 54 in which you will see the very strong lower Mount forming a pad just above the Mount of Venus.

In order that you may also see the deficiency of these Mounts, we here refer to Plate 55 in which the lower Mount is entirely absent, and Plate 53 in which you will see the hollow at the side of the hand showing a deficiency of the upper Mount as compared with Plate 52. From a careful examination of these four plates, it will be possible for you to fix in your mind the exact appearance of strong Mounts, and how the hand looks when the Mounts are not only absent but actually deficient. Between these two extremes, there are many degrees of development whereby with practice you will be able to estimate and ascribe the proper amount of Martian quality to any child.

The Martian is a very important type, for he represents physical strength and force of character, and mental strength as well. He is the fighter, and forces his way through the world either by the use of his physical or his mental powers. In any combination found in the hands of a child, Martian qualities must be reckoned with.

We find as we study the Martian that he is not always good. He does not belong to the criminal types, but in the lower grades he easily becomes violent, and many of his type are constantly in trouble with agents of the law mostly from brawls, in the largest number of cases arising from jealousy.

In our study of the Martian type, we shall follow the plan of considering him as a pure specimen of the type, and as an adult male, and shall use the pronoun "he" though there are an abundance of Martian women who follow the male in appearance, and in all of his characteristics.

In our original study of the Martian type, covering a period of years, we located many pure specimens both in men and women. In the years that have followed we have located them in great abundance, and have completely verified the composite description of their appearance as originally made.

DESCRIBING THE MARTIAN

From this description the Martian is of medium height, very strongly built, muscular looking, carries himself erect, shoulders back, and has the appearance of one ever ready to defend himself. His head is small, with unusually large development at the base of the brain. The back of the neck is broad, and in a pronounced specimen developed much above the average. The face is round, the skin thick and strong, red in color, and often presenting a mottled appearance. The hair is stiff, sometimes curly and of an auburn or red color. The beard is short and harsh.

The eyes are large and bold looking, dark in color, and with the whites often bloodshot showing the great strength of his blood supply. The mouth is large and firm, the lips thin with the under one slightly thicker. The teeth are small, regular, strong, and yellowish in color. The brows grow thick, straight,

and low over the eyes, often giving the appearance of a
scowl. His nose is long, straight, or of the Roman type, the
chin firm and strong, often turning up slightly at the end.

The neck is short and thick, connecting the head with a
finely developed pair of shoulders, broad and muscular with
large muscles running down the back and a big expansive chest
which sends forth a commanding voice full of resonance and
power.

Martian Characteristics

There are two forces which have as much to do with success
as any others. They are the two forces which acting directly
at the command of will, furnish the impulse, and the steadying
qualities which make the human engine operate. These two
forces are *AGGRESSION*, indicated by a large development
of the lower Mount of Mars, and *RESISTANCE*, indicated
by the upper Mount.

The aggression of the Martian, if the lower Mount be
largely developed, does not mean a passive state, but it means
that the child will at all times force the fighting, he will expend his physical and mental strength in causing to happen
what has been decreed by the will; so aggression, as exemplified by the lower Mount of the Martian type, is one of the vital
indications upon which we rely in an estimate as to what the
child is going to make of himself.

This lower Mount of Mars is the single exception where
one characteristic only is indicated, but its aggression is of
such supreme importance that it is enough.

Let us for a moment turn to Plate 54 where we see an
extreme development of lower Mars. Here we have one who is
overly aggressive. He is of the "rule or ruin" sort who will
have his way at all cost.

On the other hand when we look at Plate 55 we see one who
is utterly lacking in aggressive qualities. He will, often when
he *knows* his ideas are the best, let the one with a Mount such
as is shown in Plate 54 have his way. We do not wish to find
either of these two extremes in our child, but we wish to find
a good average between the two, where he will not fail to assert himself on the one hand, and where he will not be hopelessly
weak on the other.

The upper Mount of Mars (Plate 52), indicates primarily resistance, which acts as a cushion against defeat. This is the quality which enables you to stand firm when things are going against you, to endure punishment, to withstand pressure but not to acknowledge defeat. Those children who have the upper Mount strongly developed never know when they are beaten but defying obstacles they press forward to attain their objective. Many brilliant people after a struggle succumb to discouragement, often just at the moment when success is within their grasp, but those with a strong upper Mount of Mars never do. Many times when hopelessly defeated, apparently, they achieve success because they did not give up.

The Martian being the fighting type, we find that if the upper Mount be strong the child has *COURAGE*, and this means both physical and moral courage which makes him brave in moments of danger, lacking fear, and such an one makes the best kind of a soldier. He also has the quality of *COOLNESS*, so that in moments of danger he is self-possessed. *CALMNESS* is another of his qualities which means poise. All of these qualities combined make him the Warrior, which is to be taken as the superlative of the Fighter. A Fighter may engage in a brawl, a Warrior leads armies, and this is the Martian child of the pure type.

We now assemble the characteristics of the Martian type and find that he has,

Aggression
Resistance
Courage
Coolness
Calmness

which make him

THE WARRIOR

THE MARTIAN AND MARRIAGE

In his wooing and his marriage relations the Martian is a strenuous lover. He has an abundance of health and great muscular strength, and his nature is intense. He is very fond of the opposite sex and is predisposed to early marriage. Very fine specimens, while ardent, hold their passions within bounds, but as the grade becomes coarser, the passions become more violent and in the very low grades they become quite coarse. Such children are easily aroused to jealousy when grown, and sometimes commit murder in the heat of passion.

The Martian likes women of a feminine type and Venusians strongly appeal to him. There are, however, many women of the Martian type who are of fine quality, and these have a commanding presence, they are handsome, vigorous, lithe, and withal feminine, and many marriages of these kinds of Martians are made within their own type. The Jupiterian women are also handsome, have a fine presence, great dignity, and these are universally admired. They attract a fine specimen of Martian if he be of fine grade, and in the lower grades they are equally attractive to Martians of their own grade.

The real preference of the Martian is however for a Venusian wife.

MARTIAN HEALTH

The Martian is a heavy eater and drinker, and this means that he is fond of alcoholic beverages and consumes much coffee. He loves and eats rich food. Red meat, pork, veal, game of every kind, fish, crabs, lobsters and all sea foods, eggs, bread, and the heavy vegetables are his main diet. This consumption of food taxes his stomach and makes him liable to the ills arising from heavy eating. He is prone to have fevers and intestinal disorders. He has also a tendency to throat trouble, bronchitis, laryngitis, and various disorders of the respiratory tracts, high blood pressure, and arteriosclerosis.

MARTIAN QUALITIES

The Martian child as an entity represents in the highest degree the qualities of the fighter. He is brave and does not fear to engage in physical strife. Having robust health, he is a formidable adversary either in personal combat, as a business competitor, or at the head of any unit of an army. He is extremely energetic, restless, active and athletic, forceful and untiring. None of the Mount type of people make as good soldiers. In the various grades he can succeed in a military life, the finer grades as commissioned officers, and the lower grades as noncommissioned officers and privates.

He is domineering when his Mounts are very strong, he is fond of all athletic sports, especially those which require physical strength and skill. Polo, hockey, football, wrestling, boxing, and all rough sports are his favorite forms of recreation. He is popular, and well esteemed as a fair foe.

In no type is the grade more important, for as the grade decreases and the child becomes more common, it is difficult to keep him from the excesses of this type. There is a very coarse Martian child, and we must hunt for him as well as for those of fine grade, for this low grade child must have especial care when we find him.

THE SECONDARY TYPE

The secondary types play an important part in the success of a Martian child, his type qualities being largely those of strength, embodying as they do, the important attributes of aggression and resistance which give him a fighting spirit. When he has behind these fighting qualities such distinctive qualifications as are found in one of the other Mount types, it makes a wonderful combination.

JUPITER SECONDARY TYPE

When we find a strong development of the Mounts of Mars, or either of them, and in addition a high Mount of Jupiter with the apex centrally located (Plate 8), the finger straight and standing erect, and the other fingers leaning toward it with their apices deflected in the direction of Jupiter, we may decide that the child is a Martian with Jupiter as the secondary Mount.

This is a powerful combination, for when we put Jupiterian qualities behind Martian strength, the combination of the two will produce very positive results.

To review them, the Jupiterian has as his leading characteristics ambition, leadership, religion, honor, love of nature, pride, and dignity, and the Martian has aggression, resistance, courage, coolness, and calmness.

Thus the Jupiterian secondary type has added to the Martian child ambition, desire for leadership, and political ability which he did not possess before, and as the Martian child already had aggression and resistance, which means that he can aggressively pursue an objective, and that he will acknowledge no such thing as defeat, we see that the addition of the Jupiterian qualities to those of the Martian child has made him almost impossible to overcome.

In the Army and Navy

There are many excellent opportunities for the Martian child in the military service with Jupiter secondary type, and this does not mean that this service relates only to fighting, for some of the largest accomplishments of the past century have been made by men in the military service in both the medical and engineering branches of the army. For example the building of the Panama Canal, and the stamping out of yellow fever in the canal Zone, are two of the most shining examples.

When we say that the Martian child is eminently fitted for an army man, it means that army life, discipline, and training fit a man to fill important positions in the world, sometimes as a fighter, but some have even been Presidents of the United States, and many have graduated from the Army into the most important positions in the business and professional world.

Entrance to the army may be gained through the regular army, through the Military Academy at West Point where thorough training is given for military service in all branches, or it may be through the national guard, or the organized reserves which are federal bodies. For all branches of the army, the Martian child with Jupiter as the secondary Mount is preeminently qualified, and once enlisted in the service, he rises by merit, and the Martian-Jupiterian child will surpass all others in efficiency.

The Martian child is well fitted for life in the navy, where the same things are true as in the army. There is much to do besides fighting, and the life is attractive. The Martian-Jupiterian child can succeed in the navy.

In Politics

The field of practical politics offers great opportunities to a Martian-Jupiterian child owing to the political ability of his secondary type. This child has a fine presence, he is good to look at, he has a strong voice, not unmusical, he has great energy, he brings aggression to the combination which the Jupiterian does not have in so great a degree, and he also brings resistance, so that he does not accept defeat or become discouraged. The combination of these two types eminently fit the Martian-Jupiterian child for politics.

He can be distinctly a practical politician, that is he will go right out into a ward or precinct and organize it. He breaks heads if necessary, but he maintains a military discipline and he gets the desired results. He is not so often found as a holder of office, he puts a Jupiterian forward for that part of the work, but he is found most often to be what is known as a political "boss."

In Business

There is a fine opportunity for Martian-Jupiterian children in the business world, and many of them can hold important positions. This child will fight for business just as he does for anything else, and he can be successful on account of his aggressive disposition which causes him to push himself regardless of others often of those with more ability than himself.

Natural Resources

A field of business in which the Martian-Jupiterian child can be successful is in the development of natural resources. Here he is fitted for a prospector of oil fields, coal lands, copper deposits, bodies of iron ore, zinc, lead, phosphate, gold, silver, timber tracts, aluminum, and he is successful in securing leases or buying property outright in which any of these deposits are contained. We do not mean that he should necessarily pursue such occupations on his own account as they involve large capital, but he should identify himself with some of the large corporations to whom locating and acquiring such properties is important. In this capacity he is the advance guard of development, and his sturdy qualities fit him to be successful as none of the other types would be. Any company developing natural resources, equipped with a force of Martian-

Jupiterian children when grown, would lead all of their competitors.

There are especially fine opportunities for a Martian-Jupiterian child with the large oil companies, who are searching every corner of the globe for new territory, and who need the strongest kind of men to find it, acquire it when found, and to hold it from encroachment after it is acquired. No one can do this kind of work as well as a Martian-Jupiterian child.

When we realize the tremendous effort that is being made to gain footholds in foreign lands, Turkey, Russia, Roumania, or wherever there are oil deposits, and the difficulty of holding concessions after they are acquired, we can see the value which an industrial army of Martian-Jupiterians to hold these frontiers would be to any corporation. There are thousands of positions of every grade in the oil industry which are open to Martian-Jupiterian children. Then there is the necessity for opening new markets for products of all the companies who are developing natural resources, such as oil, coal, timber, and all the metals or minerals. Here again the Martian-Jupiterian child, the trail blazer, holder of the fighting front, is superior to any of the other types. Few who have not been engaged in it know the fierce strife there is in the development of new territory and new markets. Those who are there are trying to hold them, the many who are trying to preëmpt them are fighting as fiercely as is done in any war. For such work a fighting man is needed, and none excel the Martian-Jupiterian. So if your child is of this type combination, there are open to him abundant opportunities for success in these directions and there are positions for every grade of child.

Contracting and Construction

The Martian-Jupiterian child is well fitted for the contracting business, in the construction end of the business. If he is of fine grade he can succeed in the executive end. Those who do the figuring are usually men of other types, but these men rely upon Martians to obtain the contracts, handle the men, and do the actual construction work. Here there is open to Martian-Jupiterian children a large field, the most important position in which is as a superintendent of construction with a large contracting company. For this position a well balanced Martian-Jupiterian child is needed, for he must organize the force which is to erect the building, the dam, the railroad, the power plant, or whatever the contract calls for. Upon him will devolve the task of seeing that the men of all kinds engaged upon the work give their full time, and that every foreman under him has his crew well organized and working under proper discipline.

This superintendent will have a force of engineers, draftsmen, and technical men under him as well as the common labor who do the actual work. In this position as superintendent of construction the same qualities are needed as in the army, and for such a position no one of the types is as well fitted as the Martian-Jupiterian child. When we think of the enormous amount of construction work of every kind going on all the time, we can see what a wonderful opportunity is open to a child of the Martian-Jupiterian type combination. In the lower grades of children there will be a great many openings as a foreman of construction, for which position Martian qualities are also required, and there are innumerable positions of less importance for Martian-Jupiterian children of all grades, who on account of their physical strength and their aggression succeed better than those who are less rugged and less hard boiled.

Some of the vocations or trades which are allied with the contracting and construction business, for all of which the Martian-Jupiterian child is well fitted, are as a carpenter, brick layer, plumber, steamfitter, bridge builder, boiler maker, machinist, painter, sheet metal worker, molder, tinner, stone cutter, truck driver, welder, oil well driller, track layer, plasterer, lather, and for these positions we must assign lower grades of Martian-Jupiterian children.

Other positions in business industry to which we must assign lower grades of Martian-Jupiterian children consist of coal mine, copper mine, lead and zinc mine, stone quarries, gold and silver mine, and iron mine operatives called miners. Then there are the operatives of oil, gas, and salt wells, and employees of refineries for oil and other commodities, blacksmiths, forgemen, hammermen, firemen, furnacemen, smelter men, heaters, pourers, ladlers, and puddlers.

From the variety of occupations for which the Martian

child primarily, and in combination with the Mount of Jupiter, is best qualified, we see the great importance of determining the grade of the child, as by this factor alone will be determined whether he shall be placed in the more important positions or among those who labor with their hands.

SATURN SECONDARY TYPE

When the Mount of Saturn (Plate 46), is the secondary Mount, we determine it by finding it higher than the other Mounts, or with a fine clear vertical line on the Mount, the apex high and centrally located, and the finger of Saturn straight. At the same time we find one or the other of the Martian Mounts full and bulging. With this combination, the hot-headed impulse of the Martian child is much reduced, for the Saturnian has brought him some of his soberness and seriousness.

This will make a good combination if the child be of fine quality, for both the Martian and the Saturnian of fine grade have excellent qualities. If, however, the combination be found on the hand of a child of low grade it is unfavorable, as both Mounts in the low grades have a bad side. We shall, however, follow our custom, and treat the subject of which we speak as if the child was of fine grade.

The literary or scientific qualities of the Saturnian will not influence this Martian child to a great extent, for he is not inclined to be a writer, or to engage in scientific studies, nor will the engineering side of the Saturnian be important to him. The Saturnian's restraining influence, however, will be beneficial and his balancing qualities will be of the greatest value. Thus the Martian child will be fitted for a number of occupations where a less amount of fighting quality is necessary.

In Agriculture

The agrarian instincts of the Saturnian will open to the Martian child many lines of endeavor in which he may be successful, for instance in chemical and allied industries. He will not find his place in the laboratory end of these businesses however, but in the production end, chiefly in fertilizer factories, paint and varnish, powder, cartridge, dynamite and fuse, and soap factories. In all of these the grade of the child will determine whether he can occupy a position in the executive end of the business, which he can do if he is of fine grade, or whether he is to be in the production end as a superintendent, foreman, or in the lower grades as a laborer. Each of these positions can be determined by his grade, for he can be successful in any of them according to his grade. It will be noted that the Martian child is assigned to the producing end of each business, as his aggressive disposition fits him for the organizing and handling of workmen and his physical strength for doing the actual work, leaving the engineering problems to others who are better fitted for them. But his organizing ability also fits him for executive positions if his grade be fine. In none of the types does the quality of the child more fully determine what his position is to be in any enterprise.

APOLLO SECONDARY

If the Mount of Apollo (Plate 49), be the secondary Mount, which we determine from a prominent Mount of Apollo, with the apex centrally located, the finger of Apollo large and straight, and the other fingers leaning toward it while the Martian Mounts are full and bulging, we have an excellent combination, for the Apollonian has no very bad side and brings to the Martian child only good qualities.

This is true in the field of salesmanship where the Apollonian excels. The Martian-Apollonian child can be exceedingly successful as a salesman, for here we have the natural sales ability of the Apollonian spurred on by the aggression and resistance of the Martian, and such a child will go anywhere to make sales, he will get in to see anyone he wants to see, and he will not take no for an answer on account of upper Mars. The average grade Martian child will not be so successful in selling the finer lines of merchandise, such as jewelry and similar luxuries, this requires a pure fine grade Apollonian or Mercurian child, but the Martian-Apollonian child may be placed in the sales forces of bakeries, butter and cheese factories, candy factories, flour and grain mills, fruit and vegetable canning factories, packing houses, sugar refineries, agricultural implement factories, automobile factories, rolling mills, iron and steel industries, brass mills, lead and zinc factories, tinware and enamel ware factories, lumber and furniture industries, furniture factories, piano and organ factories, hemp and jute mills, rope and cordage factories, sail awning and tent factories, electric light and power plants, petroleum refineries, or rubber factories. In all of these assignments the Martian-Apollonian child will be selling in a wholesale way, for which he is better fitted than to sell at retail. Each of the industries mentioned has great future possibilities, and a Martian-Apollonian child should be prepared for a future in one of these lines beginning at an early age, the choice of which resting with the parents.

The other Apollonian qualities will only influence the Martian in a general way, refining him and taking away some of his brusqueness. This refining influence will however enable him to occupy a higher grade of positions than is possible to an average Martian child of the pure type.

MERCURY SECONDARY TYPE

When the Mount of Mercury (Plate 50), is the secondary Mount, we identify it by a high Mount, apex centrally located, the finger long and straight, and in appearance it will overshadow the other Mounts which will not be so well developed.

Presupposing the Martian child to be of fine grade with a secondary Mount of Mercury, the combination will be favorable, but we must remember that both of these Mounts have a bad side, and the Mercurian Mount has an especially bad, even a criminal side. These bad sides however develop only when the hands are coarse, and may be determined by the various tests which we have learned to apply. However, with the Martian-Mercurian combination present, we must at all times be on our guard.

It will not be hard to imagine what the effect will be when we add the shrewdness, the industry, the mental and physical alertness and the business ability of the Mercurian to the aggressive, forceful steam engine which is the Martian child. It will create a force that will be tireless in its activities and extremely capable; and the Mercurian qualities will direct nearly all the Martian strength in the direction of business. A child with this combination can be successful in the clothing industry, especially in the manufacturing end where there are fine opportunities as superintendents of plants, if the grade be fine, or as foremen; or when the grade is lower as machine operators, cutters, or operatives of various descriptions. Fine grades of this combination can also be successful as salesmen for the manufactured product.

They can also be successful as salesmen in corset factories, glove factories, hat factories, shirt collar and cuff factories, suit, coat, cloak, and overall factories, carpet mills, lace and embroidery mills, knitting mills, silk mills, cotton mills, woolen and worsted mills, linen mills, trunk and shoe factories. The positions in all of these mills and factories in which the Martian-Mercurian child can be successful will not be as merchandise men, designers, buyers, or in the actual business management of these industries, but it will be as salesman for, and in the production end, where their aggressive and dominant qualities will fit them to organize the factory and introduce military precision into its operation.

The Lunarian Secondary Type

When the Mount of the Moon (Plate 56), is the secondary Mount, the Mount will have to be very high, merging into the Mount of Mars, bulging, and extending outward at the side of the hand. This Mount with its mysticism and fancy is not much like the practical common sense Martian Mount, and must be very strongly developed before it will have much influence on the Martian character. It will in no way be much help to the Martian child in developing adaptability for many occupations. It is only in the very fine grades of Martian children that the Lunarian type would have an influence so far as occupations go.

There is no one of the types that has as great a vocabulary as the Lunarian, or better command of language, therefore in combination with a fine grade Martian child it will give him an ability to write which otherwise he would not have. Thus a Martian child with this combination can be successful as a general writer, an editor, a reporter, a correspondent, a publisher, a sales promotion writer, or an author of stirring tales, and as the Lunarian has great imagination together with his command of language, the Martian child with this combination can succeed as a writer of fiction.

In low grade Martian children this combination with the Lunarian is not favorable, as it makes a superstitious, cold, selfish creature, for whom few successful careers can be found. They must be placed where they do not come in direct contact with the public, and mostly at common labor in such places as a gas works, a straw factory, turpentine distillery, broom factory, or charcoal works.

VENUS SECONDARY TYPE

With the Mount of Venus (Plate 58), as the secondary Mount we find the Mount very high and full, inclined to be hard, and either a deep pink or red color. This is a very strong combination, for the Mount of Venus is the mount of passion, and the Martian child is himself an ardent person. We find it a fiery, aggressive combination which has strong desires and does not hesitate to gratify them.

The Venusian side gives this child an attractive quality which no one who has no Venusian in them has. People love to be near them, and this child can be placed to advantage where he will meet people and come in direct contact with them. Thus he may be placed in sales positions, he can make great headway in the army, in politics, and in business. If of fine grade he can be successful in retail jewelry salesmanship, and in other lines of retail trade such as pianos, haberdashery, furniture, draperies, and as a floor manager. This combination makes a good private secretary.

THE TESTS FOR GRADE

As we have seen in the course of this chapter, the grade to which a child belongs is most important if he be of the Martian type. We have seen where he may occupy the best of positions if he is of fine grade, and we have seen where the matter of grade will consign him to the ranks of common labor. We have up to the present time presented the Martian as a distinct entity, and have seen where he has a wide and varied scope of operation. But we have always heard that this or that occupation was "according to his grade."

FIRST TEST—TEXTURE OF THE SKIN

We now begin a study of the tests which we apply to him to determine his grade and in this study we begin with the skin, the coarsest grade of which is shown in Plate 11, and this quality of skin will be found on the hands of low grade Martian children. You will not find this skin on the hands of very young children even if they are to develop it later, but you will find coarse skin on the hands of Martian children at about ten which will be a warning to you that you may expect it to become coarser later on. We remind you again of the coarse skin of Plate 11 as we wish you to keep it in mind when you are examining the skin of a child, so that you can form a judgment of the skin you find, with this as a base.

When such skin is found, it will indicate a coarse common nature, and as the Martian child at best is brusque and aggressive and a fighter, this coarse skin will tell you that he will be pugnacious, hot tempered, and that he must not be placed in any occupation requiring refinement, tact, or great intelligence. We must at once conclude that only the lower grades of occupation should be assigned to him, such as day labor in street cleaning departments, "white wings," building sewers, or working in rolling mills. The secondary type must be watched, for if Mercurian it will, with this coarse skin, mean a criminal tendency.

From the coarseness of Plate 11 the texture of the skin will improve, and with each degree of improvement the child may be assigned to a better grade of employment. There are many occupations suitable for those of a medium grade of fineness for which the Martian child is better suited than any other type, and the skin will be one of the best tests of the special fitness of a child for these positions. They may be placed as policemen, firemen, guards, watchmen, doorkeepers, marshals, sheriffs, detectives, constables, probation officers, truant officers, life savers, lighthouse keepers, keepers of charitable and penal institutions, and of pleasure resorts, race tracks, as jailers, coast guards, sailors, marines, soldiers, inspectors, gaugers, samplers, conductors, railroad freight agents, overseers, athletic directors or coach; or as a door man, steam boiler inspector, steamboat captain, or postal inspector. All of which occupations you will note require the aggression and force of the Martian, but for none of which a technical education is necessary.

Fine texture of skin (Plate 10), will indicate the Martian child who can fill the better positions in all the Martian occupations. He will have all of the forceful qualities of the Martian type, but they will operate in a more refined way. He can occupy positions closer to the executive end of a business, such as office manager or vice president, or he can be successful in politics as surrogate, prothonotary, magistrate, or judge. In the army he will be fitted for a commissioned officer, in infantry, field artillery, or cavalry; as a fencing master, or with Jupiter secondary, as a lobbyist.

We have enumerated as above many lines of business in which a Martian child may be successful, and in all of these one with fine textured skin and with other tests showing him to be of fine grade should be assigned to the more important positions where he will have oversight of others.

SECOND TEST—COLOR OF THE HANDS

White Color

The color of the hands will be the next test we shall apply to the Martian child, and if we find the palms and under the nails distinctly white we shall know that not only is his physical vitality below par, but he will have his Martian qualities much reduced. He will not be so aggressive nor so industrious, and he should not be placed in the front of a battle line, nor should he be sent to explore wild places or prospect for oil or minerals. His occupation should be chosen where not so much fighting spirit is needed, nor so much rugged aggression.

This child can be assigned to the commissariat in the army, where he will look after the transportation and provisions if of fine grade; or he can be a tax assessor, a chaplain in the army, or hold an executive position in a munition factory. Such a child will do exceptionally well in the conduct of a physical culture school, for he will have all his Martian qualities though lessened by the white color of his hands. He will, however, have enough of the Martian aggression to conduct such a school, and this would make a good vocation for him where he can make a good livelihood.

Pink Color

Pink color will be found in the hands of a fine grade Martian child and he should be placed in the more important positions in the Martian occupations.

Such a child will have the virility that goes with pink color of the hands, which will make the Martian aggression and resistance operate to their fullest extent. He can be assigned to prospecting work for oil, metal, or minerals in which the Martian is successful, and can perform the most exacting duties in exploring expeditions in such territory as Alaska. Easy positions need not be sought for him. He can go to the front in an army, he can be successful in an executive position with a circus, or if of medium grade in the exacting positions with a circus where he is in charge of transportation, baggage, tents, and the ordinary rough work that goes with circus life. At the present time there is another vocation in which this child can specialize which has a great future and for which the Martian child with pink color is well fitted. This is in the development of passenger service in Zeppelin transportation. This branch of aviation is in its infancy and a Martian child who grows up with it can have a great future.

Red Color

Red color is plentiful among Martian children especially in the lower grades. Here we have the full amount of physical vigor, and the full strength of both aggression and resistance; consequently, a child with red color in his hands may be placed in a position requiring the greatest amount of courage, and such an one may be sent to distant countries, or wild places, or put in any of the many occupations which have been recommended for Martian children.

The Martian child with red color in the fine grades will be a great tactician and in the army or navy he can be very successful in conducting a school of tactics in an army or navy post; he will make a strict top sergeant. He can be successful with a lighterage company large enough to have their own tugs and barges. He can make a good observer in an airplane, or a navigator. He can engage in pisiculture, and with a state or federal hatchery he would be most successful.

In lower grades this child can be successful as a coachman, butler, longshoreman, a machine gun operator in the army, or a stereotyper on a large newspaper.

Yellow Color

Yellow color is not often seen in the hands of a Martian child but when found it will be a warning to look out for a disagreeable application of Martian qualities. Yellow color is never seen in the Martian hand until the child is fully impregnated with bile, and as he has such strong qualities, anything which causes them to operate in an excessive or distorted manner brings out the bad side of the type. Yellow color will make the Martian child quarrelsome at the least, and in coarse grades it will make him violent. Such a child even in the finer grades cannot be placed in as important positions as his grade demands. In the lower grades he must be assigned to the labor class of employment.

Here we must find a place for the child where he can take advantage of his strong qualities, and yet not develop his disagreeable side. Such a child can specialize in colon irrigation, in which there are many now successful who have had no medical training. He can conduct a circular letter mailing office, or be a typographer, run a vulvanizing shop, or a waffle shop, all of which vocations are now being successfully followed in cities.

Third Test—Flexibility of the Hands

Flexibility of the hands will be a guide to quality of the mind of the Martian child, and consequently to his grade.

The Stiff Hand

If we find an extremely stiff hand, such as is shown in Plate 12, it will indicate the lowest form of mental stagnation, and this child would have to be placed in the labor class of Martian occupations.

His stiff hands will mean a crass mental state which will make a mental occupation impossible.

He has Martian qualities, however, and in an occupation

where he can use them he can have success in accordance with his grade. He can be a blacksmith, a forgeman in a welding shop, a pressman in a printing or newspaper office, a sexton, a steel worker in the erection of large buildings or bridges, a tanner, a wood chopper.

The Straight Hand

If we find straight hands on the child (Plate 13), we shall find the mind not elastic, but it will not be stiff, and this child can be placed in positions of medium grade. In the paragraph on the skin in this chapter, we gave a list of occupations for medium grade Martian children and these are also some of the occupations suited to the straight hand. In these various vocations there is no more elasticity of mind needed than is furnished by the straight hand, and little technical knowledge is required.

This child can engage in mechanical arts and other vocations requiring skill with his hands. He can have a woodworking shop and be a turner skilled with a lathe. In such a shop he can do woodcarving or cabinet work, some of it of fine workmanship. He can be a joiner, he can operate an umbrella factory or repair shop. He can be a wheelwright, a horseshoer, or a masseur, and have his own bath house where he can cater to exclusive customers if he be of fine grade. He can be a machinist and have his own machine shop, and as such he can specialize in different kinds of work, tooling, grinding, boilers, valves, or engines.

The Flexible Hand

When we find a flexible hand such as is shown in Plates 14, 15, we will likely find the other tests are also fine in grade, and this child will have an elastic mind which will be courting activity at all times. It will be bright and keen, and such a child can be placed in a number of the Martian occupations already enumerated where mental activity is required. He must be placed in the higher positions where aggression, resistance, and a bright mind can secure their proper reward. A child with such hands will be particularly adaptible for sales positions in the luxury stores if he be of fine grade, and in the paragraphs on the secondary types you will find many Martian occupations concretely stated in which the Martian child with a flexible hand can be successful.

He can also be successful as a journalist, a metallurgist skilled in the art of working metals, and can conduct a smelter where he separates metals from their ores and refines them. As the Martian child has been recommended as a prospector for metals, the reduction of these metals as above is a natural process for him and such would be an excellent choice as a vocation for such a child. He can be successful as a manufacturer of power boats or storage batteries, or as an Egyptologist capable of heading a scientific exploring party for a museum or college, and on account of his Martian qualities particularly well fitted for such a vocation. If such is chosen for the child, he must be given a thorough education in all the essentials necessary for such a scientific occupation. If the child is fine in grade and passes all the tests, he can safely be assigned to Egyptology as his life's work.

Fourth Test—Consistency of the Hands

Consistency of the hands will show us with what energy a child will apply Martian qualities.

Flabby Hands

If we find the hands flabby, we know that he will talk more than he will act. Such children cannot be placed where they are to have command of others, so all such positions as superintendents, foremen and the like must be scratched from the list. It will be plain that a child with flabby hands cannot be assigned to prominent positions in the army where courage and initiative are required, nor can he be sent into wild country to develop mineral resources where hard work alone wins success; nor can he do any of the hard things which Martian children can do so well. We must find places for these flabby handed children however, where great energy is not required, where they can be supervised, where they cannot loaf. Such a position will be as a clerk in a department of a well supervised retail store where he will be under the watchful eye of a floor manager, or as a cashier in a hotel or restaurant, or clerk in a chain store where he cannot get away from work, or as time keeper in mills or factories if of medium or lower grades.

Such a child can serve in a cafeteria, he can be a curator in a museum or art gallery if of fine grade, he can be custodian of a building, he can run a fruit stand, he can be a bushelman tailor, he has the very qualities for a veterinarian and can find a most profitable occupation in the treatment and care of dogs in a large city, where a dog hospital is crowded at all times with the pets of wealthy people who will pay any price to have doggy treated when he is sick.

Soft Hands

Soft hands will show reduced energy, but do not indicate absolute laziness. Children with soft hands may therefore be placed where they do not have the extreme of physical exertion, they are more self reliant, and have more energy than those with flabby hands. For them we must not select the most difficult positions in which Martian children are successful, but we can assign them to crews that are being sent out to do surveying work, or they may accompany an expedition going to prospect for natural resources, but not in the positions of responsibility. Or they may be assigned to organizations for sales or promotions in subordinate capacities.

Such a child can be successful in a bureau of municipal research, either as the head if his grade be fine, or as an employee in lower grades. His success in this vocation will be more marked if Jupiter be the secondary Mount. He can be successful in a labor bureau, or as a labor organizer, or in a hotel service corporation which plans, outfits, and runs hotels. He can be secretary of a health resort, a microscopist, an optician, an evangelist, more successful with Jupiter secondary, a hypnotist with Saturn secondary, or a forest ranger who has little to do but keep watch for forest fires.

Elastic Hands

Elastic consistency will bring out the best there is in the Martian child. Here we find intelligent energy ready to be a background for aggression and the result is a child who is up and doing at all times, who does not have to be watched to keep him at work, who can be given responsibility and depended upon. Consequently such an one may be put at the head of an expedition, or have a commission in the army, or be the head of a department in a business, a superintendent, a foreman, or he may own his own business. He will do well as manager of a sales department, or of a store in one of the chains, and in such a capacity he would put all his aggression to work to control the trade of his neighborhood.

He can be successful as head of a bureau of industrial relations in a large corporation where he coördinates and brings about valuable business contacts with dealers, public officials, or foreign governments. He can be successful as leader of an expedition to photograph wild animals in their habitat, as a wild west hero in the movies, as an equestrian in a circus, as a field officer in the army, from the rank of major to colonel. He can be successful with an oil company in the establishment of filling stations or the purchase of sites for stations, refineries, or other necessary buildings, he can own and conduct a gasoline filling station, he can secure rights of way for natural gas companies and superintend the erection of pipe lines, booster stations, or the distribution of natural gas in cities and other communities. He can be very successful in securing franchises for the sales of gas to consumers in cities. A Martian child with elastic hands can find no better vocation than a connection with a strong natural gas company.

Hard Hands

Hard consistency will be found in the lower types of hands. These hard handed Martian children make a success as policemen, marshals, privates in the army, sailors, watchmen, and a large number of similar occupations. And they are needed by every organization which is exploiting new country, prospecting, or holding territory already acquired. They can make a great success in the Marine Corps.

A hard handed Martian child can be successful as an excavator, in which large companies specialize in the digging of foundations for large buildings. These companies have a full complement of machinery which enables them to excavate for foundations even through solid rock, and such do a large and profitable business for which the Martian child with hard hands is well fitted presupposing him to be of a grade suitable for an executive if he is to head such a company. Or in the lower grades, he can hold less important positions even down to the workmen who operate the machines and load the trucks.

FIFTH TEST—THE THREE WORLDS

The three worlds of the hand which are identified by the hand as a whole (Plate 16), and by the three phalanges of the fingers (Plate 1), are one of the tests upon which we rely to tell us whether the Martian child will be best developed in the mental, the practical, or the lower world.

The Mental World

If the fingers are the longest third of the hand (Plate 16), and the first or nail phalanges of the fingers are the longest (Plate 17), we shall conclude that the child is strongest in the mental world, and we should apply this information by placing him in positions where mental qualities will be of most assistance. If he is to be placed in the army, he should be a commissioned officer and we should try to get him a commission in the engineering or medical branches.

A mentally endowed Martian child can be successful in politics in many of the civil service divisions, in various bureaus, in some capacity on boards like the Interstate Commerce Commission, or the Federal Trade Commission, or in clerical positions in the embassies or consulates. All these, if he be of fine grade as most will be who have the upper worlds best developed.

The Martian child with the mental world best developed can be a business man, and an excellent field for him is that of factoring, where he finances manufacturers of silk, laces, tapestries, and upholstery materials by carrying their accounts for goods sold. This is a good business and such a child can be successful in it. Or he can organize and conduct festivals in cities for fraternal organizations, he can be quite successful as a naturalist and can teach natural history in a school or college. He can conduct a booking office for theatrical attractions, and he can be very successful in the milling business which is an extensive and important industry. In all of these vocations this child can hold executive positions if of fine grade, and he can fill the less important places if of medium or grades lower. The lowest grades can be placed in the brackets covering ordinary labor.

The Middle World

If the middle or practical world be best developed (Plate 18), the Martian child should be placed in business, and the development of natural resources will afford him splendid opportunities with oil, coal, copper, asphalt, or manganese companies. He will be fitted to go on an expedition to develop new territory for paper and pulp mills, or gold mining in Alaska, or to hold such territory after acquired. He can be placed in the construction end of a company contracting for iron work, carpentering, masonry or brick work, as superintendent of construction or foreman, or he can hold positions in the same companies of lesser importance if of lower grade. He can be a building superintendent in strictly building construction companies in which he will be more successful if Jupiter be the secondary Mount. If Saturn be the secondary Mount, he can be placed in manufacturing chemical companies in office positions, or in various capacities according to his grade in fertilizer factories, paint, varnish, powder, cartridge, and soap factories, and he will be well qualified for positions in dynamite and fuse or munition factories.

If the Mount of Apollo be the secondary Mount with the middle world dominant, the child of fine grade should be fitted for a career as salesman, and with this combination he may be placed as salesman in luxury stores where he will handle the better class of trade. If Mercury be the secondary Mount he may be placed in the manufacturing end as manager or superintendent of factories making clothing for men and women, or in factories making corsets, gloves, hats, shirts, suits, and carpet mills, lace and embroidery, knitting, silk, cotton, woolen, and worsted mills.

The Lower World

If the lower world be best developed (Plate 19), which will be shown by bulging at the base of the hand and with the third phalanx of the fingers puffy and full, the child will belong to the material world, and with this development the Martian child is usually sensual, a heavy eater, does not incline to mental pursuits, and should be placed where he will not require much education. This is true even if he be of fine grade. Thus he should be a soldier, sailor, policeman, marshal, constable, gas or telephone inspector, fireman, and in similar occupations.

Such a child can do well as a fishmonger, a furnace setter, or if of fine grade a manufacturer of furnaces. He can succeed as a horse trader, a bill-poster, a poultry raiser, and especially on a duck farm supplying a large city, as a glazier, and in the conduct of an agency for a large glass company, where he can use his Martian aggression, and as a contracting stone mason, or as a molder in an iron foundry.

Sixth Test—Knotty Fingers

Knotty fingers are not plentiful on the hands of Martian children for they are not philosophers nor analysts. But we do find them, and they must be given due consideration. They will make the Martian child slower in action, less impulsive, and such will not make as good soldiers, but can succeed in offices, and in bookkeeping departments. They can be statisticians in the employ of large insurance corporations, and also in the chemical industries for which the Martian child with Saturn as the secondary Mount is well fitted.

Knot of Mental Order

The first or knot of mental order (Plate 21), shows that the child is systematic in his mental operations. He will be careful in what he does, he will be able to concentrate, he will know how to plan, and can fill positions not possible without this knot of mental order. He will be less impulsive than usual, somewhat slower, and therefore can be successful in mental occupations of more unusual kinds. He can make an excellent meteorologist, and should be placed in that service with the government if possible, or he can be very useful in the meteorology of aviation and could be a success when attached to a flying field. He can be successful as a mineralogist connected with a mine mining for metals or minerals.

This is an especially good vocation for such a child. He can be an excellent publicist, writing on current events, matters of social interest, and on international law; not the lawyer's viewpoint but as relating to special events. He can be a good organizer in Red Cross work, or he can be a good biographer, in which branch of writing his knot of mental order would make him exceedingly accurate.

Second or Knot of Material Order

The second, or knot of material order (Plate 22), shows that the child will be exceedingly careful about his personal appearance. He wants order and system in everything about him, consequently he can make an exceptionally good man to have charge of a building which he will keep in repair, of an estate where the owner is away a good deal, and he can be successful as the manager of a large farm where he will take good care of the farm machinery, the live stock, and will always have everything in order about the place. He can be very successful in arboriculture, and can specialize in the care of and growth of trees, the selection of the best trees to plant in cities, and in contracting for large shipments. In new developments of real estate companies where the terrain is not wooded, he can find a large field for operations in tree planting. He can be a good auditor, a controller, a magician, for here he must be most exact and have everything in place, and always the same place.

Both Knots Developed

When both knots are developed (Plate 20), the child has both mental and material order. This child will analyze everything with which he comes in contact, nothing will be taken for granted. Consequently he will be adapted to engineering occupations of which there are many in these days. He can be an engineer of flood control and find plenty to do along the Mississippi River and other streams, or an engineer of air transport, water resources, or stream pollution, or in cellulose chemistry. Or he can be an engineer in the national bureau of economic research. He can be an actuary for an insurance company, or an entomologist who can find a connection with one of the large fruit growing companies in charge of their spraying and destruction of insect life in their orchards. Also in the prevention of the introduction of foreign and destructive insects into the orchards. This is a specialty in which the Martian child with both knots developed could do exceedingly well. He can be a geologist and teach in a university, and he can be successful as a statistician, in the collection of facts on any subject and classifying them, such as those relating to the condition of people, unemployment, domestic economy, health, and longevity. In such a specialty he could be placed with a life insurance company.

SEVENTH TEST—SMOOTH FINGERS

Smooth fingers (Plate 23), are most often seen, for the Martian is a quick thinker, impulsive, and does not always stop to consider the outcome of his actions. His first thought is that he is going to reach the place he started for, and he does not wait to see who is in the road to be run over. Real aggression does not mean to him that he will do a thing if the road is clear, but it means everybody get out of the way. It means a stiff fight if necessary, but it means to win. Thus the smooth fingered Martian child can make a splendid soldier, an officer if he be of fine grade, or a good sailor.

He never figures the danger in any enterprise, whether of war or in business, but he takes orders and executes them. This child can be an accurate gunner in the naval service, and with Jupiter as secondary type an evangelist who preaches hell fire, he can be a fireman in a city department, a cattle grazer, a groom in charge of a stable of work horses, or if of fine grade in charge of a stable of thoroughbreds, he can deal in forage such as grain, hay, oats or rye and mixed foods for cattle and horses. He can sell packing house machinery, oil burners for furnaces, motor trucks, butchers' supplies, fire protection equipment, or gas heating appliances. He will do better in positions where things are difficult than in storekeeping.

EIGHTH TEST—LONG FINGERS

Long fingers (Plate 24), will slow down a Martian child and while normally he cares little for minutiæ or details, with long fingers he will go into the reason for many things. This child will have a greater aptitude for studious occupations, he can make a good accountant. It will, however, be in the mechanical part of accountancy, for the Martian child is no mathematician. In the details of an office he can be most exact, and in bookkeeping where he does the actual clerical work he will be accurate.

It is likely that with long fingers you will find Saturn as the secondary Mount, and in this case the secondary Mount will give direction to the Martian strength and we will find the Martian child able to study the sciences, and enter the engineering professions, and do things he does not do with any other combination. He can do well in mining, mechanical, civil, or automotive engineering, or as a dentist, osteopath, or chiropractor, or as an abstractor, or assayer, and he can do especially well as a trained nurse.

A Martian child with long fingers can be successful as a housing counsel, an anæsthetist, as a teacher of sociology, civics, and in civic research, or in a national bureau of economics. He can be an indexer in a library, an annotator, a botanist, and with the Lunarian Mount secondary a paragrapher.

NINTH TEST—SHORT FINGERS

Short fingers (Plate 26), are quite typical of a Martian hand and bring out the full extent of Martian qualities. The child will be very impulsive, will make up his mind quickly, he will be restless, and constantly seeking to do big things, despising detail and is aggressive in the extreme. He will make up his mind quickly, and will fight or shoot at the "drop of the hat."

This child needs to be placed where he will have abundant opportunity to work off his energy and can be very successful on a cattle ranch, in a lumber camp, as a stock herder, drover and feeder, as a dairy farm foreman, forest ranger, timber cruiser, raftsman, and wood chopper. If he is of fine grade he can be successful as owner or manager of a log timber camp, as an irrigation contractor, as superintendent, foreman, or overseer of a general farm, as a fruit grower or nurseryman. The short fingered Martian child can make an excellent soldier, a commissioned officer if he be of fine grade or non-commissioned officer or private if of the lower grades.

In the business world, the short fingered Martian child can be successful in an active position in a public service construction company. He should never be placed in a clerical position as they are too confining and do not give him enough scope for his energy. If the Mount of Apollo is the secondary Mount he can be successful in a sales department in which he will be tireless in his industry, very quick in his mental activity, and persistent to the last degree.

With Jupiter the secondary Mount he can be successful as a practical politician. He is well fitted to become superintendent or foreman of a crew for drilling oil wells, and in road construction he can be most successful. Here he must organize and control bodies of workmen who are hard to manage and no one can do it as well as a short fingered Martian. In addition to this he must take part in the getting of road contracts and this requires skill as a politician of which the short fingered Martian child has an abundant supply.

If Mercury be the secondary Mount short fingers will fit the Martian child for a merchant in retail lines, and he can conduct his store with great energy and much success. The small storekeeper is often a lower grade Martian-Mercurian, but if he be of fine grade he can be successful in active positions in the big stores. This child can be successful as the head of the delivery department of a department store, or in an express company, and in the building maintenance department he can be successful as the superintendent of carpenters, painters, decorators, and other workmen employed to keep the building in repair. He can also be successful in the maintenance department of a factory, mill, or other plant.

When the short fingered Martian child is of low grade there are many occupations in the labor class for which he is pre-ëminently fitted; such as a boiler maker, furnace and smelter man, brick and stone mason, electrotyper, stationary engineer, craneman, derrick man, hoistman, buffer and polisher, filer, grinder, machinist, roofer and slater, plumber, or workman in car and railroad shops, wagon and carriage factories, ship and boat building yards, or blast furnaces and steel rolling mills.

Whenever short fingers are found on a Martian child, the

important thing is to determine his grade as soon as possible, for this will decide the question as to his place in the Martian occupations. If he be of fine grade we know that he must be placed in the more important positions, he must be at the head of the enterprise or he must be an executive, superintendent, or in charge of the operation of a number of men. His type will force recognition of his ability to fill these positions. And if he be of lower grade he must be placed in subordinate positions, and in the lowest grades, in laboring positions in the various enterprises recommended, where his brawn and muscle make him superior to men of other types.

Tenth Test—The Finger Tips

The tips of the fingers will have a great deal to do with determining what the Martian child should do. Here we do not have so much help in determining his grade, but we do learn facts about some of his mental qualities and characteristics which help us in choosing his occupation.

The Pointed Tip

The pointed tip (Plate 27), does not belong on a Martian hand, for its idealism is foreign to a Martian child, and yet we do find pointed tips on Martian children.

In order that we may understand the effect of pointed tips, we will apply them to the Martian-Jupiterian child, and we find that they take away much of his rugged strength, and unfit him for many of the occupations which have been recommended for him. He should not be the soldier who is going to be sent to the front to do battle.

He will not be able to stand the hardships which go with the opening of lands for oil or minerals, and he will not be sufficiently hard-boiled to make a good superintendent of construction for oil, mineral, or building companies. In all such enterprises he should be in office positions or where he will not have to exert authority.

Whenever we find pointed tips, the child should be given the easier and less strenuous positions to fill.

Pointed tips add a psychic quality to a Martian child. They are idealistic and dreamy and to the Martian strength which is inherent in every child of this type they add their idealism, and such children can pursue many studies which they could not with any other combination. They can be successful in many of the sciences. In these they can be professors and teachers in schools and colleges. Their mental processes will be keener than without pointed tips, and such a child can specialize in English literature, in pedagogics the science of teaching, in the science of hygiene, in psychometry, in sociology, which is social science in a study of the evolution of human society, in numismatics, as a result of which study the child can operate a shop where rare coins and medals are collected and sold. In each of these vocations the child can pursue them with all the aggression possible to his Martian type. Pointed tips will make the child fond of art, and if the grade be fine he can put his Martian strength into an art store or an art gallery or antique shop. In each of these he can be successful.

The Conic Tip

The conic tip (Plate 28), is more often found on the hands of Martian children than the pointed, frequently with short fingers. Here we have the extreme in quickness of thought and action, and as short fingers give the Martian child great impulse, conic tips are a natural accompaniment. He will rush into battle without a thought of getting hurt, and he will not hesitate to undertake the most difficult assignments, so he may be sent to wild places or put where there is something difficult to be accomplished. If the Martian-Apollonian combination is found with conic tips the Martian child will be refined and able to fill important positions. In the army he may be a commissioned officer, and in business he can be a successful salesman in fine stores.

Such a child can be successful as a coffee broker. This requires an intimate knowledge of conditions in Brazil and other coffee raising countries, and to be really expert in the coffee business, one must travel extensively through the coffee raising South American countries. Here there is more or less danger which will not frighten the Martian child with conic tips, who will travel much and establish connections which will help him in his business and which competitors who have not traveled will not have. This is a specialized business in which this child can succeed owing to his Martian type. He can also succeed as owner or employee of a store dealing in sporting goods especially in the department selling firearms. Here his natural type qualities would help him, and he could build up a trade in outfitting hunting and fishing parties, which in the better class of stores includes clothing for hunters and fishermen, as well as hats, shoes, sweaters, socks, gloves, camp outfits, and numerous conveniences for those who are to be much out of doors. In this kind of a store this Martian child with conic tips can be successful.

The Square Tip

Square tips (Plate 29), will give the Martian child order and system and are most often found when Saturn is the secondary Mount. This child is well adapted for accounting, and positions in offices where cost accounting is done. He can also be a good statistician and analyst. He can be successful as a floor manager in a department store where it is necessary to systematize stocks of goods, and he can be most successful as a stock keeper in a large mill or factory. He can do especially well in the stock department of an automobile factory where there are a large number of parts to be looked after, and for a similar reason in a clock or watch factory. As a soldier he can plan campaigns with great care, and while he will not be such a fighting force himself, he will be able to lay out the work for others so that they may fight to the best advantage.

As a politician he can be the one who defines the issues, lays out the speaking campaigns, and writes a good many of the speeches. He can make a good engineer in such lines as ceramic, automotive, mechanical, or civil engineering, and if of lower grade he can be successful as a workman in furniture or piano and organ factories.

If Venus is the secondary Mount with square tips, this child can be successful as a piano tuner, or he may be a wood carver, a cutter or designer of clothing, an upholsterer, a window dresser, a carpet and rug salesman, or salesman in a piano or musical instrument store.

The Spatulate Tip

Spatulate tips (Plate 30), will give the Martian child great activity, originality, a love of nature, independence, and of all the tips its qualities are most like those of the Martian. Spatulate tips will emphasize his love of outdoor sports and he can be very successful as a coach for football, basketball, tennis, baseball, and other sports at some college or school. He can also be a good shot and teach rifle and pistol shooting, or be skillful with boxing gloves and teach boxing, and he can be most successful in the management of horses and dogs. In a place where fox hunting is a well maintained sport he can be most successful as a master of hounds. He can make an exceptionally good soldier, fearless and brave to a high degree, and as he has the faculty of making himself liked he can make a good commissioned officer and popular leader.

The Martian child with spatulate tips is fond of adventure, and can make an excellent explorer or discoverer, and when trained, he can be most expert as a hunter of big game and a collector of specimens for some of the large museums.

His originality causes him to search for new ideas and new ways of doing old things, so he can be successful as an inventor and in whatever business he may engage he will constantly study to invent new machines or devices to improve the methods in operation. With each of the secondary Mounts spatulate tips will bring originality to the operation of their qualities, so the Martian child if he be engaged in developing natural resources will attempt to improve the methods in the mines or lumber camps. In contracting, building, and construction, he can devise many improvements in methods, and in engineering he will attempt to make new discoveries.

As a writer he can be crisp and original, and in a sales department he can devise new lines of advertising and new sales methods. There is a wide field of successful operation for a Martian child who has spatulate tips in very desirable occupations, so it is most important that upon recognizing them, steps should be taken at once to prepare the child for the one the parents may select.

Eleventh Test—The Thumb

This test is for the purpose of determining whether the child has a strong or a weak character, and whether he has the strength of will power and of reason necessary to bring out all the possibilities of his type. The thumb is the part of the hand from which you get this information and is very accurate in determining these matters, and for this reason we shall give it the attention to which it is entitled. We must proceed with the examination of the thumb in regular order, and the first thing we shall observe is the manner in which it is carried when the child does not know he is under observation.

Thumb Curled Under Fingers

If we notice that he holds his thumb under his fingers which are curled over it we know at once that his character is weak. That is, he is easily influenced, he does not dominate himself, and cannot dominate others. Thus if he is a very strongly marked Martian child, he will bluster but will lack the ability to make others do what he wants them to. Consequently he cannot be considered for the positions recommended where he must be forceful, and where his aggressive qualities are to bring about the results desired.

He cannot be a leader of men in the army, nor in politics, nor as superintendent or foreman in building and construction companies nor in other Martian occupations which we have recommended. He must be placed in subordinate positions where he can lean on someone stronger in character than himself.

If such a child is accepted for the army, he will do best in clerical positions in the headquarters at a barrack or in a camp, and of such positions one in the sergeant major's office would be best. He can be successful in building and construction companies of which other Martians are the head or are acting as superintendents or foremen. In such a position he can take care of the building plans and architects' drawings in a field office, and act as time keeper, answer the telephone, carry messages to superintendents, and perform like services.

Small Thumb

If the thumb be small as shown in Plate 32 it will strongly confirm weakness of character as first indicated by the thumb curled under, and if both of these indications are seen, we must not consider the child as one who can be relied upon to lead any kind of an enterprise. If he is of fine grade he must be placed in office positions or places where he will not have the supervision of men, and if of lower grade he should be placed in subordinate or laboring positions.

Large Thumb

If, however, the thumb is large, held erect, and is independent looking (Plate 33), and held away from the hand, we may conclude that the child has strong character, and we can go over the list of Martian occupations and select one which requires great aggression and resistance and place him in it. He can be successful in the army, or politics, or in the trades recommended in this chapter, and can occupy positions of responsibility where he has the supervision and direction of men. This condition will be emphasized if his thumb is such as is shown in Plate 31. Then we may count upon the full Martian strength that will enable him to head the most difficult and dangerous enterprises. For such an one there are innumerable positions with companies developing natural resources which will be most profitable, and positions in the building and manufacturing trades which are responsible and well paid for.

Such a child can do exceptionally well as head of a bridge building company if his grade be fine, or as superintendent of construction if it be medium. This is an important industry and calls for men made of the sterner stuff. The man who does the actual work of construction is the one who risks his life constantly in the riveting of steel beams that extend the construction across rivers, sometimes of great width. They also stretch cables with a great number of strands of wire from which the bridge hangs. This is difficult and dangerous work, and the men engaged in it are hard-boiled. To be at the head of such a crew takes a man of courage and great force and yet the position pays well. Of all the types, no one is as well fitted to keep such work going along at the proper rate of speed as a Martian child with a large strong thumb. Such bridge building firms also contract for the erection of the iron work of skyscrapers, and here the same men are employed as in building bridges. For a position as superintendent of such construction the Martian child with a large strong thumb is particularly well fitted.

High and Low Set Thumb

High Set Thumb

The thumb as it sets on the hand is either high, medium, or low set. The high set thumb (Plate 36), rises from the upper part of the Mount of Venus and indicates a weak character almost approaching the small thumb. This high set thumb is unfavorable on the hand of a Martian child, for he needs strength in order to bring out his greatest possibilities, and the high set thumb does not strengthen him. Such a child must be placed in inferior positions even if he be of fine grade. He can be a dyer, or work in a mattress factory, he can be a waiter in a restaurant, he can be an orderly in a sanitarium, he can be a clerk in a varnish store, he can be a paper hanger, or he can have charge of birds in a zoological garden. There are positions in all of these vocations where the Martian strength will be beneficial and yet which do not require much headwork or particular strength of character.

Medium Set Thumb

This thumb rises from the center of the Mount of Venus (Plate 35), and gives the child a wider range of occupations. He can successfully conduct a cabaret, for in these days it takes the Martian courage at times. He can run a print shop where he collects old prints and sells them. This is quite a business and a number of shops are doing well. He can do radiotherapy and give X-ray treatments under the direction of a physician. He can conduct a terra cotta store which sells benches, fountains, urns, vases, figures, and numerous articles used on lawns and in gardens on important estates or in public parks. Such a store can be very successful and many of them are at the present time.

The Low Set Thumb

The low set thumb rises from the base of the Mount of Venus (Plate 34), and usually spreads widely from the hand. It is a large thumb, bold and independent looking, and brings out the strongest qualities of the Martian type. Such a child should be placed with one of the large automobile manufacturing companies to represent them in one of the foreign countries. He will have the strong qualities necessary for such a post, and if of fine grade he can have great success. These foreign agencies, at this time when competition is so keen, call for the strongest kind of men, and pay large salaries. Many such men are doing exceptionally well at the present time. No better vocation could be chosen for a Martian child with a strong low set thumb than such a connection and good preparation should be given him from the start.

Phalanges of Will and Reason

The two phalanges of the thumb are the phalanges of will and reason, the first or nail phalanx being will and the second phalanx reason. These two phalanges should balance each other, as there should not be more will than reason. You will see a finely balanced thumb in Plate 38. We find that the first phalanx by its shape tells us whether the child has a brutal, stubborn will, such as is shown in the bulbous thumb (Plate 37), in which case we must use great care; or whether he has a fine grade of intelligent will (Plate 38) which fits him for places of high command.

Bulbous Will Phalanx

The bulbous phalanx of will (Plate 37), is especially significant on the hand of a Martian child, as his fighting qualities are easily inflamed, and such an one should not be placed where refinement is expected.

There are places, however, where even brutal obstinacy is desirable, and for such a position the child with the bulbous phalanx of will is well fitted. There are vast areas in Alaska which contain rich deposits of minerals, in some places gold and silver, in others deposits of iron. There are companies which are now developing these natural resources, and with such companies a child with the bulbous will phalanx can find profitable employment and a good future if he be of fine grade, and if of medium or lower grades he can find a position in accordance with his grade. When such a thumb is seen, the parent should inquire about companies with which the child might be connected and prepare him for a position with them.

A Strong Will Phalanx

The thumb most often found on the hands of fine grade Martian children is shown in Plate 38. Here is muscular vitality with an even balance of will and reason. The thumb is broad and well proportioned and the nail large and fine in texture, yet strong. This thumb is the essence of Martian strength both physically and mentally, and a child with such a thumb should be prepared for the best positions in Martian occupations. He will embody the best attributes of aggression, he will be firm and persistent but not brutal, and he will know no such thing as discouragement. He may be entrusted with command, either in the army or the business world, and in the latter is entitled to a position commensurate with his strength.

This child can find his opportunity in the railroad business. There is no place where a greater need exists for strong men. There are many departments in this business where Martian qualities are absolutely necessary, where great aggression is needed, and where resistance to pressure often prevents defeat. In the large cities there are real estate problems involving huge sums both in the buying and selling of realty which call for strength of character and will. In the handling of these this Martian child will have all the qualities necessary. There are depot sites to be acquired, where great pressure will be exerted to obtain large prices for land, there are roundhouses, machine shop sites, and terminal facilities to be bought, and in all of these the Martian aggression and resistance can be a source of great strength to the railroad. There are rights of way to be secured, there are roads still to be built in undeveloped territory, and these are only a few of the places where the Martian child with the thumb shown in Plate 38 can find his true vocation.

A Fine Phalanx

A very fine thumb is shown in Plate 41, which is balanced, and this is a more refined thumb than the one just considered but not as muscular and vigorous. The phalanx of will is long and well shaped, and that of reason also in good proportion, which makes this child very determined and dependable, but he should not be placed in as strenuous positions as are assigned to the child with the thumb shown in Plate 38. He can be successful as a salesman, especially with Apollo as the secondary Mount, and should be placed in the best stores in luxury lines, and he can be very successful in the diplomatic service. This child can be particularly successful in a museum of natural history, and if at the head of it he will plan expeditions to most unusual places where rare animals are to be found and scientifically valuable objects obtained from excavations of the sites of old cities. There is a vocation here for a Martian child well worth good preparation for it. If this child is not at the head of the museum, he can be valuable and hold a position in charge of exhibits, organizing the force of attendants, supervising the care of the exhibits, avoiding congestion, and seeing that everything is cared for and kept scrupulously clean. He can care for the grounds and supervise gardeners and workmen, so from the head of the museum through many departments there are opportunities for a Martian child with the thumb we have been considering.

A Short Will Phalanx

In Plate 39, you will see a short will phalanx, which is a poor companion for a Martian child. It shows that he is weak in character, easily influenced, and cannot be given responsibility nor be placed in prominent positions. Often he knows what ought to be done, but if pressure is put upon him he gives way. It is hard for such a child to meet the competition in the business world, and some position must be found for him where he can carry out routine duties. Such a child can run a branch office for a telegraph company. In such a position he will not send the messages himself, his duties will only be to receive them and send them to an office from which they are sent. This would entail no great responsibility, nor the exercise of will power. He can run a ticket office for a railroad in a suburban station. Here he will only have to sell tickets at the hours when trains run, and this does not need will power. He could be quite successful if he has the usual Martian appearance, as doorman for an apartment hotel, in which position he can make many friends and a living.

Phalanx of Reason Long

It is quite as important that the second or phalanx of
reason be long, as that we find a strong first phalanx. Such
a phalanx is shown in Plate 38, and from it we know that this
child will have a good reason for whatever he does, he will not
plunge blindly into anything, and with this strong second
phalanx supporting a good phalanx of will, we can place the
child in important positions and be sure he will succeed in
them. Such a child can enter the ministry, his logical ability
will make him good in debate, and if his grade be fine he can
fill the pulpit of a large church, and in the medium grades he
can be an assistant minister, a vicar, or a curate. In his sermons he will be an exhorter, and such an one will make friends
among ordinary people and thus have considerable influence.
Such a child can successfully occupy a chair in homiletics in
a theological seminary.

Phalanx of Reason Short

A short phalanx of reason (Plate 40), will have the same
effect as a weak thumb. It will be out of balance. The child
will have the will to do, without reason to back it. He can
only be put in positions which do not require strength of
character. He can run a shop selling greeting cards, he can
be an upholsterer, he can be a helper in a dental laboratory,
he can run a soft drink shop, he can have an agency for
distributing circulars, he can have a shop and sell artificial
flowers and decorative plants. He can be an exterminator, he
can sell kindergarten supplies, or run a kindergarten. He can
be a barber or a hair-dresser in a beauty parlor, a show card
writer, or run a towel supply service for office buildings, barber
shops, and hotels.

The Thumb Tip

Usually the tip of the thumb follows the tips of the fingers,
and they may be considered under the head of finger tips though
in some cases the tips of the thumb will not be like those of
the fingers. When they are the same shape as the finger tips
their indications are the same. But when they differ from

the shape of the finger tips, they must be read as applying only to the qualities shown by the thumb.

The Pointed Tip

If the thumb have a pointed tip (Plate 27), it will reduce the amount of will power even if the will phalanx be long, and the child should be placed in less strenuous positions than usually belong to the Martian type. He will, if his finger tips be pointed, be studious, and can succeed in scientific studies, but if his finger tips be square or spatulate, his pointed thumb will reduce his possibilities in the occupations which naturally belong to those tips. The pointed tip always shows a leaning to idealism, and this child will do well in the psychic sciences.

The Conic Tip

The conic tip on the thumb of a Martian child (Plate 45), will not reduce his will power as much as the pointed. Still it will not be as strong as with square or spatulate tips. He will do best in store positions, and if his grade be fine he can be placed in the better class of stores. If Mercury be secondary he can succeed in a department store, best in the men's departments both in clothing and haberdashery. He will do well in the sports department, and he can succeed with a summer camp for either boys or men. This is a good business and this child can specialize in it with success.

The Square Tip

A child with a square tip (Plate 44), will be set in his ways and intensely practical. It is assured that he will have plenty of will power and may be placed where the going is not so easy. He will do well as the purser on a steamship, he can do exceedingly well in charge of the supplies on one of the Arctic or Antarctic expeditions, or he can conduct one of the expeditions for a geographic society, and would have the stamina to go through the hardships many of them have to.

The Spatulate Tip

The spatulate tip (Plate 43), gives an enormous strength to the will. It takes a refined child not to have this thumb an obstacle to his progress. But under control, it means a determination that will not let anything stand in its way. This child should be handled carefully so as not to develop stubbornness. At least he will not let anything overcome him, and he should be placed in such a contracting company as will build the Hoover dam, where tremendous natural difficulties are to be overcome owing to the deep gorges that must be conquered and the character of the installation that must be made. He can also succeed with a company developing iron mines in mountainous regions, where the work is hard and the hours long, and where the labor problem is difficult to handle.

CHART NOTE: The two Martian Mounts must be judged by the manner in which they bulge into the palm, and in the case of the upper Mount by the protrusion at the side of the hand. In many cases, when they are exceedingly prominent, the other Mounts will be found to be low with the exception of the secondary Mount which is well developed. With the Martian Mounts, be particular to note whether the upper or lower is the leading Mount of the two, as we seek to know whether the child will do best in a position when he must attack, or whether he will be stronger on the defense. In some cases this will be important evidence which the chart reader should know about. Please remember at all times that the more accurate the chart is, the more accurate will the opinion formed from it be. The reader will be guided exactly by what the chart shows.

TEST CHART

Types

    Primary

    Secondary

    Others

Tests

    1. Texture of skin

    2. Color

    3. Flexibility

    4. Consistency

    5. Three worlds

    6. Knotty fingers

    7. Smooth fingers

    8. Long fingers

    9. Short fingers

    10. Finger tips

The Thumb

    11. How carried

        How set.   High.   Low.   Medium.

Will Phalanx

    Bulbous.   Short.   Very short.   Long.

        Very long.

Phalanx of Logic

    Long.   Very long.   Short.   Very short.

    Will longer than logic.   Will shorter than logic.

    Will and logic balanced.

    Large thumb.   Small thumb.

    Elementary.   Medium.   Fine

    Tip of thumb.   Pointed.   Conic.

        Square.   Spatulate.

Age of Child.   *Sex.*   *Date.*

CHAPTER SIX

The Writer

The chart is vital. It means the future of your child. The care you use means his success or failure. His type tells of inherent qualities, the tests his grade, and his thumb the presence of will to succeed. Your interest, some study, and a little effort mean a well prepared chart. The success of your child is worth the effort.

CHAPTER SIX

THE LUNARIAN MOUNT TYPE

THE LUNARIAN HAND

THE Lunarian Mount type is identified by the Mount of Luna, or as it is more commonly called the Mount of the Moon. The location of this Mount is shown in Plate 1, and at the beginning of a study of the Mount it is advisable that you get its geography well in your mind. This is the second Mount which has no finger to aid in its identification, which therefore must be made from the manner in which the Mount bulges outwardly at the side of the hand, and also from the size of the pad it forms in the palm of the hand. In Plate 56, we show a *strong* Mount, and in order that you may judge all of the various degrees of Mount development we insert a *deficient* Mount of the Moon (Plate 57).

With these excellent specimens as a guide, showing as they do the whole range from excess to deficiency, you will be able to estimate the strength of any Mount you may encounter and as the Lunarian is a peculiar type it is necessary that you have, at the outset, a clear idea of the appearance of the various developments shown above, from which you can accurately estimate the child. Inasmuch as we have no finger to assist us with this Mount, we must pay especial attention to any vertical lines which may appear on it. A strong, clear vertical line on the Mount will show nearly as much strength as a strong finger.

The Mount is divided for our use into three worlds as we did with the phalanges of the fingers. The topmost third of the Mount is the mental world, the middle third is the practical world, and the lower third the material or lower world. These worlds indicate either the mental, practical, or material mind of the child.

While we do not encounter a large number of pure Luna-

rian children as compared with other types, still they are frequently found. The hands from which the plates used in this
chapter were made are rare specimens of adults, and it required
the location and examination of a great many hands before
we came upon them. They do exist, however, and you may
encounter one in any day's examination of children's hands.
They are quite typical in appearance and qualities and as
usual we shall speak of them as a pure specimen of the type,
using the pronoun *he*, though there are just as many women
as men.

Describing the Lunarian

From a composite description of the Lunarian type prepared from living specimens, he is tall in stature, fleshy in
build, with the lower limbs thick and the feet large, he is often
quite stout, but his flesh is not firm and his muscles are not
strong. He is soft and flabby and instead of muscular vitality
his flesh has a spongy feeling. His complexion is white, marking him as the victim of a weak heart action, anæmia, kidney
trouble, and often dropsy.

His head is round, thick through the temples, bulging over
his eyes, and with a low forehead. The hair is not thick, but
straggly and fine in quality, blond or chestnut in color, and
quite straight.

The voice is thin and often pitched in a high key. The
ears are small and set close to the head. The abdomen is large
and bulges forward, giving an awkward look, and the legs are
not graceful but thick and heavy, having a dropsical appearance.

The feet are flat and large, and the gait is shambling like
the gait of a sailor when he walks on land. The hand is often
puffy in appearance, flabby in consistency, white in color,
fingers short and smooth with tips pointed or conic. The thumb
is small in size with the will phalanx often pointed or deficient
in length.

Lunarian Characteristics

The primary characteristic of the Lunarian is his gift of
IMAGINATION, which at the first glance does not seem to

be an important thing, but when we analyze imagination, we find that it is one of the most important qualities possessed by the human race. And when we look at the Lunarian, we find that his very lack of physical strength best fits him to develop his imagination. The fact that he is not attractive in looks and has no magnetism tends to isolate him from social contact and gives his imagination full play, he has few distractions.

Imagination is the faculty that gives us the ability to understand the meaning of words, and it is only because of imagination that we have words or understand them. If we had no imagination we would have no power of speech and no words, for imagination enables us to form a mental picture of the appearance and attributes of an object to which we give a name, and when we hear this name pronounced we visualize this object, and its name is a word; and this is speech. Every word spoken must bring to our minds a picture of something or the word has no meaning, and the only faculty which will enable us to form mental pictures is imagination, therefore imagination is the faculty which gives words a meaning, and it follows that imagination is necessary to the powers of spoken or written speech.

Language is a collection of words, each of which imagination visualizes, and to which it gives a meaning through this power of visualization, and a vocabulary will be large or small in proportion as the imagination makes more or less words understandable. So the Lunarian, who most easily of all the types forms a mental picture through his inherent gift of imagination, has the greatest gift of words, he best understands the meaning of words, the study of language is natural to him, and his vocabulary is large. Thus he is a writer.

Imagination is so purely a mental quality that its best operation takes place amidst quiet surroundings, noise and bustle does not invite it, and so nature has created the Lunarian in such a way that his characteristics repel rather than attract, he is not sought out, and much of his time is spent in his own company. He is fanciful, and idealizes and dreams to such an extent that he is not practical in a business sense, and *FANCY* becomes one of his strongest characteristics.

He is always introspective, his mind is ever alert on abstruse problems, he is a mystic, and so *MYSTICISM* is another strong characteristic. His physical heat is below par, his color is white, his hands and flesh are flabby, so *COLD-NESS* becomes one of his strong qualities. And all of these inevitably lead to *SELFISHNESS*, which is always marked. So we may classify the leading characteristics of the Lunarian as:

> Imagination
> Fancy
> Mysticism
> Coldness
> Selfishness

and with this collection of characteristics, we must place the child in his proper vocation.

THE LUNARIAN AND MARRIAGE

Marriage does not mean a great deal to the Lunarian as a type, and while he does not shun it entirely he is not eager for it. His is a cold nature, his physical make-up does not generate heat or ardor, he knows little of physical passion. He is incapable of strong affection, he is fickle and capricious, and next to the Saturnian cares least for matrimony.

Yet he does marry, and nearly always makes an incongruous match. Sometimes it is with one much older than himself, sometimes with one much younger, never does it seem to be a well considered choice, and these marriages turn out to be most unhappy.

LUNARIAN HEALTH

The Lunarian as a type is not robust, and is predisposed to have many diseases. His white color shows a poor blood supply, and his flabby muscles show that he has no physical strength, so he is a fertile field for the propagation of bacilli. His paunchy abdomen is an indication that the internal organs and intestinal tract are of the same flabby consistency as his muscles, so here we find many disorders arising from infection. Peritonitis, appendicitis, and other inflammatory affections find the Lunarian child an easy prey to their inroads, and all forms of bowel degeneration and inflammation find lodgment in his intestinal tract which lacks muscular tone.

The Lunarian type is also liable to severe attacks of gout and rheumatism, kidney and bladder trouble, and in women female diseases. The importance of mentioning these health defects at this time is because these diseased conditions often interfere with the success of the Lunarian child in his efforts to earn a livelihood, and they play a great part in the opinion we form of the proper occupation for him. It is manifest that no child burdened with ill health should be placed in strenuous occupations.

Lunarian Qualities

The Lunarian child, being controlled by imagination, is dreamy and idealistic. He is indolent, a prey to his imaginings, and thinks he is ill or mistreated. He is restless and changeable, and always wishing for something just beyond his reach. He does not want to remain long in one place. This is one of the strong tendencies of the type, and the more the Mount is covered with lines running in all directions, the more restless he is. This restlessness expresses itself in a love of travel, which is his greatest passion. He loves to travel on the water best, and will spend his last dollar in this way. The Lunarian child is exceedingly selfish, and is lazy both physically and mentally except when it comes to the enjoyment of his imagination. At such a time his mind becomes very active.

He is fond of poetry and music and can be both a poet and composer, and in many cases an expert performer on some instrument. He lacks self confidence, energy, and perseverance, and consequently is illy fitted for the business world or the battle of life. It requires a fine grade of Lunarian child to be successful, for with his peculiarities he cannot readily find openings in the world of practical affairs.

The Secondary Type

The secondary Mounts are most important to the Lunarian child, for upon them will depend largely what he is going to be able to do. We have in this case practically the *one attribute* of imagination and what it brings him to build upon, but imagination alone will not bring success to a child, it must have the basis of a secondary type upon which to rest in order to develop it and put it to use.

Jupiter Secondary

If we find the Mount of Jupiter full (Plate 8), with a clear vertical line running over the top of it, with the apex centrally located, the finger standing erect and the other fingers leaning toward it with their apices deflected toward Jupiter, we may be sure that this is the secondary Mount.

Jupiter being one of the leading Mounts in importance supplies many strong qualities to the Lunarian child, and the first of these is ambition which is a quality entirely lacking in the Lunarian child.

The thought of leadership never occurs to him in his pure state, but with Jupiter the secondary Mount supplying ambition, this desire follows. He now awakes to the fact that he may be a leader, and the honor and religion of the Jupiterian acting upon his selfishness and coldness pave the way for the exercise of other Jupiterian qualities.

Pride follows desire for leadership, and dignity follows pride, and with all these, the Jupiterian secondary Mount arouses an entirely new set of qualities in the Lunarian child, which spur his imagination, mental pictures new to him begin to form, which results in a desire to write.

A Writer on Religious Subjects

The Jupiterian being inherently religious lends this flavor to the newly aroused mental pictures of the Lunarian-Jupiterian child, who now has the desire to write on religious subjects. So in the production of religious books, sermons, essays, theses, hymns, stories, or arguments of every description, no one can equal him for beauty of language, breadth of view, or convincing presentation. For such a child a wide field can be opened in editorial work on religious or church magazines, or on publications of every sort dealing with religion, or as special writer on religious magazines or in newspapers, or in the production of syndicated articles on religion and kindred subjects for newspapers and magazines. He will be eagerly sought in religious publishing houses as reader, reviewer, literary editor, or author. On one of these papers or magazines he can find his vocation.

A Political Writer

Following the aptitude of the secondary Mount for politics, the Lunarian-Jupiterian child can be most successful as a political writer or correspondent. He can write the most convincing political speeches, extolling either party with equal facility, and in editorial work for newspapers he is unsurpassed. He can write articles for magazines on any political subject, or syndicate articles of general character or as partisan arguments. He can write the political history of individuals or parties, and he can write convincing literature for campaigns, or upon special laws or enactments, and he can prepare arguments to be used in furtherance of the passage of bills before legislative bodies.

In this field he can have great success by specializing as a correspondent, either in a state or the national capital, where as a political writer he will have access to the most important information on all subjects of state or national interest. Or he can be successful as a foreign correspondent in a foreign capital, or on special assignment, in which capacity correspondents are making a great success today. For such work the Lunarian-Jupiterian child is well fitted and this may well be chosen as his vocation.

A Business Writer

While the Lunarian child is not himself an adept in business matters, when he has Jupiter for the secondary Mount he acquires some business sense from the secondary Mount. As many of the business occupations for which Jupiterians are fitted require that they come in direct contact with the public, we do not find that Lunarian children can fill these positions, for nowhere do they do well in positions requiring direct contact, but they can prepare the *literature* which will enable the Jupiterian and all other types who have sales ability to increase their sales. No one can write more convincing sales arguments than a Lunarian-Jupiterian child, and though he could not use them to good advantage himself, in the hands of the sales types they are potent.

Thus he can be most valuable as a copy writer in an advertising agency, or in the same capacity in a department store, an automobile factory, for a hotel, a bank, or a real estate promoter, and he makes a wonderful press agent for a dramatic or movie star.

SATURN SECONDARY

When Saturn (Plate 46), is the secondary type, it will be when we find the Lunarian development strong enough to overbalance the Saturnian, and become the primary Mount, and we must find the Saturnian type stronger than the other types. As the Mount of Saturn is very often identified by a clear vertical line on the Mount rather than a prominent Mount, we must look for this marking in addition to a high Mount. We must find the apex centrally located and the finger standing erect with the other fingers leaning toward it; in which case Saturn will be the secondary type. This will be a combination of two peculiar people, and both types have a bad side. You are familiar with the bad side of the Saturnian and the Lunarian child has a bad side equally as disagreeable. He is apt to be untruthful, often allowing the imagination to run rampant which is the basis of lying. He is mean, cowardly, deceitful, a hypocrite, and is universally avoided. So when we have a combination of the Lunarian and Saturnian types we need to use great care to determine the grade of the child, for fine specimens of both types are talented and useful, but low grades are vicious and undesirable.

The principal characteristics of the Saturnian, wisdom, soberness, sadness, superstition and gloom, when secondary to the Lunarian child who has many of the same qualities, produce a child who if not properly placed will have a life of unhappiness and failure. It requires a great deal of will power and a fine child to achieve success with this combination, but there are certain things which the Lunarian-Saturnian child can do well and be happy when he is doing them.

A Writer on Mining and Occultism

It is in the field of writing that he will always do his best work, but there are special fields where he does better work than in others, and these fields depend upon the secondary

Mounts. If Saturn is the secondary Mount, he will write best on the subjects in which Saturn does best. So we find that the Lunarian child will be interested in mining of all sorts, and that he can write valuable treatises on the mining of coal, salt, silver, gold, aluminum, copper, zinc, or iron and find a good position with mining companies. He will read much on these subjects, and he can write voluminously and most convincingly upon the mining of all these various minerals. He can also write well on the subject of mining operations, and mechanical engineering and mathematics, all of which are subjects in which the Saturnian is proficient. The Lunarian child is also deeply mystical and delves into the occult sciences, and as these are also subjects in which the Saturnian is proficient, the Lunarian-Saturnian child can write intelligently about spiritism, hypnotism, mesmerism, and psychology, and low grade Lunarian children become fortune tellers, seers, clairvoyants, and fakers in all of these subjects.

The Lunarian-Saturnian child can find in hypnotism, or mental suggestion as it is now more often called, a field in which he can be successful. There are many practitioners who are doing a great deal in this direction just now, and with the talent for occultism inherent in both the Saturnian and the Lunarian, this child can be exceptionally good in the practice of hypnotism for the cure of nervous diseases, and as head of an institute or in private practice he can have success.

As a Teacher

The Lunarian-Saturnian can make an excellent teacher or professor in schools and Colleges, especially in languages, where his large vocabulary and great command of the written and spoken word make him superior to any of the other types. He can be very proficient in all foreign languages, and learns them without difficulty, thus he can become a writer and teacher of foreign languages, and a great linguist himself. In this capacity he can be most valuable as an interpreter in foreign legations, embassies, and consulates. He can be exceptionally good as a translator, and in this capacity he can secure positions with publishing and business houses engaged in foreign trade.

A Writer on Medicine

As the Saturnian has a talent for medicine, he will impart some of it to the Lunarian child, who can become a good writer on medical subjects for large drug houses, manufacturing chemists, chemical companies, sanitariums, asylums, health resorts, and for medicines and remedies of all sorts. He can find medical writing a good vocation.

A Composer of Music

The Lunarian-Saturnian child is a lover of music, and his powers of imagination make him par excellence a composer. Here he has the same mental pictures that make him so proficient with the spoken word. The same imagination that enables him to write well brings beautiful pictures to his mind which he does not always express in words, but in sounds, which we call music. This is composition, and often the Lunarian-Saturnian child can become famous through his ability as a composer. He can also be a good instrumentalist and voice his mental pictures through his instrument. So in the field of music and composition there are excellent openings ready for him.

As a composer, the Lunarian-Saturnian child can write classical music, his imagination runs to the heavier forms, and he produces sonatas, symphonies, nocturnes, suites, or tone poems, either for piano, orchestras, violin or voice. He has great talent in orchestration, and Lunarian-Saturnian children have produced some of the most startling effects in the history of musical composition.

A Writer on Music

He is also a ready writer on the *subject* of music. Here is indeed one of his best fields for writing, for not only does he understand music as the language of the soul, but he understands composition, and he understands technique, so he can be successful as a music critic for newspapers and magazines, and in addition he can write books on music and edit musical magazines.

APOLLO SECONDARY

When Apollo (Plates 48, 49) is the secondary Mount, it is a combination of the grave and the gay, for the Lunarian child is cold and distant, and the Apollonian gay and happy. The Apollonian does much to draw the Lunarian child out of himself and make him more human and to tinge his imagination with the brighter things of life. His natural love of nature is increased and the result is that the Lunarian-Apollonian child can become a poet and his themes are those of beauty and of love.

A Dramatic Critic

With Apollo secondary we have brought *to* the Lunarian child *from* the Apollonian, artistic sense, brilliancy, a knowledge of happiness, and a record of success. Still all of this does not make the Lunarian child one who should be placed in positions of direct contact with the public, he will not make a good salesman, which is the Apollonian's strong point. But the Lunarian child can use his gift of language in Apollonian directions, his mental pictures are of those things which are a part of the Apollonian type, and thus he can write convincingly and intelligently about the stage.

His mind seems to visualize the requirements and needs of the actor, he can see the play from his standpoint but at the same time from that of the public, so he can make the best of dramatic critics. There are openings for good dramatic criticism on the daily papers of all cities.

There are also unusual opportunities for those who can write interestingly about actors or the theater for the dailies of the leading cities, and there is a ready market for intelligent articles in many magazines not connected with the theater. Then there are the theatrical magazines who welcome such articles as the Lunarian-Apollonian child can write.

As a Playwright

He has a large field in the writing of plays. Here imagination is the essence of the art, for not only does it enable him to write and command the language that will express the idea, but in the matter of plots no faculty is as necessary. No profession brings greater financial rewards than that of a successful playwright.

A Translator

In the dramatic field as a playwright, the Lunarian-Apollonian child has a field as a translator of plays from other languages. In this connection he will also be able to become an adapter of plays, especially those translated, and this field offers an unusual opportunity as there are so few who can do this character of work.

In Art

The Lunarian-Apollonian child gains from his secondary Mount a talent in the direction of *art*. Here imagination has full sway. He forms mental pictures which he translates to *canvas*. He does not confine himself to portraits of those he sees, but he paints faces that are the counterparts of his mental pictures, and many of the old paintings of Madonnas and Saints are such.

It is not, however, in the line of painting pictures that we expect to place many children, we want to place them in more practical avenues for the development of their talent such as mural decorators, designers, commercial illustrators, etchers, and engravers, and there is a big field for artistic criticism which may be done for newspapers or magazines, and for the writing of books on art and illustration, or for magazine articles on painting, sculpture, or other of the arts.

A Scenario Writer

The moving picture industry, which has developed to enormous proportions, offers unusual opportunities to the Lunarian-Apollonian child. Nowhere does imagination and the ability to write pay larger returns. The production of scenarios is more desired by the producers than are actors. There are many good actors who have not had an appearance for a long time, because they have not had a scenario which fitted them. To meet such a case requires that one be written which emphasizes the peculiar talents of the actor. There are few scenario writers who can meet such an emergency, for it requires that he should build the scenario bodily from his imaginative faculties. The only one who has this gift in a large degree is the Lunarian-Apollonian child. This will be his most profitable field in the moving picture industry, but there are many other positions in the movies which require a good writer, and he can fill all of these.

There is much advertising matter to be written for the movies, there are titles for the pictures, there are booklets, folders, press notices, and write-ups of the industry, all of which this child can do much better than an ordinary writer. It only requires that a Lunarian-Apollonian child get started with a good company to insure his success.

Business Literature

In the business world, the Apollonian secondary Mount will make the Lunarian child more practical, and he can turn his talents to productive occupations in this field. This is particularly true of the banking business, and while he can not often occupy positions in the actual banking departments, he is the best man that can be found to prepare the literature of a bank. Most of the banks are trying to get new business, and much is being written in an effort to direct deposits and customers toward these banks, so there is a need for this class of literature. No one can produce it with such telling effect as a Lunarian-Apollonian child.

In the business of salesmanship, which is the strongest qualification of the secondary Mount, the Lunarian-Apollonian child can be of immense help to any business organization in the preparation of their literature and their selling campaigns. No department of any business is of more importance than the selling end, and selling is done in many ways. There is the direct salesman which the Lunarian can never be, and there is mail order selling, the selling by pamphlet, circular, and through newspapers and magazines, and in all of these the Lunarian-Apollonian child can be of great help. Not only does he write well but he has original ideas, his imagination conceives certain situations and ways to capitalize them in the preparation of advertising matter. What he writes will have more "pulling power" than the copy of any other type, so here is a great opportunity for him to locate with the best companies in lucrative positions.

In Foreign Trade

In an importing and exporting house in the field of foreign trade, he can be useful, for here are required many carefully prepared letters, for the writing of which the Lunarian-Apollonian child is especially qualified and many booklets, newspaper and magazine advertisements, and other pieces of literature for the preparation of which no one is as well fitted as he.

In the Advertising Business

In no place in the business world will the talents of the Lunarian-Apollonian child be more valuable than in the advertising business. In this field probably the largest amount of money is expended that goes into any single expense item. Successful returns depend upon the results derived from the advertising copy, and this child can write the most convincing copy of any of the types. The number of different positions in the advertising business is very large, and in some of them, according to his grade, the child can find a brilliant future. The advertising agency, through which most of the money of the big advertisers is spent, is constantly on the lookout for men and women of original ideas who can write the kind of copy which will induce people to buy merchandise. Here the imaginative faculty of the Lunarian-Apollonian child, together with his command of languages and his power of forceful expression, can gain him a good position in the copy department which he can fill with great success.

There is also an open field in newspaper work in the preparation of articles on salesmanship which owing to his secondary Mount this child can write about as if he were the best salesman in the world. And he will also find a demand for magazine articles on the same subject.

MERCURY SECONDARY TYPE

A strong combination is the Lunarian as the primary Mount, with Mercury (Plate 50) as the secondary. This is identified by strong Lunarian markings, and with the Mount of Mercury high, extending not only into the palm, but at the side of the hand. The finger will be long and stand erect, and the apex is centrally located. The Mercurian brings to this combination shrewdness, industry, quickness, business ability, and scientific attainment, all of them qualities which the Lunarian child has not.

The Law

One of the outstanding qualifications of the Mercurian is his talent for the law, and this talent added to the Lunarian imagination makes a strong combination. It· requires great shrewdness to be a good lawyer and this is furnished by the Mercurian, and it requires imagination to think out almost impossible points of contention and arguments to support them and this quality is furnished by the Lunarian child. So the Lunarian-Mercurian child can make an excellent lawyer of the shrewd type, who can help with desperate cases, and find, in a seemingly hopeless situation, a logical defense, but he will not always be a good trial lawyer.

Where children are of fine enough grade to be placed in the law, they should specialize in certain branches. Lunarian-Mercurian children can be excellent in criminal practice and in the preparation of cases for trial. They have not the gift of oratory, but they have the gift of writing, and as partners in a law firm where they prepare the cases and write the arguments they will be most successful. In real estate practice or where they have merely to deal with figures they will not be brilliant.

Medicine

One of the qualities which the Lunarian child lacks is industry, but the Mercurian who is so strongly endowed with it makes up a part of the deficiency when secondary. This makes him a better student, and as the Mercurian has a strong talent for medicine, the Lunarian-Mercurian child can also become a medical writer. One of his most conspicuous successes will be in the preparation of medical books, papers on various diseases, and he will be able to prepare articles on medical subjects for not only medical journals, but for newspapers and magazines.

These articles will be readily accepted because of the attractive manner in which they are expressed.

In Business

There is a wide field of operation for the Lunarian-Mercurian child in the lines of business carried on by the Mercurian. This will not apply to the low grades, for in the small stores operated by low grade Mercurians the Lunarian will have no place. But the finer grades of Mercurians are mostly engaged in the conduct of department stores on a large scale, and in these stores many places will be available in the advertising departments.

There is work in the preparation of copy for booklets, for which the Lunarian-Mercurian child is admirably adapted. Then there is a great deal of copy to be prepared for newspapers and magazines. This work he can do with much success. There are many letters to write to customers and prospective customers, and these he can prepare which are full of drawing power. With one of the large stores he can find permanent employment.

In Manufacture and Retail Distribution

In the field of manufacture and distribution of men's and women's clothing, in which the Mercurian engages so largely, there are innumerable positions in the advertising departments of these companies for the preparation of letters, booklets, circulars, and copy for the large amount of advertising carried by such companies. Much money is spent by them for advertisements in the magazines, and these must be good enough to create the demand of the public for their particular lines of manufacture. Here the imagination of the Lunarian-Mercurian child goes to work, with the result that he can produce something original and striking. Once his copy is seen, he is sure of a good position.

Then there are the individual retail stores which deal in the same lines of merchandise which is men's and women's clothing. Some of these stores are very large, and do a great amount of advertising. In all of these stores there are positions where the Lunarian-Mercurian child can be placed with safety as copy writer.

Chain Stores

In the field of the chain stores there are many which do a considerable amount of advertising, and here again the talent of the Lunarian-Mercurian child for the production of good advertising copy will be available. Nothing safer could be done for such a child than to place him in a good chain system and let him grow with it.

Jewelry

Fine grade Mercurians are largely engaged in the jewelry trade, and here the best of advertising is necessary. We are speaking now of the expensive stores which have a fine clientèle. There is no greater opportunity for the imagination to have full play than in a store stocked with beautiful gems. Fascinating booklets can be written about the special story connected with different stones, and a world of lore is available which may be worked into sales-impelling tales; all of this the Lunarian-Mercurian child can do better than any one else. A connection with such a store would be a fine vocation.

MARTIAN SECONDARY TYPE

For the Martian to be the secondary type, it is necessary that the upper or lower Mount of Mars be well developed (Plates 52–54), and that the four Mounts under the fingers be rather flat, and it will make a difference which of the Martian Mounts is the one from which we classify Mars as the secondary Mount, for from this Mount we shall know whether aggression or resistance is the force behind the Lunarian child.

It means a great deal to this child to have such strong forces as those of the Martian behind him, for it makes him do things which he would never have thought of doing in a pure state.

A Historian and Biographer

He can become a good historian, especially of the wars of various nations, and he can write of expeditions of discovery where great bravery was displayed and hardships were undergone. He is fitted to accompany the Martian on some of his tours of exploitation as secretary and correspondent and keeper of records.

He can make an admirable biographer for a soldier of distinction and none of his exploits will lose in the telling. The Lunarian child imbibes the spirit of adventure from the Martian, whose prospecting for gold, silver, iron, and other minerals he loves to follow, sending back reports to headquarters well written and illuminating. In construction or contracting work he can write convincing articles for newspapers and prepare excellent booklets and pamphlets for new buildings which will either sell them or rent space in them.

Venus Secondary

The Mount of Venus (Plate 58), as secondary Mount of the Lunarian child requires very close analysis in order to read it correctly. These two Mounts lying at the base of the the hand both suggest a development of the lower world or the world of material affairs. We have told you how to divide the Mount of the Moon into three worlds, and we must so divide the Mount of Venus as we cannot class this Mount as belonging solely to the lower world, and there is no finger from which to judge the three worlds. As a matter of fact we have found from many experiments that the qualities of the three worlds are accurately shown on the three divisions of both the Mount of the Moon already explained and the Mount of Venus divided in a similar manner.

For Venus to be the secondary Mount it must be high and full, and the Mounts under the fingers must be flat and the Mounts of Mars as well. Thus we find the Mount of the Moon strong and the Mount of Venus also strong, and we diagnose the case as a primary Mount of the Moon with Venus secondary.

The Mount of Venus is not what can be called a Mount of strong qualities. It is primarily the Mount of love, and its characteristics are love, sympathy, music, grace, and passion. The only quality which is common to the two Mounts is music, and this Venusian quality will materially strengthen the ability of the Lunarian child for musical composition. If a child is found with this combination, he should begin as soon as possible to cultivate his musical taste, not only by study but by hearing all the good music possible; when old enough, he should have thorough training in harmony and counterpoint, and musical composition. From these he will acquire a good technique, but his inspiration will be from his power of imagination which speaks through music just as it does through words. This child will be sure to write music, and the better preparation he has the better music he will write.

The musical quality of the Venusian will also help the Lunarian child to express himself in poetry, and the combination of his musical nature with the strong imagination of the Lunarian child will produce songs and poetry which will appeal to the emotions. It will be real music, and real poetry.

It is very necessary to determine the grade of the Lunarian-Venusian child. Both the Lunarian and the Venusian have bad sides. The low grade Lunarian is mean, cynical, and hateful, and the Venusian will be vulgar, licentious and a libertine, and the combination of the two will make one whose tastes are low, who is in every way degraded. When anything approaching a combination of the low Lunarian and Venusian is found, apply our tests carefully, and from them we will find a way to do the child the maximum amount of good.

THE TESTS FOR GRADE

FIRST TEST—TEXTURE OF THE SKIN

The skin on the hands is the first test to which we shall look for information as to the grade of the Lunarian child. Grade is vital with this child. We must bear in mind the appearance of the hand shown in Plate 10, for from this as a basis we will judge the grade of the skin, and if we should find one as coarse as Plate 11, we will know that this child will have none of the elevating characteristics of the Lunarian type. We will have to place him somewhere where he will not have hard work to do, yet a place which does not depend upon mental effort. One such place is as an elevator man in apartment hotels, or as janitor in such a hotel, or he may be elevator starter in the same kind of a hotel. He can be a motorman, or guard on subways, a shoe shiner, meat cutter, laundry worker, work in a broom factory, paper box factory, and because of the Lunarian's love of travel and especially by water, he will be able to occupy positions as boatman, canal man, or lockkeeper.

From this very coarse skin the quality of the skin on hands becomes finer, until we reach the very fine skin found on the hand of a baby or a refined woman. All these degrees of refining in skin texture show that the nature of the child is becoming finer, and we must place him in better positions as the skin improves in grade.

We have enumerated in this chapter many things a Lunarian child can do successfully, most of them depending upon the use of his imagination and his command of language. The finer his skin, the more elevated his thoughts, for fine skin shows a fine grade, and such an one thinks fine thoughts, and these will produce fine language. So let us be watchful and grade the skin carefully, then give the child work to do in conformity with his grade. The Lunarian child of a medium grade tends to develop the mystical qualities of the type, and can become a psychologist, a spirit medium, a clairvoyant, hypnotist, and various sorts of healers.

Second Test—Color of the Hands

White Color

Color of the hands is our second test, and we begin with white which is the natural color of the Lunarian child. In our estimate of him all the way through this chapter, and of the positions he can fill, we have taken his white color into consideration in the positions we have recommended for him.

Pink Color

We do not often find pink color in the hands of a Lunarian child, for he seldom has warmth. It is only when his secondary type is strong, and this type is one which has pink color, that we find his hand showing any sign of pink. When this is the case, we find the Lunarian child who is able to do, successfully, the various things we have outlined for him under the head of the secondary types. While in his pure state he writes only in a cold and mostly pessimistic manner, when we see pink color we know his mood will be more lively, his imagination much more active, his command of language greater, and his possibilities of occupation much extended.

Such a child can make a good director of music in a conservatory if he be of fine grade, or he can be a director of an orchestra. If the various tests through which we shall put him show fine grade, he should be prepared for such a vocation beginning at an early age. He can be successful as a dramatic producer with Apollo as the secondary Mount.

Red Color

When red is seen it is unusual, for seldom do we find in a Lunarian child as much heat as is indicated by red color. If we do find it, he will be extremely lively, talkative, and such a child will make an excellent teacher of languages. He will be a natural linguist from his type qualities, and the red color will give him the desire for personal contact, so he will gratify this desire and exert the energy given him by the red color in imparting knowledge to others. He will also make a good teacher or professor of literature, psychology, or occultism, and will be a good speaker.

He can be successful as a corporation counsel, or as a historiographer which is an official historian employed by various governments to correctly record their history. He can be an excellent correspondence secretary to an official of a large corporation, bank, or a government official. He can write upon or teach inductive philosophy, or he can specialize in ideography, the recording of ideas by symbols. In this study he will be exceptionally proficient, and if properly prepared can write books on the subject or teach the same in a college or school.

Yellow Color

Yellow color is a poor combination for the Lunarian child, and makes him irritable, unsociable, and repellent, and it is hard to find anything for which he is well suited. He has all the talents of the Lunarian who can make a success, but he cannot make himself use them, he cannot make people want him. He cannot under any circumstances come in direct contact with the public, he must be isolated and allowed to work by himself. The only kind of work he can do successfully is pure routine, such as copying, typing, abstracting, stenography, as shipping clerk, weigher, cemetery keeper, librarian's assistant, railway mail clerk, paper hanger, filing clerk, stock or record clerk. When yellow color is found in the hands of a Lunarian child, a physician should be consulted to see if medical treatment might not improve his condition.

THIRD TEST—FLEXIBILITY OF THE HANDS

Elasticity of mind is most essential for the success of a Lunarian child, and fortunately we have an accurate guide to this quality in the flexibility of the hands. Where we depend so much on the mental quality of imagination for the success of the child, it is plain to be seen how much he will be handicapped by an inelastic mind, indicated by a stiff hand.

The Stiff Hand

We have a most unusual example of a stiff hand shown in Plate 12, and the mind connected with this hand is entirely inelastic, is totally unadaptable, and its owner is densely ignorant.

The only occupation open to such a child will be manual labor and this of a most inferior kind, such as is found in tanneries, stockyards, livery stables, street repair work, chimney sweeping, slaughter houses, stone yards, brick kilns, or pulp mills.

The Straight Hand

The straight hand will show a great improvement in the grade of the child, and an excellent example is shown in Plate 13. This hand will indicate a much greater elasticity of mind, but its owner is never brilliant.

On another type there will be many things which he could do successfully, but as he has the background of the Lunarian type he is limited by the peculiarities of that type and as we cannot expect any lofty flights of imagination from him nor any great vocabulary with a straight hand, we must find him an ordinary position where his shrinking nature and idiosyncrasies will not handicap him. Some such occupations are as a telegraph operator, or teacher of sign language, or shorthand. The inherent linguistic tendency of the Lunarian child will fit him for the last two. He will also be able to do typing, copying, or to keep cost accounts. He will make a good time-keeper.

The Flexible Hand

We look, however, to the flexible hand (Plate 14), or to the super-flexible hand (Plate 15), to bring out the full powers of the Lunarian child. Here we have extremely elastic minds which can grasp the full meaning of his mental pictures and turn them into word pictures.

Lunarian children with flexible hands can be poets of first rank, authors of books written because they had something to write about, essayists, and no other type can produce such books of travel. They can originate new cults and give new turns to old religions, they can write textbooks on literature, they can teach it, they can edit magazines, newspapers, encyclopedias, and with Apollo as the secondary Mount they can become creative artists and sculptors who express their mental images in paint and marble; or composers of music in its various forms in accordance with the type that is secondary. They can write on anthropology or evolution, either side of the question, and such children will be fine grammarians and can write successful books on philology and teach the same most successfully. In the world of business they can do much by the preparation of literature for the promotion of sales.

We have enumerated in this chapter positions which the Lunarian child can fill in various fields. The child with flexible hands can occupy all of these positions better than anyone else. For immediate results and profit, positions in the business world will bring quicker returns than poetry, literature, or art; it is a matter of choice which it will be. This should be the choice of the parents while the little one is too young to choose for himself, and then it should be thorough preparation for whichever field is chosen.

FOURTH TEST—CONSISTENCY OF THE HANDS

Flabby Hands

We start into the consideration of consistency of the hand with that of the pure Lunarian child determined, which owing to his type is flabby, and we have found him running true to form, and consequently lazy. The flabby hand, if unsupported by strength from some quarter, will not furnish energy enough to bring this child success, so we must look to his secondary Mount, from which he will have to receive whatever energy he has. The Jupiterian, Apollonian, Mercurian, and Martian types are all vigorous and energetic, and with either of them as secondary Mounts, the laziness of the flabby handed Lunarian child will be partially overcome. The Saturnian or Venusian types will not give strong support in this direction. At best a flabby handed Lunarian child will not go very far when it comes to competition with physically strong, energetic, determined people. He must be placed in some occupation for which his secondary type is adapted, and in a position which will not require much will power or energy, and where he can work by himself.

If Jupiter is the secondary type, this child can write political literature, or he can be minister of a small church where he will be a better preacher than pastor. With Saturn secondary, he can write on agricultural subjects for a farm journal, or on cattle breeding, or on subjects of interest to the dairy industry. With Apollo secondary he can write on art, either painting, sculpture, engraving, embossing, woodcarving, or on the theater, or about actors or moving pictures. With Mercury secondary, he can write on advertising questions for advertising magazines, on textile manufacturing, or on sales promotion, but in all of the occupations mentioned, it has not been suggested that he take an active part in the management, he is only to write.

Soft Hands

The secondary type must also be depended upon for help in the case of soft hands, which do not mean as much energy when found on a Lunarian child as on any of the other types. They do, however, mean more energy than flabby hands, and will not require so high a degree of support. They can take positions requiring more work, but they will have to be in some of the enterprises for which their secondary Mounts are adapted.

Such a child will on account of his type be a bibliophile,

and can succeed in a library as a buyer of books, he can be especially good as a collector of old books for a library or store which deals in old and rare books, he can write excellent articles on old books, pictures, or sculpture. He can collect folklore of different countries and write books and articles for magazines and newspapers on the subject, and with Saturn or Venus as secondary types he can write musical settings for many of these folklore legends or myths. He can be a lexicographer and assist in the compilation of encyclopedias or dictionaries.

Elastic Hands

Elastic consistency marks a great advance in the amount of energy possessed by the Lunarian child, and such a child can be the writer who makes his mark. He will have not only a better grade of imagination with its accompanying benefits, but he will have more energy to develop it. Much may be expected from a child with elastic consistency in the character and amount of work they will turn out, and they may be placed in positions requiring mental power and writing of the best quality.

With elastic consistency the child can take up serious studies. We have told you that with Mercury as the secondary type the child can take up medicine, both on account of the aptitude of the Mercurian for medicine, and on account of the energy he possesses. Thus the Lunarian child with elastic hands can also study medicine, having the energy to pursue the study diligently. He will do best if he specialize in some particular branch. He can be successful in physiology and can write well on the subject or teach it, and as there is much interest today in microscopic anatomy or histology, he could do well to specialize in this subject where he might help solve some of the questions now puzzling the medical profession. He will also find a fertile field in neuropathy, as the present mode of living produces many nervous cases, or he can be an embryologist.

He can also write well on futurism in art, on humanism which has gathered a considerable following lately, he can write interesting articles on ethnology and as the world is rapidly becoming all one family this subject is timely and such articles will find a ready market with newspapers and magazines. This study of races, and articles on the subject, in view of the problems in China, India, and Russia, can well occupy the time of any serious student. And as a correspondent for some prominent paper, a Lunarian child with elastic hands who has been well prepared can find his great opportunity.

Hard Hands

Hard consistency of the hands of a Lunarian child does not mean the same excess of energy as on the other types. The Lunarian child has so much deficiency to start with that even hard consistency does not bring the energy much above normal. But when we find it, if the child be of fine grade, it may be taken as an excellent indication. A fine grade Lunarian child can accomplish much if only he have the energy in his hands to back his will.

He will be a great traveler, one who can write the best books on travel. The energy of his hard hands will bring out his Lunarian love of travel, and his imagination will paint wonderful word pictures of scenery and places. If Apollo be the secondary Mount he will also paint with pencil and brush, many pictures of the places where he has been.

It is a fair estimate to say that a large part of the success which a Lunarian child has will be due to the energy shown by hard hands.

FIFTH TEST—THE THREE WORLDS

The three worlds, in the case of the Lunarian child, must be judged from the hand as a whole (Plate 16), and we have divided the Mount of the Moon into thirds inasmuch as there is no finger. From these two sources checked against each other, we learn whether he will be strongest in the mental, practical, or lower worlds.

The Mental World

With the mental world developed (Plate 16), he can better employ his talent as a historian, and with the present day demand for biography, he can with great profit employ his

ability for writing in preparing accounts of the lives of soldiers, diplomats, captains of industry of the present generation and those of bygone days, as well as kings, princes, or
any whose lives have anything of romance or particular
strength in them. He can also write on scientific subjects,
geology, hydrography, or zoölogy, and can make spectrum
analysis most interesting. He can be a rhetorician and teach
in a college or school, and if of particularly fine grade, he
can be secretary of an academy to which belong men eminent
in science, literature and art. Such a position requires a very
bright mind, and offers the right person a vocation well worthy
of considerable effort to secure. For such a position, however,
great preparation is required, but for a Lunarian child of
fine grade with the mental world predominating, it offers a
fine future. Here he will have the best kind of opportunity for
exercising his talents as a writer of distinction, and in such
a position it will be his mental ability that will attract, not
personal appearance or magnetic qualities.

The Middle World

If the middle or practical world (Plate 16), be best developed, he can write on business subjects and be able to take
positions in an advertising agency, or a department store in
the advertising department, or in the sales promotion department of large corporations.

There are many trades or classifications of business which
desire good literature, pulling advertisements, pamphlets that
will sell the articles they make or handle, letters, and circulars,
and these can all be made very attractive, and create the desire
to read them, without costing any more than an ordinary
job for printing, illustration, and paper; provided they are
prepared by one who has the gift of impelling language. We
already know that the Lunarian child is a wizard in word
selection, and from his pen can flow just the business literature
these firms and corporations want. A Lunarian child with the
middle world best developed can adapt his work to the lines
of goods handled by piano manufacturers, or manufacturers
of furniture, refrigerators, jewelry, fur goods, chocolate, underwear both men's and women's, glassware and china, paints,
confectionery, electrical goods, radios, shirts and collars,

bread, drugs, knitwear, silks, tobacco products, especially ciga-
rettes, automobiles, and for hotels, publishing houses, tailors,
coffee companies, milk companies, and fruit coöperative associations. From such a list can be selected a reliable firm or
corporation with whom a good position can be secured for a
fine grade Lunarian child with the middle world best developed.

The Lower World

With the lower world (Plate 16), best developed, it is most
likely that the tests will show a lower grade child who cannot
be placed where mental efforts are required. The two upper
worlds both show that success can be had through mental
occupation, viz., writing. The lower world does not show that
success can be reached in this way as the imagination will
not be elevated, nor the command of language good. We must
find ordinary and routine occupations for this child, and try
to keep him away from the things that low grade Lunarian
children often do, viz., become impostors and cheats, through
preying upon the credulity and superstition of unintelligent
people.

He must be placed where he does not have to come in direct
contact with the public, and such positions are to be found
in jobbing houses, or with wholesale distributors of various
classes of merchandise. He can do well in a jobbing house for
shoes as a packer or stockman, or with a coal dealer as a
weigher and in charge of delivery trucks, or with a whole-
saler or jobber of dairy products, in the stable of a company
which delivers milk and ice cream at retail, with a jobber of
plumbers' supplies, coffee, hardware, iron and steel, or woolen
goods.

SIXTH TEST—KNOTTY FINGERS

Knotty fingers (Plate 20), which indicate an analytical
mind and consequently much slower mental processes, are quite
distinctive in their effect upon a Lunarian child. All of his
mental pictures will be subjected to analysis, with the result
that he will be more exact in his statements, and while he
has no less ability in expressing himself, he will incline to
write upon subjects which do not give such opportunity for
flights of the imagination but are more practical.

Knot of Mental Order

The knot of mental order (Plate 21), gives a distinct ability to write well on engineering subjects, more especially if Saturn be the secondary Mount. There is a great demand from public service and other engineering corporations for good work in their publicity departments, and this kind of work can be done better by a Lunarian-Saturnian child with the knot of mental order than by any of the other types. This publicity takes the form of illustrated booklets showing the territory served by the companies with pictures of plants both interior and exterior, and the mechanical and other processes by which their products are manufactured and distributed. Often with pictures of the executives. Also newspaper articles which from the pen of a Lunarian child with the knot of mental order read like a fairy tale. There are feature articles for Sunday issues, pictures of laboratories where wonders are being worked by companies engaged in chemical, mechanical, electric, and hydraulic engineering, and there is much publicity work for the big steel mills, telephone, telegraph, radio, cable, or wireless companies and a large number of manufacturing companies.

There is the romance of paint, from a chalk mark to duco, of rayon and the silkworm, the possible story of concrete, asphalt, radium, aluminum, the automobile, the adding machine, the typewriter, or an infinite number of wonders which are daily being accomplished by manufacturing companies; all of whom want these stories told by one who can visualize the accomplishments and who has a power of expression equal to the subject. No one is so well fitted for the kind of work for which these large companies are willing to pay as the Lunarian child with the knot of mental order.

Second or Knot of Material Order

This knot (Plate 22), when developed so as to be noticeable, shows that the child has material order which will fit him for positions in an office where everything must run smoothly and be well systematized and orderly. If not in an office, in the conduct of a store or factory, or wherever order in the daily surroundings is required. An especially good position for such a child is as a train dispatcher for a railroad. Here there must be no mistake made. Too many lives depend upon the accuracy of the man who is directing the movement of trains, and for a fine grade Lunarian child with the knot of material order no better position could be found either for himself or the railroad. He can also make an excellent locomotive engineer where great exactness of operation is required. He can succeed in the assay office of a mint, as a weigher of bullion, in a manufactory of machine tools where the greatest exactness is required often to the thousandth part of an inch, or in a manufactory of lenses for telescopes where similar exactness is essential.

Both Knots Developed

The child with this hand (Plate 20), can succeed as a writer on many philosophic subjects, and he will be especially fitted for the study of hierology where he can become an authority on the deciphering of hieroglyphics which engross the attention of scientific men who find them in the excavations now being so widely carried on in the former seats of civilization in the old world. This child owing to the Lunarian gift for language can excel in this study and cannot only write upon it but can teach it in colleges. It is worthy to be the vocation of a fine grade child.

SEVENTH TEST—SMOOTH FINGERS

Smooth fingers (Plate 23), do not give the child an analytical mind as do the knotty, they supplement conic tips and show a love for art which may be expressed through writing, painting, or sculpture. Such a child will be extremely sensitive and can make an especially good music critic, and a general writer on musical subjects. This will open many avenues of employment on newspapers or musical journals which he can fill with great success. He can also be a good writer of fiction, and as a novelist can have a successful career. What he writes will be tinged with romance which makes him a good short story writer or poet. He can be successful as a collaborator in the writing of plays and with Apollo as secondary type he can be a successful playwright. He can be exceptionally successful

as a writer of burlesque, and a good librettist. With Saturn
secondary he can write well on floriculture, and in the preparation of the large catalogues issued by nurserymen and seed
stores can be valuable to a large firm. This is a specialty for
which few are adapted and one who can do the work can
have a good salary. This child can do well as a composer of
music, especially in orchestration. He can write the words and
music for songs both grave and gay, and in a music publishing house he can find a successful future. If he develops his
talent for painting, he can do best in portraiture if he be of
fine grade, and if of lower grade he can be a scene painter or
an illustrator for advertisements or for panels used for window
dressing. In large stores there is a good position for a child
who can do this work and in addition card writing and other
decorative work now much used in such stores. He can also
do well in porcelain painting which is a specialty needed by
the manufacturers of fine china.

Eighth Test—Long Fingers

Long fingers, which are well illustrated in Plate 24, give
the Lunarian child a love of detail and minutiæ, which will
make him extremely careful in everything he does. He will be
slow, but when he makes up his mind he will have all the facts
and this makes him an exceedingly exact writer. He has some
peculiar traits which influence his work; he is retiring, he has
an excellent memory, and nothing will hurry him. Thus in
the preparation of scientific works he can have considerable
success. This child with Saturn or Mercury secondary can
do well in medical research and laboratory work, and in specialties in medicine. He is peculiarly well adapted to be an
anatomist, and as professor of anatomy in a medical college
he can make a name for himself. In this study, his love of
detail will give him a great advantage over any other type,
and it is well worth while for the parents of such a child to
give him every advantage possible in preparation for such a
vocation. He can be successful as a specialist in gynecology,
osteology, and particularly in the subject of helminthology
the study of parasitic worms, which requires the closest application and is much used in medicine today. In all of these
specialties he can lecture, be a professor in a medical college,

and write able articles for medical magazines and textbooks on all of these subjects. With Saturn secondary he can succeed in scientific studies, and is well adapted for work in a chemical laboratory connected with an ore reducing company, or a research laboratory with a tuberculosis society or foundation, and in a research laboratory for cancer study. He can write books on these subjects which will command attention. In all of these studies, laboratory tests, or medical specialties, this child will have his data correct and his conclusions will be well thought out and accurate. A vocation can be chosen for him from this list.

He can also find a vocation as a teacher of theology in a seminary, and while his personal views may not always be strictly orthodox, he can adapt himself to the tenets of the body with which he is connected as a lecturer on the subjects taught. He can be most successful as well in the writing of books and articles on theology, which will closely follow his lectures.

NINTH TEST—SHORT FINGERS

Short fingers (Plate 26), on a Lunarian child make an odd combination. Here we have a child who is naturally slow in his movements, to whom a dynamo has been attached with the result that he has been speeded up and that some of his ideas have been changed. Instead of moving in his naturally deliberate manner, the Lunarian child with short fingers becomes much more alert both mentally and physically, and is also less self centered and retiring. He will retain all of the Lunarian qualities but their operation will be accelerated, and in addition he will acquire some of the big ideas which are always present with short fingers.

This child must be placed where the spontaneity of short fingers can be used to advantage. Their faculty of making up their minds quickly, and the fact that their first impressions are the most correct, give children with this combination an urge which expresses itself in their writings. There is no place where this child can find a better opportunity for self expression than with a hydraulic company such as one at Niagara Falls. The Lunarian child with short fingers would find a great opportunity with their publicity department where he would

have the inspiration of the mighty cataract to stir his imagination. For such a company he could write the most impelling
literature. In the department of publicity of a trunk line
railroad he would also find a great opportunity, and nowhere
do they strive harder to get out the best of stories about the
points of interest along their lines than in such a department.
There are also expensive booklets about special trips and an
endless variety of advertising matter which a Lunarian child
with short fingers could write successfully. There are the big
steel and iron companies, the copper mining companies, silk
manufacturers, textile mills, and an endless number of large
companies all of which have departments where this child can
be successful. He can also write short snappy stuff for retail
stores of all kinds as he has the faculty of adapting himself
to whatever is to be written about. When a Lunarian child
with short fingers is found, he can safely be placed in the
publicity department of one of the industries above enumerated.

TENTH TEST—THE FINGER TIPS

We need to study the finger tips of the Lunarian child
with a great deal of care, as their qualities when applied to
this type fit him for a number of occupations.

The Pointed Tip

This tip with its idealism (Plate 27), found on the hands
of a Lunarian child who already has a large supply of the
same quality, produces one who has little that is practical
about him. Unless we find strong secondary Mounts, it is
difficult to find an occupation for such a child. It will help
a great deal to find a strong thumb. With Apollo the secondary
type a fertile field will be the painting of stained glass windows which is a specialty in which some of the best artists
are engaged. With a studio devoting itself largely to church
work this child can have success and a good vocation. Such
a child can be a caricaturist if he is properly prepared, which
profession offers large financial returns. He can successfully
conduct a curiosity shop which deals in curios from foreign

lands such as Russia, India, China, Turkey, Persia, and those made by our own Indians. He can be a fresco painter and specialize in murals for the many large buildings now being erected. Preparation is needed for all of these occupations, but with a difficult problem to solve with such a child, the parent had better go a good deal out of his way to get him ready for one of them. Good companies exist where a place for him can be found in all of them.

The Conic Tip

The conic tip (Plate 28), shows an artistic temperament, and is more practical than the pointed. This child can be a philatelist and conduct a shop where he sells the postage stamps he collects, which is not a large business enterprise but one which is capable of being a good vocation for such a child. He can also be the cataloguer for a library which he can do well on account of his love for books. With Apollo secondary he can be a writer of scenarios for moving pictures, and he can be very successful in writing advertising and booklets for thrift promotion for banks, insurance companies, and building and loan companies. There is a large field for advertising and sales literature with the tobacco companies. Here the Lunarian child can be very successful, for all of this advertising is of an extremely artistic character and the conic tip is the "artistic tip." With this help and his talent for trade impelling writing, the child can find in some large tobacco company a fine position where he can express himself and win success. With a steamship company he can also find a great opportunity. These companies are spending a large amount of money in advertising their regular travel schedules and special trips all over the world. They issue the finest kind of literature, profusely illustrated and executed in the highest style of the printer's art. For such, advertising and booklets are needed, the very best copy that money will buy, and for such work the Lunarian child with conic tips is especially well fitted. We are presuming in all this that the child will have the proper preparation, and if he has, a place can be found for him in the publicity department of a large steamship company where he can make for himself a vocation that will be well worth while.

The Square Tip

Square tips (Plate 29), give a distinctly practical turn to the Lunarian child. His mind will have a mechanical ability which enables him to visualize the possibilities of machinery. Thus he can do well in a publicity department for a company building engines, turbines, boilers, elevating machinery, water purifying equipment, drilling and hoisting machinery, or welding equipment. These companies are many of them very large and spend a great deal of money in trade journals and other forms of advertising. The copy for all of this can be prepared with great success by this child. He can write the best of copy for a typewriter company, his square tips showing him the advantages of such a machine, or it may be for a dictating machine company, or an adding machine company, a telephone company, or a sewing machine company. He can study and teach social science in a school or college or in an institute of technology. With Saturn or Mercury secondary he can compile statistics for state or federal health boards, or for insurance companies on the death rate for various diseases, the length of life in different occupations, the birth rate in different states and cities, or collect facts and tabulate them on finance, the rise and fall of commodities, the cultivated acreage in states, and vital statistics on any subject, and he can through his Lunarian talent for writing present these facts so that they are interesting reading. These are all serious and worth while occupations and in one of them according to his grade the Lunarian child can find his vocation. Those who cannot occupy the best positions can find one to suit their grade in the enterprises we have mentioned. They are all big enough to have a large number of positions to fill.

The Spatulate Tip

Spatulate tips (Plate 30), will almost make a new person of the Lunarian child. The activity of these tips, their enthusiasm, their love of sports and games and their skill in them, their love of nature, their independence, their originality, are all so different from the qualities of the Lunarian that they give him a new viewpoint, and they open to him a largely increased field of operations.

He is first of all practical and while he has a unique viewpoint on many questions he will not be so visionary. He will be much more agreeable in his contact with people, not so shy and retiring, and better able to come in direct contact with the public.

The spatulate tip will make the Lunarian child very original as a writer. He can write on almost any subject. He can write volumes on the subject of religion from every angle. He can prove or disprove evolution. He can write histories that will prove anything he wants to about any nation. With such a child the preparation should be, to give him as much language, English, grammar, and literature as possible and the widest reading.

Such a preparation can make this child successful in newspaper work of all kinds, and he can be especially adapted for sports departments owing to the love of spatulate tips for such pastimes. The sporting section of any newspaper is its most widely read department, and a child who can write good sporting columns can command a good position and a good salary. This is a well worth while occupation for a Lunarian child.

When properly prepared this child has a field for his talents as what is commonly called a "hack writer." This means one who can write a story to order, or who can take a manuscript and improve the style, correct the spelling, grammar, and English, and put it in shape for publication. Or he can revise a play and adapt it for stage presentation.

Spatulate tips indicate an inventor, an explorer, a discoverer, and with the Lunarian love of travel they make a strong combination. This child can go to the ends of the earth and write delightful accounts of his adventures. There is a great demand for such books, which he can prepare better than anyone else.

Such a child will be practical in engineering and scientific subjects. If properly prepared, he can build a rheostat himself, he can teach or write on all branches of electrical operations, he understands seismology, and delights when he sees the vibrations on the seismograph and reads the account of the earthquake in the papers, he can write about it and teach it. He loves all the studies that relate to birds, fish, reptiles, and all members of the animal kingdom, and can write entertainingly about them and teach zoögraphy, ichthyology, or herpetology, and as a vocation he can find an opportunity with some prominent zoological garden where he can be successful.

We now reach a consideration of the driving force which is in each child; that force which is going to be either strong enough to bring about the development of his talents, or so weak that they will come to naught. This force is will power, and the thumb is its indicator on the human being.

Thumb Curled Under Fingers

First we note the hand when in repose, when the child is not conscious of observation, for we wish to see if the thumb curls under the fingers or is held erect. If we see that it folds into the palm of the hand and the fingers curl over it, we know that the child is weak in character. He will not be bold and self confident, and thus he will not write vigorous and vital literature, he will incline toward poetry and will produce only by fits and starts, and his output will be of an emotional nature.

This child should not be placed in business. What he writes will not be adapted to business. He can write for newspapers and magazines as the mood strikes him, selecting his own subjects, and if he is of fine grade and well educated what he produces will be salable.

Size of Thumb

Large

If the thumb stands erect, away from the hand, is large and independent looking (Plate 31-33), the child has will power, a strong character, will write in a vigorous manner about practical things. He may be placed in advertising departments, or write for business sections of newspapers, or articles on business, historical subjects, biography, or short stories for magazines, or he may write works of fiction and romance.

With this large thumb, the child can be a successful financial editor of a newspaper, and if his grade be fine it should be on a prominent daily in a large city. This is a field where there are great possibilities, as the child will meet important people, and usually after a service with a paper of this kind he is offered a good position with some financial house which is greatly to his advantage. Such a child can find a place as corresponding secretary in an international banking house, where correspondence is always couched in the most perfect English and is dignified and courteous. In the same house he can attend to foreign language correspondence, and can be successful as the assistant or secretary of the head of this department, for the Lunarian child is naturally a linguist. For these positions, which are very desirable, the child needs good preparation especially in the languages.

Small

A small thumb, which is well illustrated in Plate 32, has the same meaning as one curling under the fingers, a weak character. The child is deficient in will power. He cannot assume responsibility, but he has imagination, and in a position where he can work by himself he can get along very nicely. It is not that he has no ability, it is only that he has not the will necessary to dominate others, so he can be a student of various sciences and teach them and write upon them for scientific magazines, newspapers, and popular magazines. What he writes, while carrying the stamp of the savant, will at the same time be interesting to the layman, and in this way a child who otherwise might have a hard time to find his vocation can be successful. One of the branches of scientific study which will be best suited to his talents is the science of language, or glossonomy to use its technical name. Here he has full play for the display of his powers of language and his vocabulary and as a professor in the subject in a college he can have his opportunity. For this career he must have good preparation.

High and Low Set Thumb

High

The high set thumb rising from the upper third of the Mount of Venus (Plate 36), shows weakness of character, and such a child must be placed very carefully if he is to have success. He can neither take responsibility nor do work with his hands, so many occupations are closed to him. In spite of this, however, there are things he can do very well if the vocation is carefully selected and he is properly prepared. Such children need greater care than those with more strength, but they should have this care and be put in the way of success. There is quite a business done at the present time in preparing the genealogy of families who want their ancestors traced as far back as possible. In fact there are a number of specialists in this line who are doing exceedingly well. The Lunarian child with the high set thumb can make quite a success of such a business, which requires only mental work and does not entail responsibility nor much will power. He can work by himself and take his time. He can be prepared for and practice optometry which requires only technical training and involves no responsibility in the way of having people under him. He has only to know how to fit the proper glasses for customers, and this requires no exercise of will nor does he have to be a mechanic.

Medium

The thumb which has a medium setting (Plate 35), rises from the center of the Mount of Venus and gives the Lunarian child more will power than the high set thumb. He can take more responsibility and hold better paying positions. He can also be in business for himself. One business in which he can be successful is as a steamship agent among a foreign population for travel in foreign countries. His linguistic ability will enable him to converse with his customers in several languages, and if he locates in a foreign locality in a city he can do well. He can also conduct a bookstore in the same locality for readers of foreign language books and such a business can be made to pay. He can do well in the publicity department of a food product company, in writing advertising for cereals which are now so widely used, and with such a company, of which there are many large ones, he can use his imagination in the design of new packages for their product which is a specialty by itself in which there are what are known as product development engineers, marketing directors, color engineers, and merchandising counselors. The kind of a package in which a product is put up has a great deal to do in its sale, and in a position of this kind with a good company a Lunarian child with a medium set thumb can have a successful vocation.

Low Set

The child with a low thumb (Plate 34), has an advantage over children with a medium setting. If his grade be fine, he will be exceedingly practical, he has strong will, and he will have good reasoning faculties, all of which will fit him for positions in the business world and as a mechanic, and in mechanical arts. His low set thumb enables him to do work with his hands and opens up a number of good vocations. With Saturn or Mercury secondary Mounts he can study medicine and should specialize in orthopædic surgery where his strong thumb will be a great help to him, and in such a profession he can be a professor in a medical college or an assistant professor if his grade be fine. This child can also be a surgeon, as his low set thumb will make him skillful with his hands. He can be successful as a bookbinder, and in the hand tooling of leather bindings, he can be a cigar maker, an engrosser, a glass carver, a professor or teacher of orthography and a writer on this subject. He can be a compositor, and with Apollo secondary a frescoer. For all of these trades and professions the low set thumb will materially help this child, and he can safely be placed in one of them.

Phalanges of Will and Reason

The first phalanx of the thumb, or the will phalanx, should be of the same length as the second or phalanx of reason or logic, that is, these two phalanges should balance each other, in which case it will be a strong thumb and the child will have many avenues open to him (Plate 38).

The balanced thumb is the best thumb that can be found on a child, but the will phalanx is sometimes found so short that the will is deficient, and sometimes so shaped that it indicates qualities which will interfere with his development.

Bulbous Will Phalanx

In the study of the thumb we must consider these different formations, and the first is the bulbous phalanx of will shown

in Plate 37, which is so coarse and common that the child
with this thumb must be assigned to inferior positions as he
is so stubborn that he cannot be placed in the higher brackets.
If his grade is fine, which is not usually the case with this
will phalanx, he can be a stock man in a furniture store which
sells at retail, he can run a boat house either power or sail for
the Lunarian loves water, he can be a circular and sample
distributer, he can assist in compiling a telephone directory,
but if he be in the coarser grades he can only fill positions
in the labor class. He can be a deck hand on a river steamer,
a cleaner in an apartment house or office building, a gateman
in a railroad station, he can be porter with a company selling
marine engines.

Short Will Phalanx

Sometimes we find a short phalanx of will, such as is shown
in Plate 39, which indicates a weak character and weak will.
This child need not be placed in as low a grade of employment as with the bulbous phalanx, but he cannot be put in
positions needing courage or strength. In fine grades he can
be a refolder and stock man with a wholesale dry goods firm
or jobber, he can be a compiler of codes for business; legal
codes, foreign codes, or cut rate codes, for which he is well
fitted owing to his type qualities in the command of language,
and this is a business in which a number of large companies
are engaged in one of which this child can find a position
and a vocation. On account of linguistic ability he can be successful in an employment agency for foreign labor, and can
specialize on hotel labor, rough labor for railroads, or household servants, also in office help among foreign houses. He
can superintend a department of rare books, book plates,
letters and manuscript in a museum, and his fondness for such
articles will make him careful and useful, and such a position
offers a specialization in these valuable literary relics which
can be made a vocation. This child can be successful as a
proof reader, and be very successful as a literary agent where
he will correct manuscripts for authors as to style, grammar,
spelling, paragraphing, and English. And he can do the same
for foreign authors, playwrights, or scenario writers.

Long First Phalanx

The thumb which will do the most for the Lunarian child is shown in Plate 38. You will see by its broad well shaped first phalanx, of the right length to balance the second, with a clear open nail and with a strong second phalanx, the thumb which will give the child fine reasoning qualities, a strong will, and good physical strength. Such children can occupy the editorial chairs of magazines and newspapers, they can be on the reading staffs of publishers, they can edit departments of music, drama, literature, and language, they can teach all of these subjects. They can write short stories or novels of fiction or romance, histories, biographies, advertising, and in all of these they can occupy the first positions with publications and corporations. Throughout the entire range of occupations which we have recommended for children in this chapter, this thumb will make their success more certain.

A Fine Strong Thumb

Plate 41 shows a thumb which is not so robust as the thumb just described, it is well balanced as to length of phalanges, and in every way it shows refinement. This child can be a writer of beautiful verse or prose. His work will be of the dainty kind, beautiful imagery, lacy fabrics of the mind delicately woven, and no matter what the subject on which they are engaged, the work will be carefully and daintily done. Such a child can make a success as a writer of stories, books, and verses for children. There is a big demand for such literature and a Lunarian child who can specialize in children's stories will have a great demand for their services especially from the large houses which issue Christmas cards and books of verse and stories for children. There is a constant demand for new material of this kind and new characters taken from the animal, bird, flower, and other kingdoms, which a lively imagination can develop into delightful stories for children. In such a field the Lunarian child with this thumb can find a vocation.

The Phalanx of Reason

The second phalanx of the thumb, or the phalanx of reason, should balance with the first phalanx (Plate 38), for will needs a reasonable and logical mind behind it to insure the best results. If the phalanx of reason balances that of will the child will be logical in what he writes and on any of the many subjects which he can handle with success he will give a reasonable presentation. This phalanx means more to a Lunarian child than to the other types for his success is mental. With the balanced phalanges the child will be especially valuable in the writing of business literature, for what he writes will be solid; thus for companies selling standard merchandise he can be effective. With a company selling standard plumbing fixtures he can be successful, and with companies selling modern improvements in building material and devices for adding comfort to homes he can have success. With companies manufacturing and selling machinery which reduces man power requirement, or aids in sewage disposal, or sells marketing machines, improved laundry equipment, ice making machines, lubricating devices, button covering machines or can making machinery, he can be placed in the publicity departments with an assurance of his success. We must place children of the higher grades in the best positions, but in all of the above mentioned industries there are many places which those of lower grades can fill successfully.

In the writing of medical or scientific books, or teaching these subjects, the child with a strong phalanx of reason will be the most successful. He can write successfully or teach applied physiology, dermatology, biochemistry, laryngology, ophthalmology, otology, anæsthesia, roentgenology, or pediatrics. In each of these specialties the Lunarian child with a strong phalanx of reason can be successful in writing or teaching especially with Saturn or Mercury as secondary Mounts.

We sometimes find a child whose phalanx of reason is short, and such an one must be assigned to subordinate positions in the enterprises in which the child with a strong phalanx can be successful. He will have the type ability even with a short phalanx, but will lack strong reasoning faculties as an impelling force to develop his ability.

The Thumb Tip

Pointed

The tip of the thumb will show the same characteristics as when seen on the fingers, but in this case it will apply to will power alone. A pointed tip on the thumb (Plate 27), even if the will phalanx be long, will weaken the will and make it impractical. What this child writes will be lacking in force, and we must place him among the poets and idealists who write chiefly of their emotions.

Conic

There are many conic tips on thumbs (Plate 45), and they are stronger than the pointed. Such a tip will indicate a considerable degree of determination, and such a child can write excellent musical and dramatic criticism, reviews of art in various forms, and good advertising for stores dealing in pictures, sculpture, antiques, oriental rugs, period furniture, and art treasures of all kinds.

Square

The square tip (Plate 44), seen on the hand of a Lunarian child, will indicate that he will have sufficient will power to bring out his talents. He will have a practical turn of mind which will enable him to write for the professions and for business. In various engineering fields he can find a demand for his services as he will write well on the subjects of chemical, electric, or radio engineering. He can also be successful as a historian, biographer, or composer of classical music.

Spatulate

A spatulate tip on the thumb (Plate 43), shows a tremendous strength of will and when such a thumb is found, all the tests should be applied to determine the grade of the child. If he be of fine grade he will be very practical, determined, and forceful owing to the length and breadth of the will phalanx.

Thus as a news writer, a writer on religion, a sports writer, a traveler and writer on travels, or a general or hack writer he not only has the talent for such writings, but he has the will power to develop them and the sooner we begin his preparation for a career of general writing the better it will be for him.

CHART NOTE: A correct estimate of the Mount of the Moon will be made entirely from the manner in which it bulges into the hand. Excellent examples of a number of developments are shown among the illustrations. These plates should be visualized, so that in any case where similar formations are seen, they may be recognized at once, and properly charted. When this type is identified as the primary type, great care should be used, in order that all the markings charted as relating to the secondary type and all of the tests shall be exceedingly accurate. The Lunarian depends so much on the combinations present when he is the primary type that an accurate judgment cannot be formed as to his best occupation unless great care has been used in preparing the chart. This is an exceedingly difficult type to place properly, but no difficulty will be experienced if the chart is properly prepared.

TEST CHART

Types

    Primary.

    Secondary.

    Others.

Tests

    1. Texture of skin

    2. Color

    3. Flexibility

    4. Consistency

    5. Three worlds

    6. Knotty fingers

    7. Smooth fingers

    8. Long fingers

    9. Short fingers

    10. Finger tips

The Thumb

    11. How carried

        How set.   High.   Low.   Medium.

Will Phalanx

    Bulbous.   Short.   Very short.   Long.

      Very long.

Phalanx of Logic

    Long.   Very long.   Short.   Very short.

    Will longer than logic.   Will shorter than logic.

    Will and logic balanced.

    Large thumb.   Small thumb.

    Elementary.   Medium.   Fine.

    Tip of thumb.   Pointed.   Conic.

      Square.   Spatulate.

Age of Child.   *Sex.*   *Date.*

CHAPTER SEVEN

THE VENUSIAN MOUNT TYPE

The Lover

There is no need to memorize the indications in this book. The principal need is to know where the Mounts are located and how to identify them. Once this is done, the chapter on that type will tell you what the child can do best if you will read it carefully with the hands of the child before you. In order to avoid memorizing, answer each of the inquiries on the chart; it will tell the whole story.

CHAPTER SEVEN

THE VENUSIAN HAND

THE Venusian Mount type is identified by the Mount of Venus, the position of which is shown on the map of the hand in Plate 1. It is not difficult when Venus is the primary Mount to identify the type, for the Mount will be high and full, showing either pink or red color, while the other Mounts are flat; with the exception of the secondary Mount which will be well developed, showing plainly that it is stronger than the other Mounts.

As the Mount of Venus has no finger, for we do not consider the thumb as a part of the Mount, it will be identified by the manner in which the Mount bulges into the hand, perceptibly to a greater extent than the Mounts of Mars or the Moon, and once a primary Mount of Venus is seen it will never thereafter be difficult to recognize.

In order that there may be no difficulty in identifying a primary Mount of Venus, we present Plate 58, which shows a large development, and Plate 59, which shows a deficient Mount. It will be noticed in Plate 58 that all the other Mounts are flat, with the exception of the lower Mount of Mars, which in this case is the secondary Mount. This is an exceptionally plain case of the primary and secondary Mounts, and such cases will not often be encountered. In most cases, however, the secondary Mount will show itself plainly enough to be recognized. With the strong case shown in Plate 58 in mind, and the equally plain case of deficiency shown in Plate 59, there will be no difficulty thereafter in estimating the various degrees of development which lie in between.

The Venusian is the opposite in every way of the Lunarian whom we have last considered. Instead of the coldness, the lack of sympathy, and the dislike for his fellowman which are so strongly marked in the Lunarian, the Venusian is the embodiment of love, sympathy, warmth, and attractiveness. It is a healthy type, a happy one, and Venusian children are filled with the joy of living. They are unselfish, generous, and in every way desirable.

In combination with the other types the Venusian softens the asperities of each of them, and into each occupation in which they engage they bring a more desirable outlook, they are the leaven which makes business less hard, which makes life easier to live.

Though there are a vast number of Venusian women, we shall as formerly consider the Venusian type as an adult male, and shall in describing him use the pronoun he and shall speak of the Venusian child when referring to occupations. This is merely a matter of convenience which will facilitate our study of the type.

The Venusian has, with his strength and beauty, and his love and sympathy, a very strong side, which in the children of fine grade means the use of these splendid qualities for the benefit of all who surround them. In the coarse grades they descend to the greatest sensuality, profligacy, and license.

Describing the Venusian

From a composite description prepared from many pure specimens of the type, the Venusian is always attractive and handsome. He is graceful, shapely, well balanced, and easy in his manner. He is of medium height, and presents graceful curves of form from head to foot. His skin is pink, fine in texture, soft and velvety to the touch, transparent in its fineness through which a pink color glows showing normal health and blood supply. The face is round or oval in shape, is finely proportioned with no high cheek bones, thin cheeks, prominent temples, or square jaws to make it angular or mar its beauty. The cheeks are well rounded and often show dimples when the face breaks into a smile.

The forehead is high, well proportioned, gracefully rounded in front, perfect in contour. The skin on the forehead is tightly drawn and does not wrinkle. The hair is abundant, long, silky, fine, and wavy.

The eyebrows are well marked, abundant, and form graceful curves on the forehead, well pointed on the ends. The eyes are round, brown or dark blue in color, and have a tender expression of human sympathy.

The nose is shapely, full sized, but with fine curves. The chest is large, full, round, and expansive, the voice is full, musical, and attractive.

VENUSIAN CHARACTERISTICS

There is no one of the types who has as great a love of humanity in general as has the Venusian. Whether it be men or women, they feel attracted to those with whom they come in contact; there is never the feeling of repulsion which is present in a Saturnian. This may be partially accounted for by the fact that the Venusian is a vigorous type and that he has rich warm blood coursing through his veins; he is himself magnetic and feels drawn toward both his own and the opposite sex. He is passionate and full of fire, and his first great characteristic is *LOVE*. This extends from warm mating love to the platonic love he feels for mankind in general.

His instinctive love brings in its train *SYMPATHY*, which is his second principal characteristic. This quality extends even to the lowly, and the Venusian of all the types feels most for those whose path in life has been difficult and filled with obstacles. He is entirely unselfish and hearing a tale of distress he forgets himself and seeks only to help the sufferer.

The very soul of the Venusian responds to the love of *MUSIC*, which is the third characteristic of the type. The Mount has been aptly called the Mount of melody and this nomenclature describes the kind of music which the Venusian most likes and produces. He is too full of the joy of life to love or write somber music, and thus he runs little to the classics. His compositions are full of lilting harmony, and the music he loves to hear must be the perfection of rhythm and full of the sparkle of life.

He is graceful, and *GRACE* is his fourth characteristic. He dances well, he makes a fine appearance on the tennis court, when he rides or drives, even in his walk he is the personification of grace. It is natural grace, too, never affectation. It is the expression of his mind, which has all the graces of natural beauty, a fine attitude toward those around him, a love of humanity, and these are reflected in the grace of his body, a lithe sinuous grace, that makes him charming and irresistible.

He has passion, the white heat of *PASSION*, which is the fifth characteristic of the Venusian. This is inescapable in one with his characteristics. He could not be the embodiment of love, sympathy, music, and grace, without having passion. And passion as exemplified by a fine grade Venusian means more than animal heat or attraction of the sexes—it means that intangible thing which produces immortal poetry, that sings immortal songs, that dies for its country or its friends.

Thus we find the Venusian characteristics to be:

> Love
> Sympathy
> Music
> Grace
> Passion

And we shall see what these qualities are going to do for the child.

The Venusian and Marriage

To the Venusian marriage is the natural state. He cannot think of "Single Blessedness" as a desirable condition. Always filled with the attraction of the opposite sex, most Venusian children think of marriage at an early age. They mature early and are healthy, so the natural qualities of the type predispose them to listen to overtures looking to an early entrance into the marriage state. The women like men of the strongest types best. To them love is romantic, courtship a ceremony. Those men who regard love casually, and express their devotion in feeble utterances, need not hope to win a Venusian bride. The suitor who comes urgently, presses his suit with heat, and if necessary carries the lady off willy nilly is the one who wins. The men are the same. They do not desire a mate who merely acquiesces. Their passion is intense, they want the same kind of a response, thus Martians, Jupiterians, and Apollonians mate best and most acceptably with Venusians. Their homes are always filled with cheer, and no repining is ever heard over the arrival of little strangers. Few catastrophes occur with well mated Venusian marriages.

Venusian Health

The Venusian has no diseases peculiar to the type. They are a healthy type and strong. Only the acute diseases which are peculiar to all persons in this germ ridden world attack them. They have febrile diseases, colds, sometimes hay fever and asthma, and they fall ill when the epidemics of influenza and other similar epidemics occur. These ailments do not arise from any particular weakness of any of the organs, but they are such as fall to the lot of mankind in general. The Venusian is sometimes prone to nervousness, but he has no chronic ailments.

Venusian Qualities

The Venusian sees life from its bright side. He is healthy and his bounding pulses speak to him of the pleasures that life affords. His is never the gloomy side of anything, even amidst the most discouraging circumstances he will laugh and sing and in the end things generally come out right for him. He is always gay, and his happy disposition makes him universally popular. He does not take life seriously, each day answers its own questions, thus he is carefree and often improvident. He does not court responsibility, nor does he seek riches. Money means the pleasures it will buy or the help it enables him to give to those less fortunate. He is not a great student, and unless with a good secondary Mount is not ambitious, but he has no trouble in getting along and enjoying life.

The Venusian Entity

As we have presented the Venusian in the preceding paragraphs, he stands revealed as a distinct person, plainly different from all the types which have gone before. He embodies noble qualities and many lovable ones, but he also has a low side which makes him actually bestial. It will therefore be apparent that the tests which we are to apply to him will be most important, and that the secondary Mounts will largely determine what he can make of himself. Purely a pleasure lover, and one whose principal claim is of attractiveness and charm, he can only take a place in the battle of life in company with a strong type who will furnish the qualities he lacks. And in every case his grade

will determine his place in the various occupations which will
be assigned to him.

THE SECONDARY TYPE

In enumerating the qualities of the Venusian, it will be
noted that his principal attributes were charm and grace of
manner, good looks, and a kindly sympathy arising from his
boundless love for humanity. None of the stronger qualities
that make engineers, explorers, big business men, or chemists were enumerated. Thus it appears that in his case the
secondary type will largely determine what he shall make of
himself, but it means a great deal to have all the desirable
qualities of the Venusian child to coöperate with a secondary
type. These will increase the strength of any of the types, for
even a Saturnian or a Lunarian will be less harsh and severe
if combined with a Venusian child.

JUPITER SECONDARY TYPE

If Jupiter (Plate 8), be the secondary type, which will be
indicated by a strong Mount of Jupiter, a large and upstand-
ing finger, the apex centrally located, and the other fingers
leaning toward the Mount, all the attractive qualities of the
Venusian child will be added to those of the already attractive
Jupiterian. In the ministry such a child will be intensely human,
and his ministrations will bring comfort wherever he goes.
The Venusian-Jupiterian child can be immensely successful in
the ministry. He can be the candidate in politics who leads
his ticket and who is acclaimed by the populace. He will not
be as profound in knowledge of statecraft as some of the other
types, but the voters will love him and elect him. His very
frailties will endear him to them. This child can be successful in artistic occupations, such as a decorator, in many
capacities in stores handling art objects, if of fine grade in the
exclusive art stores dealing in old masterpieces. In such stores
he will not be the one who knows the imitation from the real
old masters, but he will be the one who can enthuse the buyer
with the beauty of the object to be sold, often calling upon
someone of another type to close the sale. He can be successful
in haberdashery, retail automobiles, banks, fine bake shops, exclusive stores for women's apparel, in jewelry stores óf fine

grade, in a bookstore, and in more ordinary grades as a trained nurse or social worker.

SATURN SECONDARY TYPE

Saturn (Plate 46), will not often be the secondary Mount, his austere qualities will shun the gay Venusian child. But we *do* find Saturn as the secondary Mount to Venusian children. When this combination is found, it will generally develop the musical talents of the Venusian child. Thus he can be a composer, and in this case he will compose a better grade of music. While naturally the Venusian child can compose and loves only light music, the Venusian-Saturnian child can write classics. Both types have the urge of composition and in the expression which this combination gives to it comes a deeper, more heart-searching form than is possible to either of the types alone. The Venusian-Saturnian child will have no aptitude for any of the engineering occupations, nor those of chemistry or agriculture in which the Saturnian is so successful, but he may partake of some of the Saturnian talent for writing. A child with this combination can produce poetry that will bring tears to the eyes, that will stir the fountains of emotion, and for a literary calling he should have his preparation begin early and be thorough.

This child can be successful in stores selling antique furniture, period furniture, or in stores selling old books, back numbers of publications, books with rare bindings, first editions, or in shops specializing as baby shops. He can be successful with firms making and selling band instruments, or he can conduct a business making blueprints, or be salesman either wholesale or retail in the coal business, this in view of the Saturnian's love for mining and the ability of the Venusian child to use his pleasing personality in selling. He can succeed in the business of selling dairy products, equipment for dairies and supplies for same, this again with the help of his secondary Mount. He can successfully conduct a detective agency.

APOLLO SECONDARY

Apollo (Plate 48), is often the secondary Mount, and makes a happy combination. All the fine qualities of the Apollonian are strengthened by the Venusian type qualities, and the Venusian child has the fine qualities of the Apollonian to aid him. Thus he may become a high grade salesman in all the luxury lines in which the Apollonian is so successful. In jewelry, precious stones, house furnishings, and tapestries he can be successful, and in window trimming and designing; and he can specialize in draperies, stained glass, upholstery, men's furnishings, china decorating, or as buyer for millinery, gloves, women's dresses and cloaks.

He can be very successful in conducting a musical bureau which manages leading singers or the many pianists, violinists, 'cellists, orchestras, or choruses. He can successfully manage a billiard hall, a soft drink establishment or chain of stores selling the popular beverages, and he can be most successful as a manager of a nightclub or popular dance hall. He can, if properly trained, become a first grade entertainer. He can be successful in the conduct of his own or as an employee in a fur store, catering to a fine trade if his grade be high, and to a medium grade clientèle if his grade be coarser.

MERCURY SECONDARY TYPE

Mercury will add much shrewdness to the Venusian child. Thus he can be successful in the department store business. He can be most successful as a department manager, a floor walker, a buyer in many luxury lines where good taste and the beauty of the goods to be bought are a consideration. He will have the best of taste in dress, so he can be very valuable in a store or department handling men's wear, especially of the better sort, and in all departments of women's goods he will be a success either as a salesman or as buyer, or department manager. His fine appearance and charming manner will attract much trade, and the Mercurian shrewdness will enable him to turn his personal charm into money. The Venusian-Mercurian child can be successful in the music business. Here his love of and ability as a musician will be of great assistance to him, and the Mercurian business ability will direct him in the way to make a profit out of it. The Venusian child has no ability as a scientist, so none of the Mercurian strength in this direction will come to him. That is, he will not be able to make a doctor of himself even with the added ability of the Mercurian for this profession.

There is one direction however, in which the Mercurian secondary type will help the Venusian child into a profitable business, and that is in brokerage. Here is a wide field, where his charming manner will enable him to be successful. He readily attracts a following wherever he goes, and in the good company he finds in brokerage offices it is not long before he has a well established clientèle. This brokerage may be in many lines. It may be stocks, bonds, wheat, corn or other grains, in insurance where it may be life, fire, liability, accident, surety, or indemnity. Or it may be lumber, iron, coal, steel, or any of the standard commodities, or it may be as a custom house broker. The Venusian-Mercurian child can make the best sort of a manufacturer's agent, and in this field a child with this combination can be most successful. He has all the qualities for success in dry goods, cloaks, suits, men's clothing, hats, shoes, underwear, and he can be successful in foreign trade in all these lines. While the Mercurian has many qualities which fit him for foreign trade, he has not the personality of the Venusian-Mercurian child, and such a combination presents the strongest possibilities of success. Much depends on personality in foreign trade which the Venusian-Mercurian child has in abundant supply. For this line of work, the same preparation must be given the child as has been heretofore recommended for foreign trade.

MARTIAN SECONDARY TYPE

When the Martian Mounts (Plates 52, 54) are secondary, it will add an unusual set of qualities to the Venusian child. He is not supposed to be aggressive, which he will be to a more or less extent if the lower Mount of Mars be the secondary Mount. Unless this Mount be excessive in height, red in color and hard, the aggression will not be of an extent which will do more than spur the Venusian child to greater effort. But if the Martian lower Mount be as above described, the child will be coarse and will not operate on the highest plane of his possibilities. With a moderate development, which means that the lower Mount of Mars is less developed than the Mount of Venus, the Venusian child will be very active and in all the occupations which have been recommended for him this will be a help; for he will exert himself to make the most of his opportunities. While he cannot be recommended for the strenuous occupations that have been mentioned for the Martian, he can take part in them, in positions that do not require the agressive domineering qualities of the Martian. The Venusian-Martian child is splendidly qualified to be a business ambassador of the highest grade, and if a child of fine quality is recognized as a Venusian-Martian he should be put in training for this, which is one of the most important and best paid positions in the business world.

The Venusian-Martian child can make a success as a tailor, where he caters to fine trade. He can be the one who deals directly with customers where his pleasing manner will help him and his taste in dress will prove an asset. He can be most successful as a secretary of a club which has a membership among the better class, and in such a position he can make many friends for the club and be popular among the members. He can also be successful as a clerk in a hotel of the better class. This position is called a "greeter," as the incumbent comes so directly in contact with the guests of the house, and in such positions today a good salary can be commanded and the acquaintances made often lead to offers of better positions from those who have been pleased by the attention received.

This child can also be very successful in the commercial agency business, and can conduct an agency of his own if his grade be fine. These agencies report on all lines of business, and a paying agency can be established in different groups or trades. He can also successfully organize various business agencies, or trade organizations specializing in particular lines of trade, or he can organize groups for different purposes such as the peace society movements and others. He can very successfully operate concessions at resorts, fairs, or wherever there are to be gatherings of people for any purpose. He can succeed in securing members for fraternal organizations, social organizations, and the like. He can succeed in the directory business, getting out directories for towns, villages, or cities, or business directories, or directories of the membership of fraternal organizations, lunch clubs, insurance organizations, and others. He can run a modern drug store successfully.

LUNARIAN SECONDARY TYPE

A combination of the Venusian and the Lunarian is quite uncommon, but it does occur. We have in this combination two quite opposite sets of qualifications, but as we are considering the Venusian as the primary type and the Lunarian as the secondary we have the charming Venusian child to begin with, backed by some of the difficult qualities of the Lunarian. We will have to consider the disagreeable qualities of the Lunarian as overcome by the pleasant qualities of the Venusian.

This, if the grade be fine, will bring to bear the Lunarian gift of imagination, his ability as a writer and his large vocabulary, and we find that the Venusian-Lunarian child can be successful in sales promotion campaigns for the lines of industry which have been recommended for him. He can excel in the preparation of sales literature for department stores, music stores, gents' furnishing stores, art stores, decorators' shops, for schools, or he can be a teacher of language, a composer of delightful music where his human qualities will blend with the fanciful imagery of the Lunarian mind; and such a child can be successful in sales promotion, a field of business which presents great opportunities for large salaries.

The help which the Lunarian gives the combination will be, in every case, that he enables the Venusian child to put into words the ideas which will influence sales. He can successfully write sales promotion literature for a high grade confectioner either wholesale or retail, for a beauty parlor, a real estate developer or broker, a corsetière, for landscape architects, for picture framing stores, for newspaper subscription agencies, for laundries, millinery houses, piano stores, medical institutes, office equipment companies, for new books, radio, phonograph, and sports goods stores, for magazine subscriptions, for ice cream parlors or wholesale ice cream companies, for ladies' tailors, for humidors and smokers' supply houses, for boat builders of all kinds, for an electric bath house and the numerous Russian and Turkish bath houses, for a cabinet maker, or for hosiery stores. In each of these cases the Venusian child's love of beauty and luxury and his ability to meet and please the public will assist him in his work, aided by the Lunarian's gifts for expression.

THE TESTS FOR GRADE

FIRST TEST—TEXTURE OF THE SKIN

We have spoken in the foregoing paragraphs of many things which the Venusian child can do well, and all of these statements have been based on the assumption that the child was of fine grade. All children will not be of this grade however, many will be coarse, many common, many low in all their tastes. All of these grades of children can find places in the Venusian occupations mentioned, but they will not all of them be in the higher brackets. The grade of each child examined must determine what *his* exact position can be in the various enterprises, and for this purpose we begin with the coarsest texture of skin on hands, using Plate 11 as the basis from which we begin to judge texture, in an ascending scale. We do not find skin as coarse as Plate 11 on the hands of a very young child, but we will find degrees of coarseness, which we must carefully estimate.

It is unfortunate if we find coarse skin, for the Venusian has a bad side if he be of coarse grade. Thus we cannot assign this child to first grade positions, even in industries for which his type fits him; we must be content to have him fill the less desirable and less responsible ones in these industries in which his brothers of fine grade are likely at the head. But there are many positions ready for the Venusian child of lower grades in some capacity in all of the enterprises for which the Venusian child is best adapted. There are positions with landscape gardeners, architects, and contractors, with motion picture companies in all of their various departments. With mail order houses, furniture stores, perfume manufacturers, at soda fountains, in pool rooms, with caterers and restaurants, in music stores, gents' furnishing stores, and while the positions he may hold in these lines of business are not at the head of the companies, there are good and medium positions available for lower grade Venusian children as shown by the texture of their skin.

Fine velvety skin (Plate 10), will show us that the child is fine in grade, and we may therefore so chart him and go over the list of things a fine grade Venusian child can do well, among which we will find one that our child can do better than other people. This is the one we should choose for him and we should at once begin to prepare him for it. We will not reach a final conclusion as to his occupation however from the skin alone, this will be the *first* straw that will lead us, but we will at once determine, upon seeing fine texture, that this child is likely fitted for the best grade of Venusian occupations. Other tests will confirm this opinion.

SECOND TEST—COLOR OF THE HANDS

White Color

Color of the hands will begin with white, which is not usual with Venusian children. This type is not cold, they rather incline to heat. Therefore when we find white color in the hands of a Venusian child, we must first of all think that he is not altogether normal. This color indicates a lower degree of vitality than we expect to find, and this reduces the ardor of the child and he becomes more backward and less filled with the exuberance of the type. The charm of his personality is reduced and he will not be able to fill as important a position as he would with pink color. He may be successful in a position with a bookstore, an art publisher, a theater ticket agency, a store selling toilet articles, an information bureau, with a decorator, a milliner, an upholsterer, a haberdasher, florist, a jewelry store, or a travel bureau, but he should not be given the best positions.

Pink Color

Pink color is the natural color for a high grade Venusian child. Here we have the indication of health, it brings out all the ardor of the type, and this produces one of the most charming personalities of all the types.

He is the one who should be placed in the front of a store where he can meet the public, for no one attracts people to him to a greater extent than a Venusian child with pink color. If there is such a thing as "IT" this Venusian child has it, he can galvanize the coldest customer and put him in a buying mood. He can be most successful as a floor manager, a hotel greeter, an actor, a promoter, a salesman in a fine jewelry store, a carpet, rug, or drapery store, an art store, and many with this combination are highly successful as automobile salesmen in one of the stores situated in principal locations in large cities. Here he has a considerable field for the exercise of his talent as a salesman among the class with which he can be most effective. He can also be successful in all the various stores and lines of trade recommended for Venusians.

Red Color

Red color is often found in the hands of the Venusian child for he is an ardent type. There is always the danger that this color may mean too great ardor, and when seen it should cause you to determine at once the grade of the child from the other tests. If all of the tests show him to be of fine grade, then the red color will only mean that he is intense. If the tests show him to be coarse, red color will intensify the coarseness. This child with red color, if of fine grade, must be placed in the most strenuous part of all the enterprises recommended for Venusian children. He must be in the production end of an art publisher, he can have charge of window displays, he can do outdoor advertising, he can conduct sightseeing trips in large cities, or own sightseeing bus lines. If with Martian secondary Mounts, he will do well as a ticket seller for theaters or a circus, as a radio announcer, and he will be successful in dealing with certain difficult types of customers in all the stores recommended for Venusian children. It does not mean that the Venusian child with red color will be brusque, or disagreeable, he will only be intense, and will do best where all his Venusian charm can be utilized in the most intense manner.

Yellow Color

Yellow color is most unusual in the hands of a Venusian child. His is not a bilious type and when yellow is seen it means that something is wrong with the child. A physician should be consulted and his development should be carefully watched. It will be best to place him where he does not come in as direct contact with the public, but he had better be in one of the list of occupations recommended for Venusian children but not in the leading positions. In stores carrying lines in which Venusians do well the child with yellow color should be placed as stock clerk, buyer, file clerk, stenographer, buyer's assistant, merchandise man, supervisor, inspector, traffic manager, manager of postal department, personnel director, supervisor of buildings, or as assistant to the treasurer, or secretary, in all of which positions he can be successful without coming in direct contact with the buying public.

THIRD TEST—FLEXIBILITY OF THE HANDS

Flexibility is a reliable test as to the elasticity of the mind, and in order that you may visualize different degrees of flexibility we show an extremely stiff hand (Plate 12), a straight hand (Plate 13), a flexible hand (Plate 14), and a super-flexible hand (Plate 15). These excellent examples will enable you to judge the degree of flexibility of the hand of any child, and to determine the flexibility of his mind.

The Stiff Hand

The extremely stiff hand (Plate 12), is not often seen, and seldom in children. If present, it will tell you that the child will be coarse, common, and unintelligent and cannot be placed in any of the refined occupations open to the Venusian child. This child must be placed in the ranks of common labor where no mental elasticity is required. It will be best to place him in stores or enterprises recommended for Venusians, but in positions such as porter, delivery driver, watchman, packer, window cleaner, or in other positions of similar grade. He cannot fill any of the positions which relate to stock, buying or selling. Such a coarse hand as is shown in Plate 12 will likely have the vices that belong to the type, and though these may not be criminal they are too often degrading.

The Straight Hand

The straight hand (Plate 13), will tell you that the child is of a much better grade than the one just considered. He will be able to fill positions of more importance in the Venusian occupations. He can succeed in positions such as buyer's assistant, stockkeeper, manager of an office building, newsdealer, window dresser, sign writer, printer, building superintendent, personnel director, dealer in oriental goods, welfare worker, decorator, or as assistant to merchandise men, and officials. This child has made a distinct advance over the stiff hand in the quality of positions hich he can fill successfully, and in all the occupations recommended for Venusian children he can be used to the best advantage in medium grade positions, but he cannot reach the full measure of possibilities open to those of the finest grade.

The Flexible Hand

The flexible hands shown in Plates 14–15, indicate the flexible mind. This child will be versatile, sympathetic, lovable, and most attractive. He can be placed in positions where he meets the public and can be depended upon to create the most favorable impression. He can be business ambassador in foreign trade, the salesman who is put to the front to meet the best trade in stores, he can succeed in leading positions in music stores, fine grade haberdasheries, in the best of stores dealing in men's ready to wear clothing, and in tailor shops catering to the most exclusive trade. In all of these he will attract and hold a following, he will be universally liked, and he will sell the most expensive merchandise with ease. He can conduct schools for music, language, dancing, and will be most sucessful in conducting a girls' school of the better class and boys' academies. He will do exceptionally well as salesman in high class automobile distributing agencies, and as broker for stocks, bonds, sugar, wheat and other grains, lumber, iron, cement; and with oil companies he will be most successful as negotiator of leases, or in dealing with governments.

Fourth Test—Consistency of the Hands

Consistency of the hands is the test we use to find out the amount of energy the child possesses. We may find that he has all the qualities necessary for success, but if he is lazy they will come to nothing.

Flabby Hands

If we find that he has flabby hands, which means that they crush as you press them and seem to have no firmness, we shall know that the child lacks energy, and that we must find a place for him where he can utilize his type qualities without much exertion. Flabby hands reduce the chances of success, but do not make it impossible. This child can do best if he be devoted to music and art, for often what we call the artistic temperament is found possessed by those who do not work very hard. They have their fits and starts, and in the intervals when the mood is upon them they can compose delightful music, but they are not capable of sustained effort. The flabby handed Venusian will seldom succeed in business, but if placed in a position where he can utilize his inspiration when it comes, he can often do things that will gain him a reputation, and in popular song writing, much money. This is a field that is very profitable when the child can write song hits, but those who grind steadily only write a hit occasionally. He can also write music for revues and this is a profitable field.

Soft Hands

The soft hand is a grade above the flabby in energy. This child can be placed where he will have to work steadily. He will not do more than he has to, but he will not be so lazy that he is ineffective. He can be quite successful in conducting a beauty parlor, and a large business can be done in this speciality, his charming personality will bring him many customers. He can conduct a high class grocery catering to a fine trade who do not care much about price if they get novelties and unusual delicacies for their table. He can be very successful as manager of an exclusive country club, or of a resort hotel. He can specialize in old Americana and be very successful in a museum collecting the same. He can succeed as manager or owner of a chop house which has unusual decorations, food, and music. No more genial host can be found for such a place. With training he can be a designer, and among other things make a specialty of coats of arms, and he can conduct motor tours.

Elastic Hands

These hands do not crush in your grasp, they are resilient. When you press them they respond with a firm feeling, they have spring, and seem virile and alive. Such hands show the most effective kind of energy, not intermittent, not lacking, but ever present ready to do the day's work. A child with such hands can be placed in exacting positions with the assurance that he will use his ability to the utmost. He can be success-ful in business in important positions. He can be manager of a telephone company, he can be an official in a bank. He can be sent to foreign countries as a diplomat, or an agent for a large corporation. He can manage an office for a public utility company, or be a credit man for a large hotel, manager of a piano store, be secretary of a race track association, casting director of a radio company, a vaudeville booking agent, a casting director for a moving picture company, and with proper training an elocutionist and impersonator.

Hard Hands

With hard hands, the Venusian child can do the utmost in labor that is possible to a child of this type. He will have unusual energy, and can be placed in positions where real work is needed. He can be a cutter in a wholesale clothing manufacturing company, conduct a physical training school, canvass from house to house for the sale of insurance, carpet sweepers, vacuum cleaners, washing machines, rugs sold on the instalment plan, or electric household appliances. He can be a suburban real estate broker, he can be a census enumerator. With some of the better grade of clothing manufacturers he can be production manager, or in a factory making lingerie, hosiery, men's collars, neckties, shirts, or lounging robes. He can conduct an exclusive pipe and tobacco store, or a store for novelties in leather goods, baskets, bridge sets, and games. In all of these vocations the Venusian child with hard hands can be successful.

Fifth Test—The Three Worlds

The three worlds as shown by the hands as a whole and by the phalanges of the fingers (Plate 1) will tell us whether the Venusian child can be most successful in the mental, the business, or the material world. The method of separating the three worlds has been fully covered in a former chapter and an illustration of the hand as a whole divided into the worlds is shown in Plate 16.

The Mental World

When we identify the child as belonging to the mental world (Plate 16), we know that he will, if the other tests show that he is of fine grade, succeed best in vocations where he can use his mental qualities. This will be more surely indicated if the hands be flexible and of a good color, and the texture of the skin be fine. The secondary types will at this time be of great assistance, for if the Mount of Jupiter be secondary we know that the child can be most successful as a lecturer, an art publisher, in concert management, an entertainment bureau, as an advertising counsel, a teacher, a librarian, in art galleries and schools, amusement enterprises, and in the grade of stores which we have enumerated which deal in merchandise appealing to the better classes.

If the Mount of Saturn be the secondary Mount with the mental world best developed, the Venusian child can excel as a composer of good music, not only of light melodic forms, but of the more serious kind. He will have the basis of the severe classical style of the Saturnian, and to this will be added the rhythm, sparkle, and harmony of the Venusian. This child can write well on musical subjects, and can teach privately or in musical schools. He will be more serious in everything he does, and can be successful in occupations such as dealing in stained glass, in clay modeling, in the conduct of a teachers' agency, as a publishers' agent, a cartoonist, in a school of design, a press clipping bureau, as a dentist or as manager of a bowling alley.

If the Mount of Apollo be the secondary Mount with the mental world dominating, the child can be an exceptionally good writer of advertising for department stores, suit and cloak houses of the better grade, men's furnishing stores or stores selling gloves, hats, or shoes, and he can be a successful salesman handling these and other lines of merchandise which have been recommended in this chapter for Venusian children.

If Mercury be the secondary Mount with the mental world best developed, the child will be successful in the executive end of factories manufacturing clothing, suits for women and men, and in the better positions in other firms or corporations which have been enumerated in this chapter. He can be successful as a lawyer, and will be effective before juries on account of his charming manner. The Venusian child *per se* has no ability as a lawyer, but with Mercury as the secondary Mount he acquires the skill of the Mercurian to which he adds the charm of his Venusian type, thus winning all with whom he comes in contact. He can be successful in stores selling fine jewelry, laces, tapestries, rugs, and art objects of all kinds. He can also conduct a collection agency, a mercantile reporting agency either general or for special groups, he can succeed as an electric contractor either for heating, lighting, or as an electrician, he can do well with a firm engaged in the sale of electric refrigeration machines, and can successfully conduct a secretarial school. He will be valuable with the best class of art dealers, where they handle paintings of great rarity or sculpture at high prices. But great care must be exercised that his grade be fine, for the Mercurian in the coarse grades has a very bad side.

The Martian Mounts secondary and the mental world best developed make a successful combination. The vigor of the Martian will push the charm of the Venusian child into many successful undertakings. He can excel as a second to the Martian on many of his expeditions, and can aid him greatly in his dealings with men. Thus in securing oil concessions or preparing literature for the Martian undertakings this child can be of great service and successful. Owing to the sturdy qualities of the Martian, the Venusian child who has Mars as his secondary Mount can succeed as the operator of an armored car service, in the conduct of a garage, in the business management of a baseball park or team, he can conduct a store selling army and navy goods, he can successfully conduct a bath house at a summer resort and in cities, he can be successful as the manager of an air port, in charge of power plants, as a political organizer, especially the organizing of political clubs, in the conduct of a military academy, in the organization of secret and benevolent societies and the securing of members for same. He can succeed in second hand stores if his grade be only medium, and he can manage a fleet of taxicabs or a bus line. He can manage a storage warehouse and fleet of moving vans, or he can organize and manage an automotive express and freight service between cities or confined to one city.

The Lunarian as secondary Mount brings to the Venusian child with the mental world longest his gift of language and his vocabulary, which makes the Venusian-Lunarian child eloquent in addresses before conventions, as an after-dinner speaker, and will enable him to write well on any subject dealing with Venusian occupations. This will make him successful as an advertising writer, or as a designer of outdoor advertising, in direct mail advertising, in conducting an advertising service, and in the preparation of sales literature for stores or manufacturing companies making or dealing in fine clothing for men and women, for art publishers, banks, silversmiths, stores selling tapestries, for clubs, wall decorators and wall paper stores, architects, iron, electric, glass and other signs, cash registers, and in all the luxury lines enumerated in this chapter which the Venusian can sell so well.

The Middle World

If the middle or business world (Plate 16), is the best developed, which means that it is the longest part of the hand and that the middle phalanx of the fingers is the longest, the Venusian child will be most successful in the business world. This means that he can in some cases do best in the *manufacture* of the lines of merchandise for which the child has been recommended, and in other cases he can do best in the *sale* of the merchandise *after* it is manufactured. Secondary Mounts like the Saturnian or the Mercurian will show his talent for manufacture, and Mounts like Apollo, Jupiter, and Mars will show that his best qualifications will be for selling. In each case, however, he will do best in the practical side of any business enterprise. He will not have much desire to write, nor will he have great ability to do so with the middle world dominating, but he will have a strong business instinct, and the secondary Mounts will show the best direction for it to take. In each case, review the things the secondary Mount can do best which we have now covered completely in this and former chapters, and add to these the desirable qualities of the Venusian type, and you will know in what lines the child should engage, and as his middle world is best developed it will be in the practical parts of these businesses that he can succeed best.

The Lower World

The lower world (Plate 16), on the hands of a Venusian child signals danger. This world indicates that the animal part of the child is best developed, and as the tendency of the Venusian is toward the indulgence of his passions, with the lower world best developed he will have great temptations. We must therefore judge this child according to his grade and place him in positions requiring a less degree of mental effort and refinement. The secondary type will indicate the lines in which he will be most successful, and in these lines the child must be placed in lower grades of positions than if either of the upper worlds are dominant. Thus the Venusian-Jupiterian child will not make a good minister, but he can do well as a political boss in a ward or precinct. In such a position he can be very successful. He can be a leader or foreman of workmen on contracts in shipbuilding yards, or in the construction of buildings. If Saturn be the secondary Mount this child can be the helper in laboratories, the foreman or salesman in factories producing fertilizer, and in a similar position in dairies or the factories producing dairy products. If Apollo be the secondary Mount with the lower world strongest and the grade coarse, the child cannot make a salesman who meets the public; he can, however, be the one who keeps a store clean, opens and checks the stock, looks after the building, sees the windows are washed, and he can be generally useful in capacities in the lower brackets. With Martian Mounts secondary he can be a private or noncommissioned officer, the man in charge of the baggage and equipment of the expeditions which the Martian leads, and in all of the Martian activities this Venusian child with the lower world dominant can occupy the subordinate positions.

The Venusian child with the lower world strongest and the Mount of Mercury as the secondary Mount can be a factory superintendent if of fine grade, and the porter if his grade be common. He cannot be the lawyer, but can be the man who cares for the lawyer's offices. He can drive the doctor's car but he cannot be the doctor. He can run a small store but he cannot head a department store. Many times he will be the push cart peddler and have a stand on market, and for such positions this Venusian-Mercurian child with the lower world dominant will be qualified.

He can be an operator in a shoe factory or fill other positions in the factory such as superintendent if his grade be fine, or he can be salesman either on the road or in the house. He can be a coffee blender or roaster, have an agency for vacuum cleaners, he can be an embalmer, operate a swimming school or natatorium in a city, be a commission merchant for fruit, vegetables, nuts, dairy products, or eggs, or he can operate a feed store, store for pets, a dog hospital, hardware store, sell parquet floors, sell tailors' findings and textile mill supplies, confectioners' supplies or conduct a store selling fish and sea foods.

If the Mount of the Moon is the secondary Mount when the lower world is dominant, it will not be a favorable combination. The lower side of the Venusian child can receive little support from the cold, selfish, superstitious Lunarian, consequently this child can fill only the most ordinary positions. He can be a bookbinder, operate a clothes pressing establishment, or a seed store, or be a hat renovator, barber, a carpet layer, masseur in a bath house, conduct a place for colonic irrigations, or operate vending machines.

Sixth Test—Knotty Fingers

Knotty fingers (Plate 20), on a Venusian child are a rarity. He is not one who analyzes. He acts by impulse and this is not a quality of knotty fingers. We do however find Venusian children with well developed knots, and for this reason must give them careful consideration in these paragraphs.

The greatest effect of knotty fingers will be shown in combination with the secondary types.

Knot of Mental Order

In this case we will have analysis shown by the mental knot (Plate 21) added to the qualities of the Venusian child and the secondary type. We have found when the Jupiterian is the secondary type that, almost universally, smooth fingers are present. When, however, we find a mental knot on a Venusian child with Jupiter as the secondary type, it will have the effect of slowing down his operations, and also the support which he receives from the Jupiterian. In this way we will have a child whose best field of endeavor will be as an advertising counsel, in connection with a travel bureau, as a librarian, literary agent, social worker, play broker, in stores dealing in optical supplies, as a foreign exchange broker, commission merchant, or in the conduct of a business school.

If Saturn be the secondary type with the mental knot, the child can enter a number of the engineering professions or can be successful in laboratories for pathological research. This child can also be a good writer on scientific subjects and especially successful as a writer on all agrarian topics. If of high grade, he will be able to come in contact with the public and may thus be an excellent salesman especially well qualified in the selling and manufacturing of products used in agrarian occupations. This will include farm machinery, fertilizer, feeds, and dairy equipment, the conduct of a grain elevator, and if the child be of a low grade he can be successful in occupations of less importance in the factories manufacturing these products.

If Apollo be the secondary Mount, the child will have great ability as a salesman, as the charming qualities of the Venusian type will be added to those of the Apollonian, and with this combination the child may occupy leading positions in luxury stores selling diamonds and jewelry of the best quality, oriental rugs, draperies, laces, works of art, and sculpture.

If this child be of high grade he can find a wide field of operation in the automobile industry, first in manufacturing operations, from which he can graduate into a connection with the sales departments either as direct factory agent or with high grade distributing agencies for the better grade of cars. If the mental knot be identified when the child is quite young, which may be done, and the primary and secondary types also identified as well as the grade of the child from the tests which we employ, his education for the sales field in the automobile industry should begin early, and preferably he should take a position in the mechanical and manufacturing departments and fill the various situations in factory production. Knotty fingers will make this Venusian child especially proficient in the latter line of endeavor.

If we find the mental knot on a Venusian child with Mercury as the secondary Mount, it will be a fine combination for a career in the business and mechanical lines in which the Mercurian succeeds best, and he will be very successful in all of the scientific endeavors in which the Mercurian is so proficient.

He can be successful as a publisher, or in the conduct of

a store selling medical or law books, and he can operate a company furnishing service to lawyers and doctors through reports of medical or law cases in all the various states. He can be successful as an auctioneer either of merchandise or real estate, or in conducting a store or agency for sewing machines and the supplies for same. He can successfully operate a store for the sale of typewriters and supplies for same, he can be a dealer in precious stones, he can be a manufacturer or whole-sale or retail dealer in ribbons, he can successfully conduct a steamship agency, he can operate a store for the sale of auto-mobile tires and supplies, he can be a lithographer. In each of these occupations some of the qualities of either the primary or the secondary Mounts will make the child especially fitted for them.

The mental knot with the Martian type secondary will make a child extremely pugnacious and will accentuate the Martian qualities of aggression and resistance. This child will be especially proficient in positions of command where he may hold commissions in the army or navy or be at the head of oil prospecting and developing companies. A great deal will depend upon the grade of this child. In the fine grades he can be in occupations which are of a sturdier sort. The Martian backlog to the Venusian type will make the child a more ag-gressive person and the mental knot will supplement the Mar-tian strength. This child can have the agency for the sale of fire hose and fire apparatus where the Martian strength and the Venusian personality will enable him to get business from aldermen and city councils. He can be a hotel broker, a labor organizer, have an agency for the sale of heavy machinery, take dredging contracts, operate warehouses, be a loan broker, conduct a leather store either in a retail way through the sale of bags, purses, traveling bags, trunks, or in a wholesale way through the sale of hides and leather findings for shoemakers. He can be a masonry contractor, and if his thumb be low set, a woodcarver.

When the Mount of the Moon is the secondary type the child with the mental knot will be most successful as a musical or dramatic critic, or in the production of literature for music schools, and he can be successful as a composer where the Luna-rian qualities of imagination will blend with the Venusian har-monic qualities enabling him to produce most successful popular music. He can also be a musician and proficient as a pianist or violinist and if this combination is identified while the child is young a musical education should be begun at once.

Second or Knot of Material Order

If only the second or knot of material order (Plate 22) is found on the hand of a Venusian child, it will emphasize his love of dress and his desire to be at all times well groomed. Such a child will be more systematic in his immediate sur- roundings than is usual with Venusian children; thus he can succeed in the financial department of a company manufac- turing clothing, hats, lingerie, gloves, or sport clothes for men and women. He can be successful as an office manager in such companies, and can have charge of a department in a factory where there are many parts to be cared for. This may be in automobiles, farm machinery, with telephone companies or electric manufacturing companies. He can be successful with radio companies, in the management of a haberdashery store which he will keep in perfect order and in which the stock will be well chosen and selected with good taste. With both knots developed, the child will have an extremely analytical mind.

SEVENTH TEST—SMOOTH FINGERS

Smooth fingers (Plate 23), are expected on the hands of a Venusian child. This type is so thoroughly a creature of impulse and inspiration that smooth fingers with their artistic tendency will be found in almost every case where the Venusian Mount type is identified. Smooth fingered qualities add to the attractiveness of the Venusian child and his quickness of mind. If the grade of the child be fine, he can be most successful as a dramatic reader, an actor, a composer of popular music, a pianist, violinist, accompanist, but in these cases will have little inclination for classical music and will attain his best success by expending his efforts on music of the popular kind. The charm and attractiveness of the Venusian child will make him able to come in direct contact with the public, and he can be a salesman in stores handling the better class of ladies' suits, millinery, sport clothes, shoes, men's furnishings and haberdashery, and in stores dealing in fine furniture, silver, glass, china, tapestries, unholstery, and in tailoring establishments catering to the finer trade. He can succeed in art stores handling high grade art objects, in antique shops, jewelry stores, in art galleries and schools, and in stores dealing in artists' materials. In judging the child with smooth fingers they must be regarded as increasing the desirable qualities of the type which reaches its best operation from the qualities of impulse and inspiration. The Venusian child does not gain in efficiency or charm from an analytical turn of mind.

Eighth Test—Long Fingers

When we find long fingers on a Venusian child care must be used to determine whether they are merely long or extra long. In Plate 24, we show especially good examples of long fingers, and in Plate 25, a most unusual specimen of extremely long fingers. Until proficiency has been gained by practice it will be best to measure the fingers, and in this way determine exactly the *extent* of long fingered development present in the child under examination.

Extremely long fingers are not a good combination with the Venusian child. The extreme slowness in movement of children with these extremely long fingers reduces the spontaneity of the child and he becomes slow and even sluggish.

When normally long fingers are identified, this child should be placed in offices in some capacity such as filing clerk, installing filling systems, stock keeper, or where the qualities of detail shown by the long fingers may be brought into their best operation. This child will be intelligent though slow and can be of great assistance to an executive of some large corporation in handling the details of office management and having charge of research departments, analytical departments, and in supervision of departments preparing estimates for contracting.

He will not have great ability for mathematical work in such departments but he will be careful in collecting the facts worked out by others engaged in these departments, developing them, and preparing them for proper consideration. In positions of this character the Venusian child will be very successful. He can be successful in classifying and arranging a research department in an importing firm, technical school, and other scientific institutions. He can be an efficiency engineer, can be successful in conducting a teachers agency, a reporting bureau of which there are many who do more than the kind of mercantile reporting done by the regular agencies, who investigate the character and antecedents of any firm or individual, giving a complete history going back for years. These kinds of research bureaus are used by firms and corporations when considering connections or business engagements. The long fingered Venusian child can be eminently successful in the conduct of such a bureau. He can be successful as an industrial engineer, as an embosser, enameler, in the thrift department of banks, as a timekeeper for a large manufacturing corporation, in the conduct of a tourists agency, as a circulation auditor or circulation builder, as a draftsman, with a firm selling adding, duplicating, or other machines which reduce labor in offices, or he can manage or own a store selling all manner of engineering instruments.

NINTH TEST—SHORT FINGERS

Short fingers (Plate 26), are natural to the Venusian child. They add in every way to his charm, to his quick thinking, and to the activity which is natural to the type. This child becomes more spontaneous and the short fingered qualities will give him the ability to undertake larger operations and carry them through successfully. Short fingered Venusian children if of fine quality can be most successful as promoters of water power development, distribution plants where chains of gas, electric, and water distribution are linked together many of them extending over a very wide territory. He can also be the conceiver and *planner* of large storage dams which provide for the impounding of water supplies and their distribution to cities and factories, but he can do none of the engineering or technical work. He can *plan* and promote transportation lines in cities, and in many of these various activities the Venusian child with short fingers can be most successful. He will receive from the Venusian type the charm of manner necessary to make him successful with city councils, boards of trustees, and others with whom these public utility corporations must come in contact, and the short fingers will give him the activity, impulse, and inspiration to carry forward these enterprises.

The finger tips will play a most important part in assisting the Venusian child to his best occupation.

The Pointed Tip

Beginning with the pointed tip (Plate 27), we find this child highly imaginative but impractical. He will be most attractive, charming in every way, and can be successful if his activities are directed into the proper channels. It would be most unfortunate if such a child were placed where he was called upon to deal in figures or with scientific subjects. These are beyond his capabilities to master.

He can, however, become expert as a linguist, and in this connection would be highly successful as a teacher of languages, or as a translator of plays or volumes of fiction, and can be especially successful in dealing with the romance languages and in using these languages as a medium for the expression of his own emotions either as an actor or writer. Many celebrated playwrights in the French and Spanish languages have had these pointed tips. This child can be successful in a store of fine grade dealing in antiques, imported laces, oriental rugs, draperies, tapestries, or sculpture. Such children can also be successful as guides in foreign cities, and in conducting departments in stores handling a fine grade of table delicacies, bags, or costume jewelry. As writers they can produce excellent poetry of an emotional character, and they can write short stories dealing with pastoral subjects and natural history.

The Conic Tip

The conic tip (Plate 28), will give the Venusian child great love of beauty, and if such a child can be properly educated from the beginning, he can achieve success as a commercial artist, painter, interior decorator, and as a composer of popular music. Such children will have a large amount of musical talent but not of a classical kind. From a money making standpoint, however, their music will be far more saleable than that of the musical composers who write a better class of music. In business lines, this child can be successful in stores selling needlework, artificial flowers, steamer baskets, infants' wear, lamps, decorative linens, as a dressmaker, in the conduct of a gift shop, and in a store selling pianos, radio sets, victrolas, and all the luxury lines to a good class of trade. He will have no scientific ability and no ability in mathematics and should not therefore be placed in any technical school or forced to engage in any technical occupations. His success will lie in using the charm of manner which belongs to the Venusian type to which is added the artistic temperament of the conic tip. This child will be highly successful in the management of music bureaus, lecture bureaus, or in directing concert tours. He can be successful as a literary agent, theatrical agent, and in the conduct of a casting agency where the business consists in casting players for parts in different productions. A child with this combination should be thrown with prominent people in all these amusement lines during the early years of his life, and should be furnished books and literature tending to arouse his musical and artistic tastes and an early choice should be made as to whether he shall be in business, paint, or be a musician or actor, and his education should follow the decision in these matters.

The Square Tip

Square tips (Plate 29), found on the hands of a Venusian child give him more ability for scientific and practical pursuits. This child, if his grade be fine, can be successful in stores dealing with articles which though practical still have attractiveness and charm, and such a child should never be placed in stores dealing in hardware, machinery, or merchandise of similar character, and should never be placed in factories manufacturing such goods. He can be successful in the conduct of chain stores and is well adapted for the management of such. He can be successful as *manager* of stores dealing in show room furniture, men's hats, shoes, clothing, women's apparel, as a tailor, stationer, shirt manufacturer, with a school of design, a secretarial school, and can be successful in the conduct of a decorative china store, and in amusement enterprises. The Venusian qualities of this child will give him the impelling force necessary to acquire a following, and the square tips will give him the practical qualities necessary to make such stores successful. In all these recommendations it must be noted that it is as manager not salesman. Such a child can be very successful in companies handling theatrical draperies.

The Spatulate Tip

The spatulate tip (Plate 30), on a Venusian child will add originality, love of nature, and will make him most successful as an inventor but his inventions will rarely be connected with technical subjects. He will be active and highly successful as a director of athletics in schools and colleges, as a teacher of riding, golf, tennis, fencing, and shooting. This child can be most successful as a writer on natural history subjects and of stories for children dealing with animals, birds, and flowers. When the Venusian qualities of musical composition are employed, the spatulate tip will give the child the ability to compose unusual music which universally attracts attention. The Venusian child always composes popular music, and some of the most successful song hits have come from the hands of those of the Venusian type with spatulate tips. In the business world, this child can invent new methods of advertising and create new styles. Thus he can be successful as a merchandise man in a department store or as style director of a manufacturer producing men's and women's clothing. He will be exceptionally independent in thought, and thus can be successful as originator or developer of new ideas, founder of cults or new societies, in which capacity the Venusian qualities and his charm will make him most successful.

A very important development in merchandising in recent years is the designing of the packages in which proprietary articles are offered to the public. A great variety of toilet articles are sold in drug and department stores which are known as package goods. There are many food products which are sold in packages, tin cans, and containers of all sorts. Prominent merchandise men have recently stated that a product may not sell in one package, but that if the package is changed, and has a label put on it with a different color combination, this product can be taken out of the first package and put into the second, and a large demand will spring up for it. From this psychology of the public has grown up the profession of packaging, in which there are engineers in color choosing for packages, called color engineers. The importance of packaging to merchandising makes these desirable vocations for children, and the Venusian child with spatulate tips is particularly well fitted to take up this new work and be successful in it.

ELEVENTH TEST—THE THUMB

In previous chapters we have explained the great part which will power plays in the life of the individual, and also the manner in which we may determine the extent and character of the will possessed by any child.

The thumb, which is the indicator of will and logic, is the means which we employ, and by its shape and the manner in which it is carried we determine whether the good qualities and talents of a child will be developed or whether they will lie dormant. The thumb can be used successfully in estimating the youngest child in the earliest days of its life, and many of the important things relating to his future success can be determined even while he is yet an infant.

Thumb Curled Under Fingers

When we see the hand extended with the fingers curling over the thumb we know that the child has a weak will and consequently a weak character. However brilliant the qualities which he possesses, they will not be brought to a successful issue if the thumb is carried in a folding position under the fingers.

High or Low Set Thumb

We are anxious at the earliest possible moment to determine whether the thumb is high set, low set, or has a medium setting. The manner of determining this has been fully explained, and these facts can be recognized on the hand of the youngest child.

High Set

If the thumb is high set (Plate 36), we know that the intelligence of the child is below par, he inclines to animality, his will power is largely diminished and he must not be placed in positions of responsibility or those which require skill with his hands. This child must occupy medium positions in the various enterprises and occupations already recommended for Venusian children. He can also succeed with a wholesale dealer in butter, cheese, eggs, fish and clams, meats and poultry and bread, and with a jobber of canned goods, and groceries including flour, sugar, and coffee.

Low Set

When the thumb is low set (Plate 34), the child will have greater ability for all the Venusian activities which have been recommended, and in addition will have the ability to take part in occupations requiring manual dexterity or skill with the hands; thus he may be placed in the factories of silversmiths, coppersmiths, watch and clock factories, and other factories manufacturing articles which appeal to the sense of beauty which the Venusian child possesses and which require manual dexterity. Such a child should not be placed in a factory making iron work, or those making machinery or other heavy products. His manual skill should be confined to companies making more artistic merchandise, such as a bookbinder in a shop making art books, special bindings, and publishing limited first editions, in a factory making art calendars, Christmas, Easter, New Year cards, or valentines and other art work such as books for children, in a candy factory, or a factory making display fixtures, embroideries, garden furniture and pottery, hosiery, or he can be a diamond cutter, do clay modeling, be a pattern maker, or banknote engraver.

Medium Set

A medium setting of the thumb (Plate 35), will enable the child to be evenly balanced in the matter of will power but he will have neither the lack of intelligence and manual skill of the high set thumb, nor will he have the skill possessed by the thumb set low. The medium setting is, however, a distinctly favorable marking, and may be regarded as exemplifying a well balanced set of qualities.

This child can be very successful as a mechanical draftsman. In this class of work it is best to specialize, and a very good line is the making of appropriate sketches and designs of mechanical contrivances and equipment suitable for the operations of bridges. Another good line in which to specialize is in making sketches and designs for the construction of power plants, coke plants, and oil or sugar refineries. It will help this child very much to have experience in the offices of contractors, architects, and engineers, and some shop experience as draftsman or inspector.

Phalanges of Will and Reason

The phalanx of will, which is the first phalanx of the thumb, indicates the extent and strength of the will power and also its quality.

Bulbous Will Phalanx

Beginning with the bulbous will phalanx shown in Plate 37 we have the lowest grade of will quality. This produces a stubbornness and determination that makes the child unattractive and is not a favorable indication. It may be accepted as a fact that whenever this bulbous thumb is found there is excessive determination and stubbornness which may interfere with the best operation of the good qualities of the Venusian child.

This child cannot engage in the artistic employments open to one with a better thumb, he must, in order to be safe, be assigned to ordinary vocations. But in spite of his bulbous thumb, he will have much Venusian charm, and can succeed in the proper occupations. He can do well in the sale of oils for engines, automobiles, railroads or steamships, and for greases of all grades and kinds. He will make friends in garages and the places where contracts are made, and such a child can build up a business for himself, for the bulbous thumb gives him a good deal of will power even if of poor quality and his Venusian type enables him to sell.

Short Will Phalanx

The short phalanx of will shown in Plate 39 indicates an entire lack of will power, and this child must not be placed in any position of responsibility as he will be utterly unable to have charge or dominance of either an office or manufacturing organization. Such a child must be placed in a position where he can do purely routine work.

He can succeed, however, as the steward in a dining car with one of the railroad companies. Here he will not need much will power, and his Venusian qualities will make him popular with the patrons of the road. So long as this child has this weak thumb, we cannot place him in responsible positions, and it is much better for him that he be in something he can do well even if it is not all that you might wish than to put him where he will invite failure because he lacks certain qualities you cannot supply.

Long Will Phalanx

The long phalanx of will shown in Plate 38 will give the child abundant power of will so that he can develop all of the talents and possibilities of his Venusian type. He can be placed in positions of trust and responsibility in all the occupations already recommended for Venusian children where he will have charge of large forces of employees either in offices or in manufacturing companies or in the construction of buildings, railroads, public utilities, and other enterprises of similar character in which Venusian children can and do engage successfully. This thumb will show that whatever the type developments of the child and his secondary type which shows the occupation best for him, he will have the will power necessary to develop the qualities needed for the occupation. There will be none of the weakness shown by the short will phalanx, and none of the excess shown by the bulbous phalanx. This is the best development to find on any child as an indication that whatever the type qualities indicate, they can be fully developed.

There are some fine positions open now in board of education work, connected with the building of the many modern school buildings which are going up all over the country. Each of these buildings must be furnished after it is completed, and there are many lines of school furniture which must be installed. A Venusian child with this strong phalanx of will can be successful as a superintendent of purchase, delivery, installation, and inspection of new furniture equipment which is used in such public schools, and to direct the writing of specifications for and preparation of detailed drawings of new furniture, and for the necessary repairs and replacements of furniture equipment already installed. If he is well prepared for such a position he can find a ready market for his services. He should have experience in the wholesale manufacturing trade or in a factory manufacturing such furniture. He must be familiar with the various processes entering into the manufacture of furniture and castings, and with the kinds of wood used in the manufacture of school furniture, the methods of drying and seasoning, staining and finishing, the same. There is a fine vocation here for a Venusian child with this strong will phalanx.

Phalanx of Reason and Logic

The second phalanx of the thumb, indicating as it does the powers of reasoning and logic, is of the greatest importance in considering the future of the child.

Short Phalanx of Reason

If the second phalanx be short, as shown in Plate 40, the child will have poor reasoning qualities and strong will. This will produce a condition out of balance, in which case the child will make many mistakes owing to the fact that he does not reason carefully nor does he bring matters to their logical conclusion.

Such a child will perform a task at which he is set with great determination owing to his strong will phalanx, but he will lack initiative, and can only do routine things under direction. There are some very large manufacturers of handkerchiefs who enjoy a large trade, and in one of these factories this child can succeed in the office. If of fine grade as an assistant office manager, and if of medium grade as a file clerk, telephone operator, or receptionist, for he will have the Venusian charm of personality in spite of his weak phalanx of reason. Similar positions are to be had by such a child in cotton goods manufactories, or with manufacturers of rayon.

Long Phalanx of Reason

If the phalanx of logic be long (Plate 38), it will indicate strong reasoning qualities and ability to bring things to a logical conclusion. This is a very fortunate development, especially with a strong will phalanx.

As the Venusian child is at all times artistic when of fine grade, this child with a long phalanx of reason can be very successful in the position of teacher of art in a school or college for girls. Many prominent colleges have openings for teachers of literature, history, and music, and in either one of these specialties this child can be successful. This is a fine vocation for a Venusian child. With this phalanx, the child can do well as an actor either on the stage or in the movies. He can be a dramatic reader or conduct a school of expression. He can be an assistant to a professor of music, art, or history, in a college or university, or secretary to the faculty. He can be an exceptionally successful receptionist in a bank, where his good judgment will be valuable.

Will and Reason Balanced

The development which we wish to find is that of the balanced thumb (Plate 38), where the two phalanges are of equal length and thickness. In this case we have the operation of a strong will power guided by good reasoning and powers of logic. This child will develop his charming Venusian qualities and bring out all the strong points of his type. He will be able to come in direct contact with the public, he can make the most of all of the advantages belonging to his type, and can be placed in the most responsible positions in all of the occupations recommended for Venusian children. He will have especial business ability for the type.

He can be successful as owner or employee in tobacco and cigar stores where he meets many men, in the insurance business either in life or fire where he needs a pleasing personality and good salesmanship, in introducing new accounting machines which is a good form of specialty selling, in running an addressing and letter service, as an adjuster, which requires diplomacy and a pleasing manner, in selling advertising displays, posters, or out-of-doors signs, as a photographer, agent for an air transportation service, and will do well in selling church supplies.

Elementary Thumb

The shape of the thumb as a whole will indicate the degree of intelligence possessed by the child, for we find that in some cases we have a thumb which is so thick and blunt that it bears little resemblance to the better thumb developments.

An excellent example of this elementary thumb is shown in Plate 42 and this thumb we use as a starting point, indicating, as it does, the greatest lack of intelligence and an ignorant degree of stubbornness. Few such thumbs as this will be found, and rarely on the hands of very young children. When, however, they are seen, the child must be placed in the commonest and most ordinary forms of labor connected with the various enterprises in which the Venusian child succeeds. He can be a painter but only of the rough sort, doing such work as painting barns or fences, he may be a hod carrier or rough brick layer, a truck driver, or work in abattoirs, he may be a butcher, a grave digger or a chimney cleaner.

Strong Independent Thumb

From this common thumb the quality of thumbs increases in fineness and we find in Plate 33 a strong balanced thumb of good muscular strength, standing erect and away from the hand, with broad clear nail, which indicates the power and ability to bring out in a substantial way all of the strong qualities of the Venusian type. This child can occupy the most responsible positions in the Venusian occupations.

He can be successful in one of the stores that specialize in the sale of lamps, where there are many beautiful designs, and where the lamp shades conform to his love of beauty, or in the sale of architectural bronze work, with building and loan companies, in the flower trade both wholesale and retail, as agent for one of the many bus lines where his fine personality will draw trade, or he can own or be connected with a nightclub, a café, or cafeteria. If he have spatulate tips he can be successful with boys' camps. Or he can successfully manage one of the very attractive candy and lunch serving stores, or be secretary of a chamber of commerce, or he can be successful in a store specializing in house furnishings, furniture, and stoves.

Fine Balanced Thumb

In Plate 41 we show another well balanced thumb but of a more refined quality where the size and muscular strength of the thumb is not so great as that shown in the thumb last considered. This thumb will identify a child able to take all of the finer positions in the best grade of stores and in the better firms and occupations recommended for Venusians. Here will be found good judgment, strong will, good reasoning powers and logical faculties, which combined will bring this child a certain success.

He can be successful in the sale of surety bonds, especially if Apollo be his secondary Mount, he can manage a tea room, have great success as a radio broadcaster, can conduct a store for the sale of artists' supplies of all kinds, or theatrical shoes. With Apollo as secondary Mount he can be a business broker and engage in the sale of businesses as a whole, he can conduct a store for the sale of photographic supplies, cameras and developing, with spatulate tips he can succeed in a store or department or have a store of his own for the sale of camping equipment, canoes, golf equipment and sporting shoes, hats, clothing, or he can be successful in a connection with a firm selling carnival supplies, or he can be a very successful caterer.

The Thumb Tip

The tips of the thumbs indicate the same qualities as are shown by the tips on the fingers, with the exception that the tips on the thumbs relate to will power rather than other qualities.

Pointed Tip

The pointed tip (Plate 27), will show idealism and weakness in the will and such children must not be placed in the most responsible positions. They will not have the force sufficient to overcome those who have stronger thumbs. Children with the pointed thumb tip can, however, be made successful if they are placed as clerks in barber supply stores, or they can be successful as costume decorators. They can be especially successful as clerks in stores selling Chinese goods, or Chinese or Japanese art goods, they can do well with firms specializing in church furniture, they can be successful with tailors specializing in clerical clothing and vestments, they can be successful in the office of a cleaning and dyeing establishment, not where they do the cleaning, but where they receive the goods to be cleaned.

Conic Tip

Conic tips on the thumb (Plate 45), give artistic qualities to the will and are stronger than the pointed tip. Such children can occupy more important positions and have more responsibility over the operations of other people. They can be very successful as amusement directors where they can have charge of the amusement features at summer resorts, in the big hotels in the large cities, on roof gardens, and they can hold affairs and entertainments for lodges and secret societies. There is quite an extended field for a good amusement director. They can manage and direct street fairs, bazaars, and can be successful as ring masters and directors of entertainment for circuses both large and small. They can be successful in selling hotel supplies of which there are many kinds, and can do well as owner or employee with firms dealing in hotel supplies. They can be illustrators, successfully conduct an information bureau, do well as a manufacturing jeweler, a ladies' tailor, a magician, a manufacturer of costumes and paraphernalia for lodges and secret societies. They can be a manufacturers' agent for silks, laces, gloves, hosiery, velvets, and similar merchandise, and can conduct inspection bureaus for fire insurance companies where they fix the rate charged on various buildings.

Square Tip

The square tip (Plate 44), will give all of the practical common sense ability of this tip to the power of will. These children will be most successful in the business side of all the occupations recommended for Venusian children as proprietor or employee in the various stores and Venusian occupations.

They can be successful as secretary of a library, the square tip will make them exact, and the Venusian qualities will make them popular with patrons of the library. They can be successful in the sale of adding machines owing to the square tip, or of advertising specialties, dental equipment, or as real estate appraisers, or in the conduct of a "drive it yourself" auto rent-

ing service. They can be successful in the sale of electric household appliances, in the trust department of trust companies,
as members of the stock exchange, as a mortgage broker, a
taxidermist, in the conduct of a trade journal, in the sale of oil
burners, and can be exceptionally successful in conducting
a business for the sale of office equipment of all kinds, the planning and laying out of offices, the installation of filing systems
and short cuts to office efficiency, and in the sale and conduct
of a store for the sale of optical goods.

Spatulate Tip

Spatulate tips (Plate 43), give originality and independent
character of will, which is exceedingly strong, and those with
spatulate tips are found in every case dominating their brothers
with tips of the other formations. These children can be placed
in positions of responsibility in all the Venusian occupations
and as dealers in live stock for which the spatulate tip has a
great fondness. They may conduct a commission stable where
horses or mules for draft purposes are handled on a commission basis, or it may be fancy riding horses or ponies for
children. Or this child can be a successful breeder of stock,
either cattle for dairy purposes, or beef cattle, or horses for
racing, draft, or riding and driving. Or the child can be successful in the conduct of a store for the sale of sporting goods,
sports clothes, bowling, tennis, boxing, riding, or golf supplies.
He can successfully conduct a riding academy, a botanical
garden, can specialize in the building of greenhouses, can
conduct a nursery, a gymnasium, be a physio-therapist, conduct an academy for physical culture, a moving picture theater,
sell playground equipment, or he can conduct a parcel delivery,
health resort, or be a golf professional.

CHART NOTE: The Mount of Venus is one of the easiest
Mounts to identify. Either a strong development or the deficiency of the Mount can be plainly seen, and after viewing the
plates shown among our illustrations and referred to in this
chapter there will be no trouble in properly judging the Mount.
With this Mount, the secondary Mount is very important, for
it is largely from the secondary Mount that the clue to the
Venusian's best occupation is obtained. It is what his charm-

ing manner and engaging personality add to a secondary Mount that is important. His grade is also most important, for low grade Venusians are barred from many occupations in which a fine grade Venusian can be highly successful. The careful preparation of the chart is again of signal importance when a child has been identified as having a primary Venusian type.

TEST CHART

Types
  Primary.
  Secondary.
  Others.

Tests
  1. Texture of skin
  2. Color
  3. Flexibility
  4. Consistency
  5. Three worlds
  6. Knotty fingers
  7. Smooth fingers
  8. Long fingers
  9. Short fingers
  10. Finger tips

The Thumb
  11. How carried
      How set.   High.   Low.   Medium.

Will Phalanx
      Bulbous.   Short.   Very short.   Long.
          Very long.

Phalanx of Logic
      Long.   Very long.   Short.   Very short.
      Will longer than logic.   Will shorter than logic.
      Will and logic balanced.
      Large thumb.   Small thumb.
      Elementary.   Medium.   Fine.
      Tip of thumb.   Pointed.   Conic.
          Square.   Spatulate.

Age of Child.   *Sex.*   *Date.*

READING THE CHART—CHOOSING THE OCCUPATION

Never allow your ambition for your child to force him into a vocation for which he is not fitted. A prominent scientist recently broadcast this statement: "The commonest cause of failure in life is to be found in discrepancies between the ambition of parents and the capacities of children."

A carefully prepared chart of his hands, properly read, can prevent such failure for your child. The same scientist said further:

"It is a popular delusion that because two parents produce a child they are endowed with wisdom in planning for him."

Do not think that you know your child so well that you do not need any help.

TEST CHART

Types

Primary.   *MERCURY* Plainly Marked.

Secondary. *JUPITER* Well Defined.

Others.   *MARTIAN* Mounts Medium Development.

Tests

1. Texture of skin. *FINE*.
2. Color. *OLIVE*.
3. Flexibility. *MEDIUM*.
4. Consistency. *ELASTIC*.
5. Three worlds. Mental world. *YES*. Business world. *2ND*. Lower. *NO*.
6. Knotty fingers. *YES*. Mental knot. *YES*. Knot of material order. *SMOOTH*.
7. Smooth fingers. *NO*.
8. Long fingers. *MEDIUM*.
9. Short fingers. *NO*.
10. Finger tips. Jupiter-Apollo *CONIC*. Saturn-Mercury *SQUARE*.

The Thumb

11. How carried. *INDEPENDENT*.
    How set. High. *NO*. Low. *NO*. Medium. *YES*.

Will Phalanx

Bulbous. *NO*. Short. *NO*. Very short. *NO*. Long. *YES*. Very Long. *NO*.

Phalanx of Logic

Long. *YES*. Very long. *NO*. Short. *NO*. Very short. *NO*.
Will longer than Logic. *NO*. Will shorter than Logic. *NO*.
Will and logic balanced. *YES*.
Large thumb. *YES*. Small thumb. *NO*.
Elementary. *NO*. Medium. *NO*. Fine. *YES*.
Tip of thumb. Pointed. *NO*. Conic. *NO*. Square. *YES*. Spatulate. *NO*.

Age of Child	*Sex*	*Date*
10 years.	male.	

READING THE CHART

In the preceding chapters we have outlined to you in detail various steps necessary to prepare a chart of the hand of a child, so that you might in the end use it as a doctor does in diagnosing disease. The various steps you have taken in applying the tests and identifying the types of your child represent the manner in which tests are made in laboratories for the use of a physician; and as you have passed from chapter to chapter, we assume that you have, at the end of each, noted on the chart which follows these chapters what you have found in the hands of your child as described in that chapter.

For the purpose of showing how a chart should be read when completed, we are assuming that the chart attached is the one you prepared, fully assuring you that any combination of indications, no matter what they are, can be read as easily and as accurately as those in this hypothetical chart. Furthermore, it can be done by anyone of average intelligence, it only requires the application of common sense.

Passing now to the chart before us, which sums up the results of our labors, we begin to select the occupation for which the child is best fitted, so that we may prepare him for this occupation.

It is not necessary that you shall have memorized the contents of the preceding chapters or any considerable portion of them, you need only to refer, as you reach each item on the chart, to the portion of the chapter on his primary Mount type dealing with that indication, which we shall now begin to read in the manner intended beginning with the first test.

READING THE CHART

The first test shows us the texture of the skin is *fine*. This leads us to believe that the grade of the child is *likely* to be fine, but we do not make a final determination of this question until we have examined the *other tests*.

319

The second test shows that the *color of the hand is Olive.* This at once warns us that either the child belongs to a type *whose normal color is olive,* or that if he belongs to *another type* he has the qualities that *go with yellow color,* of which olive is a modification. We at once realize, on seeing yellow color, that each succeeding test must be carefully considered, as we often find that *yellow color* is a very *unfavorable* indication.

The third test shows that the hand is flexible, but that it is *medium flexibility.* This will tell us that the child has a *flexible mind,* he readily absorbs new ideas, he can master a variety of subjects, but because his hand is only medium in flexibility, he will not be an extremist, he will not fly off on tangents, he will not be a spendthrift in matters of money or time. His mind will be keen and elastic, and whatever we may find his best occupation to be, he will have the mental equipment to master it.

The fourth test shows us that the consistency of the hand is elastic, and from this we know that the child will have *abundant energy* of an intelligent sort, and that whatever the other tests may show, he will not fail from laziness.

The fifth test shows that the *mental world* is most highly developed, and that the middle or practical business world is secondary. Thus the child will succeed best in the mental occupations of whatever the chart may show his type to be. He will not be visionary, however, owing to the secondary development of the middle world, and for whatever occupation we find him to be best adapted, he will be able to *make money* out of it, as he can be successful in it.

The sixth test shows that the knot of mental order is best developed, which will tell us that the child has *system* and *order* in his *mental processes,* thus the keen mind shown by the flexible hands will operate in the mental world, in a *systematic and orderly manner.*

The seventh test shows that the child's fingers are not smooth, our chart showing that the first knot is developed. But the chart shows that the *second knot* is smooth, which tells us that the child will *not be orderly* in his *material surroundings,* he will not be careful in his dress or his person, in his home or his office. While he will have *mental system,* he will not be orderly in his surroundings.

The eighth test shows that the child has fingers which are *medium* long. Thus he will be *rather* slow in his movements, he will have a faculty for detail, he will be careful to look after minutiæ, and as his best sphere is in the mental world, this will add to the order and system of his elastic mind (flexibility), as shown by the developed first knot. It is to be noted that these fingers on the chart are not *extremely* long, otherwise they would make the child suspicious and a martinet. They are *medium* long, which makes them a much more favorable indication in support of the other indications already charted.

The ninth test shows that the child's fingers are not short, therefore none of the impulse and quick thinking that belongs to short fingers is present. The indications so far show that this child should rely on his *analytical qualities* rather than upon *impulse*.

The tenth test shows that the tips of the fingers of Jupiter and Apollo are conic, and those of Saturn and Mercury are square. Thus Jupiter the secondary Mount will have a love of beauty (conic tips), he will have all the desirable qualities of the spontaneous type, he will, with this tip, have all the charm that belongs to the type and the magnetic qualities that make the type successful. Saturn will, with a square tip, have his scientific side prominent, Apollo with a conic tip will have his natural and most desirable qualities, and Mercury the primary Mount will develop his *serious side*, his *practical* side, and with the indications shown by the other tests, a square tip is a most favorable combination.

The eleventh test, which is the thumb, will tell us whether the child can make the most of the qualities he possesses, whether he has the *will* to prepare himself for his future occupation, and the *will to drive himself* to do the things necessary for success. It will also show whether he has a logical or clear thinking mind, is a good reasoner, and whether there is force behind the human engine which is the child himself.

Our chart shows us that the child has a *large thumb*, carried independently, not curling under the fingers, that it has a medium setting on the side of the hand: that the *will phalanx* is *long*, the *phalanx of logic* is also long and *balanced* with the *phalanx of will*. It is not elementary, but is a strong *balanced thumb* with a *square tip*.

It is only necessary to turn to the paragraph on the

thumb, in the chapter on the Mount of Mercury, to learn that the child has a *strong character, good intelligence, strong will* but not stubbornness, that he has a clear thinking *logical mind,* is a *good reasoner,* that his will is *not out of balance with his reason,* and that it will operate in a practical manner.

With all the knowledge which we have now secured from the application of the eleven tests, we come to the determination of his type and here we find indicated that the child is of a *primary Mercurian type plainly marked,* and that *Jupiter is the well defined secondary type.* We also find that the *Martian Mounts* have a *medium* development.

These types have been identified by the rules laid down in the chapter on the identification of the Mounts, and we now have the complete picture of the child as a human entity from the chart. It then becomes your task to choose the occupation for which he is best fitted.

Choosing His Occupation

From a digest of the chart, we find that the child is a *Mercurian,* of fine quality, the *olive color* which first arrested our attention being the *color natural to the type* and not sufficiently yellow to indicate the bad or unhealthy qualities of the type. He has the energy that belongs to the type which will give him industry, one of the leading type qualities. He has an *elastic mind,* his best operation will be in the mental world which dominates, but he has assistance from the business world sufficient to make him *practical* but not enough to make the business world his best field of operation. His *best occupation,* therefore, will be in one of the *mental occupations* peculiar to the *Mercurian type.* This is further confirmed by the fact that he has the knot of *mental order,* which shows that he has a systematic and analytical mind, and that the knot of *material order* is absent, emphasizing the fact that his strength is in the mental world. His long fingers show that he is careful as to *detail,* and looks after the *minutiæ* of all things with which he comes in contact, that he overlooks nothing, and the square tip on the finger of *Mercury* shows that he will *not be flighty* in his *mental operations,* but that he will be *practical.*

The *thumb* shows that he has *strong will power,* good *reasoning powers,* which make him *firm but not stubborn,* but one who cannot be dominated by others.

One of the strong characteristics of the *Mercurian* is his *power of oratory* when the *first phalanx of the finger of Mercury is longest,* so we must now add oratory to the qualities possessed by the child. This is one of the *prime necessities of one of the leading occupations* of the Mercurian type.

APPLYING THE TESTS TO THE MOUNT TYPES

From the chart we learn that the primary type is the Mercurian, and that Jupiter is the secondary type, and we learn that there is some Martian development.

From this we know that the child receives from his primary type:

> Shrewdness,
> Industry,
> Scientific ability,
> Business ability,
> Quickness.

The chart shows that he is of fine quality, has energy, normal color, an elastic mind, the mental world rules, that he has the gift of oratory, that the business world is secondary, that he has system in his mental operations, care for details, a strong character, strong will, strong reasoning powers, and logic.

We must therefore reach the inescapable conclusion that the shrewdness, industry, scientific ability, business ability, and quickness of the primary type *will operate only on a high plane.* There will be none of the scheming, trickery, or criminal tendencies of the low grade Mercurian. We must also conclude that this child will *not find* the occupation for which he is best fitted in the *business world.* In none of the enterprises mentioned in the chapter on the Mercurian Mount type in which the Mercurian succeeds best in manufacture, trade or traffic will this child find the occupation for which he is best fitted.

HE IS PREËMINENTLY FITTED FOR AND CAN ACHIEVE HIS BEST SUCCESS IN THE LAW

which, it will be remembered, is a profession strongly recommended in the chapter on the Mercurian Mount type for Mercurians when the mental world rules, and *especially* when the *gift of oratory* is present as shown by the long first phalanx of Mercury as indicated on the present chart.

If you will check over all the qualities we have found indicated on the chart, and apply them to the profession of the law, it will be found that every one of them brings added strength to the child for use in this profession. His grade, his elastic mind, his mental system, care for details and looking after the little things, his strong will, clear thinking and oratory, equip him, if properly prepared, for great success. And when we remember that all of these strong qualities are added to the native shrewdness and keenness of the Mercurian type, his natural business ability and his industry, we see again how well fitted the child is for the law.

We have, in the present instance, been able to select the best occupation for the child from his primary type alone, but we must not forget that he has a strong secondary type as well in the Mount of Jupiter, whose qualities are:

> Ambition,
> Leadership,
> Religion,
> Honor,
> Love of nature,
> Pride,
> Dignity.

Thus we have behind the already strong Mercurian qualities for success, another set of qualities equally as strong but of a different kind. Ambition will drive the Mercurian to increased effort, he will use his elastic mind and his strong will to bring his Mercurian shrewdness to its highest state of perfection. This will be invaluable to a lawyer. He will desire leadership which will be a further stimulant. The religious character of the Jupiterian blends well with the fine grade of the Mercurian child. Honor will bulwark him more firmly in the high ideals he will have and practice. Love of nature will help all of his favorable qualities, and pride in his work will cause him to use his industry and care for detail so that every case will be thoroughly prepared and the dignity of the Jupiterian will enable this child to use the oratory inherent in him with the musical voice and telling effect that the Jupiterian knows so well how to employ.

This case shows clearly the tremendous effect which the secondary type has on the primary, in this case favorable, in others directly the opposite.

This child has a third type notation on the chart:

"The Martian Mounts Medium Development."

Here is another support for the child, he will have aggression and resistance, than which there are no more necessary qualities for a successful lawyer. Thus he will be able to attack and defend with equal force. The lower Mount with its aggression will lead the attack, and the upper Mount with its resistance will defend. In this case the Martian Mounts are not strong, they are medium, so the child will have the aggression he needs but he will not be a bully, and from the upper Mount we know that he will never know when he is defeated.

These qualities, with an already strong will, and all the other forces which we have seen from the chart are to come to the support of the child, will make him well-nigh invincible in the occupation for which he is preëminently fitted:

THE LAW.

SUMMATION ON PRECEDING CHAPTERS

A List

No matter what vocation you choose for your child, no matter how well he is fitted for it, he cannot achieve the ultimate in success unless he is properly prepared.

It is now possible to know his best vocation from his hands in time to prepare him for it.

Schools and colleges and devoted teachers are waiting to give him the instruction he needs. Don't blame the schools if he lacks in success.

Blame yourself.

SUMMATION ON PRECEDING CHAPTERS

The manner in which you can use the hand of your child to select the best vocation for him has been explained in preceding chapters, and positions have been suggested for him in many industries, trades, and professions. These vocations cover most of the present-day activities of business and professional life, and many trades. Taken as a whole, they will enable a parent to select for his child, from recommendations in the chapters on the types, the thing he can do best; and find a vocation for which there is a world-wide demand. To summarize further opportunities in concrete form, we here append a list containing individual occupations, trades, lines of business, and service rendering companies, from which may be selected a vocation for which your child is fitted, as shown by his hands; using the methods outlined in preceding chapters. With a carefully prepared chart, average parents can select from the body of this book and this list the occupation for which their child is best fitted. There is a best occupation for every child that lives: over 4000 of them are contained in this book.

A SUPPLEMENTARY LIST

For Use in Selecting a Vocation for a Child by Means of
His Hands

Accountants—certified public—consulting
Acoustic engineers
Actors
Actuaries
Adjusters
Advertising agencies—advisers
Advertising copy writers—publishers
Advertising service
Aerial photographers
Agricultural consultants
Air conditioning contractors
Aircraft engineers—distributors

Aircraft flying instructors—machinists
Aircraft repair men
Ambulance service
Animal dealers—hospitals
Apothecaries
Appraisers—diamonds—industrial
Appraisers—household goods—tax
Appraisers—manufacturing plants
Appraisers—natural resources
Appraisers—public utility — real estate
Architects — industrial — house— bank

Architectural engineers
Art publishers—color
Art schools
Artists—landscape—cattle
Artists—miniature—water
Artists—portrait
Artists' supplies
Art stores
Assayers
Attorneys
Auctioneers
Auditors
Authors—prose—poetry
Automobile agencies
Automobile companies
Automobile distributors
Automobile exporters
Automobile importers
Automobile painting
Automobile repair shops
Automobile upholstering
Automobile wreckers

Bacteriologists
Badge makers
Bail bondsmen
Bakeries
Bakers
Bake shops
Band—musician—leader
Bankers—commercial—mortgage
Barbers
Barge repairing—renting
Baseball parks
Baths—electrical—hydriatric
Baths—Turkish—medicinal
Battery service
Bead dyers—repairers
Beauty shop experts
Bicycle repairs
Bill posters
Billiard halls
Biological laboratories
Blacksmiths
Blueprint operators
Boarding house keepers
Board of trade secretaries
Boiler repairers
Boiler setters
Boiler tube cleaners
Boilermakers
Bonding—surety
Bonds—investment—real estate
Bookbinders
Book indexing—stamping
Booksellers
Bootblacks
Bottlers
Bowling alleys
Brass foundries
Brewers
Bridge builders

Brokers
Broom makers
Brush makers
Builders
Building and loan associations
Bungalow builders
Bus lines
Bus rental
Business brokers
Business counselors
Business schools
Butchers
Button dyers
Button makers
Buttonhole makers
Buyers

Cabinet makers
Cafés—cafeterias
Calculating service
Calking contractors
Camera repairing
Camps
Candy makers
Candy wrappers
Canvassers
Car builders
Car loading contractors
Carpenters
Carpet cleaning
Carpet layers
Carting
Caterers
Ceiling contractors
Cement contractors
Cemetery brokers
Chair repairers
Charts—business
Check room service
Chemical engineers
Chemists
Chemists—analytical—consulting
Chemists—industrial
Chimney builders—cleaners
Chimney engineers—repairers
China decorators—repairers
Chiropodists
Chiropractors
Chlorinators
Christian Science practitioners
Cigarette makers
Cigar makers
Circulation auditors
Circulation builders
Civil engineers
Claim adjusters
Clay modeling
Cleaners and dyers
Clergymen
Clock repairers
Cloth spongers
Clothes pressers

Code makers
Coffee dealers
Coffee mill repairing
Collection agencies
Colonic irrigation
Colonic therapy
Color counselors
Combustion engineers
Commercial agencies
Commissary contractors
Commission merchants
Concessionaires
Concrete construction
Confectioners
Consulting engineers
Contracting engineers
Contractors—alterations
Contractors—general
Coopers
Coppersmiths
Corset makers
Costume rental shops
Costumes—makers
Crating
Credit rating agencies
Credit unions
Cremating
Curtain cleaners
Curtain hangers

Dancing masters
Dancing partners
Dancing schools—Oriental—stage
Day nurseries
Decorating contractors—flag—conventions
Decorators—interior—expositions
Delivery service
Dental laboratory—help—dentists
Department stores
Designers—rugs—textiles
Desk repairers
Detectives—agencies
Die makers
Dietarians
Directories—office buildings
Directories—telephone
Directory publishers
Disinfecting contractors
Dispensaries
Distillers
Distributors—circulars—samples
Divers
Dock builders
Doctors' information
Dog boarding
Dog hospitals
Draftsmen
Dredging contractors
Dress contractors
Dressmakers
Drilling contractors

Drug brokers
Drug importers
Drugstore brokers
Druggists
Duplicating service

Efficiency engineers
Electric engineers
Electricians
Electro-therapists
Electrotypers
Elevator repairing
Embalmers
Embossers
Employment agencies
Enamelers—porcelain—wood products
Engineers—cellulose
Engineers—radio—ceramic—automobile
Engineers—stationary—locomotive
Engravers—bond—photo—brass
Engravers—stationery
Engravers—steel—copper plate
Engravers—wax—wood
Engrossers
Entertainers
Entomologists
Etchers
Excavating contractors
Exchange brokers
Exchanges—stock—commodity
Exporters
Expressing
Exterminators

Facial treatments
Fac-simile typewritten letters
Fashion publications
Fashion syndicated service
Feather dyers
Feed stores
Fencing schools
Ferries
Fertilizer brokers
Filing consultants
Financial counselors
Finger print experts
Firemen
Fish markets—Wholesale—Retail
Floor layers and finishers
Florists
Flour-jobbers
Food brokers
Foot specialists
Foreign exchange brokers
Foresters
Forwarding agents
Freight agents
Freight bill auditors
Freight brokers
Freight forwarding—foreign

Freight rate service
Fumigations
Funeral directors
Fur auctioneers
Fur cleaning—Storage—Dyeing
Fur farms
Fur stores
Furnace repairing—Refinishing
Furniture stores
Furniture—upholstered

Galvanizers
Gasoline filling stations
Gasoline—wholesale
Gauge repairers
Genealogists
Geologists
Gilders
Glass benders—Bevelers—Blowers
Glass carvers
Glaziers
Glove makers
Gold refiners—Stamping
Golf instruction
Golf professionals
Grain dealers
Green house builders
Grinding service
Grocers
Guards
Guides
Gunsmiths—Gun stores
Gymnasiums

Haberdasheries
Hair dressers
Hair stores
Hair treatments
Handwriting experts
Hardware stores
Harness makers
Harness stores
Hat renovators
Hat stores
Hauling
Health institutes—Foods
Heat treatments
Heating contractors — engineers —
   specialists
Homeopathic pharmacies
Horse shoers
Hosiery stores
Hospital consultants
Hospitals
Hotel brokers
Hotels
House cleaners
House furnishing stores
House movers
House wreckers

Ice cream parlors

Illustrators
Importers
Incinerators—repairing
Income tax consultants
Incorporating companies
Indemnity bonds
Indian goods—American
Industrial engineers
Industrial relations bureau
Industrial surveys
Information bureau
Inspection bureau
Insurance adjusters—analysts
Insurance—Brokers—Credit
Insurance—fire—forgery—life
Insurance—marine—elevator
Interior decorators—architectural
Interpreters
Investigators
Iron workers

Japanners
Jewelers—repairing
Jewelry stores
Jig sawing
Junk dealers

Kerosene—retail—wholesale
Kindergartners

Label—cutters—designers—finishers
Labelers
Labor organizations
Laboratories—analytical—clinical
Laboratories—biological—bio-chem-
   ical
Laboratories—chemical—electrical
Laboratories—diagnostic
Lacquering
Ladies' tailors
Lamp mounting
Lamp and shade stores
Land clearing companies
Landscape architects
Landscape contractors
Landscape gardeners
Landscape irrigation companies
Lathing contractors
Laundries—family—hotel
Laundrymen
Law court service
Law printers
Leather goods stores
Lecture bureaus
Legal papers serving
Letter brokers
Librarians
Lighterage service
Linen supply service
Linoleum layers
Linotype operators
Lip reading schools

Literary agents
Lithographers
Live stock breeders
Livery stables—owners—help
Loan brokers
Loans—pawnbrokers
Locksmiths
Lodges—fraternal orders
Looms—hand operators
Loose leaf accounting
Luggage stores—owner—help
Lumber yards—owners—help
Lunch cars—owners—help

Machinery moving
Machinists
Magazine subscription agencies
Magic tricks stores—magicians
Magneto repairing—Magnetos
Mailing—Mailing lists
Mailing lists—automobile owners
Mailing lists—investors—stockholders
Maltsters
Management engineers
Manicurists
Manufacturers' agents
Map mounting
Marble cleaning
Marble contractors
Marble dealers—owner—help
Marine contractors
Marine electrical service
Marine engineers
Marionette operators
Market analysts
Market research service
Masonry contractors
Masseurs
Mausoleum builders—promoters
Meat markets
Meat packers
Mechanical engineers
Medical institutes
Medical laboratories
Medical research institutes
M e n ' s furnishings—retail—wholesale
Merchandise brokers
Merchandising service
Message bureaus—telephone
Messenger service
Metal finishers
Metal lathing contractors
Metal printing—sawing—spinning
Metal stamping
Metaphysical practitioners
Meter readers
Microscopists
Midwives
Milk products
Milliners

Millinery—wholesale—retail
Millwrights
Mimeograph service
Mineral water agency
Mineral water salesmen
Mining companies—Miners
Mining engineers
Missionaries
Money brokers
Monotype compositors
Monument makers—owners—workmen
Mortgage loans—brokers
Morticians
Motion picture distributors
Motion picture operators—Authors
Motion pictures—producers—actors
Motion pictures—theaters—laboratories
Motor boat sales agency
Motor bus lines—owners—operators
Moving vans—owners—operators
Multigraphing—owners—operators
Museums—curators—help
Music arrangers
Music dealers—engravers—printers
Music publishers
Music schools
Music stores—musicians
Musical bureaus
Musical instrument repairing

Napkin supply service
Natural gas companies—operatives
Naturopaths
Naval architects
Naval stores—owners—help
Neckwear stores—ladies'—men's
News dealers
News service
Newspaper brokers
Newspaper clipping bureaus
Newspaper subscription agencies
Newspapers—owners—help
Notaries
Notion stores—novelties
Numbering service
Numerologists
Nurseries—day
Nurserymen
Nurses—male—female—registries

Occulists—and aurists
Office building—help—cleaning
Office buildings — owners — superintendents
Office furniture—refinishing—repairing
Office location surveyors
Oil burner agencies—salesmen
Oil filling stations

Oil reclaiming — collecting — crank case
Oil royalty companies
Oil well engineers
Opticians — optometrists — optical goods
Orchestras
Organ instructors—tuning
Organ sales agencies
Oriental goods store—help
Ornamental iron work—workers
Osteopaths
Outboard motors—boats
Oven repair men
Oyster men—oyster bars

Packers—meat—household goods—service
Painters—house—sign—automobile
Paper hangers
Paper stores
Parcel delivery
Parquet floors—dealers—workmen
Passenger transfer companies
Patent attorneys—brokers
Patent engineers—office draftsmen
Patent protection service
Patrol companies
Pattern makers
Paving contractors
Pawnbrokers
Penmen
Perfumers
Personal service bureaus
Pet shops—owners—help
Petroleum engineers
Phonograph recording artists
Phonographs—stores—repairers
Photographers—architectural—children
Photographers —commercial — supplies
Photographers' repairs
Photographic reproductions
Photo prints—blue
Photo prints—enlargements—copying
Phrenologists
Physical culture institutes
Physicians and surgeons
Physio-therapists
Piano instruction
Piano movers—tuners
Piano stores
Picture stores—owners—help
Pile driving—contractors
Pilots
Pipe fitters
Pipe and tobacco stores
Plasterers
Platers
Play brokers

Playground specialists
Plumbers
Policemen
Political clubs
Poultry raisers
Power engineers
Precious stones—dealers
Press clipping bureaus
Pressing—clothes
Printers—banknote—catalogue
Printers—book—commercial
Printers — financial — foreign language
Process servers
Promoters
Psychologists
Public relation counselors
Public speaking instruction
Public utility companies
Publicity bureaus
Publishers—art—directory
Publishers' representatives
Purchasing service

Quantity surveyors
Quilting shops

Radio artists—broadcasting stations
Radio broadcasting studios—announcers
Radio engineers—program producers
Railroad contractors
Railroads—help
Range agencies—repairing
Real estate—acreage—brokers
Real estate—loans—mortgages
Real estate management
Receivers
Reducing treatments
Refiners—oil—metals
Refrigeration engineers
Refrigeration service—agency
Refrigerator dealers
Refrigerator installing—repair
Registers — cash — accounts — agencies
Religious goods
Reporters
Research laboratories
Resident buyers
Restaurant brokers
Restaurants
Riding academies
Road builders
Roof garden designers
Roofers
Rotogravure printers
Rubbish removal
Rug cleaners

Saddlers

Safe deposit companies
Safe movers
Safe openers
Sailmakers
Sales management engineers
Sales promotion
Sales research
Salvage—marine
Sand blasters—contractors
Sandwich shops
Sanitariums
Sanitary engineers
Sausage makers
Savings banks
Saw makers
Scalp treatment
Scene painters—theatrical
Schools—accounting—art—business
Schools—beauty culture—Chinese
Schools—chiropractic—civil service
Schools—dancing—dental—designing
Schools—drafting—dramatic—electrical
Schools—fashion—fencing—filing
Schools—for deaf—interior decorating
Schools—kindergarten—language—lip reading
Schools—massage—music—riding—secretarial
Schools—shorthand—show card—speech correction
Schools — stenography — French — Spanish
Schools—welding—motion pictures
Sculptors—architectural
Seaman's outfitters
Second hand stores
Secret society organizers
Seed stores—owners—help
Sewer builders
Sewing machine agents—repairing—supplies
Sewing machine stores
Sextons
Sheet metal workers
Ship brokers
Ship builders
Ship chandlers—registers—agents
Shirt makers—custom—repairs
Shirt stores
Shoe stores—shiner—repairs—help
Show card writers
Sight seeing busses
Sign hangers—painters
Sign painters
Silk converters
Silk stores—retail—wholesale
Silver plating
Silversmiths
Skylight engineers

Social service workers
Soda fountain dispensers
Soft drink parlors
Speedometer repairing
Sporting goods stores—owners—help
Stair builders
Stammering treatment
Stamp dealers
Stationers—supplies
Statistical service
Statisticians
Steam engineers—companies
Steam fitters
Steamship agencies
Steamship companies
Steel mill workers
Steeple jacks
Stencil cutters
Stenographers
Stereotypers
Stevedoring contractors—help
Stock brokers—exchanges
Stockyard help
Stockyards
Stokers
Stoneyards — cutters — setters — masons
Storage—cold—household goods—merchandise
Storage batteries—wholesale—retail
Street railways—help
Street sprinkling contractors—help
Street sweeping contractors—help
Structural engineers
Stucco workers
Subscription agencies
Surety bonds—agents—salesmen
Surgeons—plastic
Surveyors—city—construction—marine
Swimming pool engineers—schools
Syrup dispensers

Tabulating service
Tailors—men's—women's—help
Tanners
Tapestries—wholesale—retail
Tax consultants
Taxicabs—drivers—repairs
Taxidermists
Tea rooms—owners—helpers
Teachers' agencies
Teamsters
Telegraphers—telegraph companies
Telephones—secretarial bureaus
Telephones—switchboard operators
Tennis court contractors—help
Terra cotta workers—makers
Testing laboratories
Textile engineers—painting—printing
Theater ticket agencies

Theaters — agencies — expressing — managers
Thermographers
Threshing machines to rent—operators
Thrift promotion service
Thrift shops
Ticker service
Tile—importers
Time lock rental
Time recorder clocks—rental
Tinsmiths
Title companies—help
Tobacco—wholesale—retail
Toilet preparation agencies
Tombstones—cutters—help
Tourist agencies
Tours—motor
Towel supply service
Towing—automobile—marine
Toy stores—wholesale—retail
Trade journals
Trade mark—drawings—registering
Traffic service
Translators
Travel bureaus
Travel consultants
Tree treatment—surgery
Trucking
Truck sales agencies
Trunk store—repairing
Trust companies
Turkish bath houses—help
Tuxedo rental
Typewriter agencies—repairs
Typewriter supplies—rental
Typewriting—manuscript—legal
Typographers

Umbrella repairing
Umbrella stores—wholesale—retail
Undertakers
Underwriters
Uniforms — military — naval — fraternal

Upholsterers

Vacuum cleaners—agencies—salesmen
Variety stores
Vaudeville agencies—actors—theaters
Vending machines—agencies—help
Ventilating engineers
Veterinarians
Violet ray treatments
Violin repairing
Vocal instructors
Vocational advisers
Vulcanizing shops—help

Wall cleaning
Warehouses—help
Washing machine agencies — salesmen—help
Watch inspectors
Watch makers—repairers
Watch stores—wholesale—retail
Watchmen's reporting agencies
Watchmen's time clock agencies
Water—mineral—carbonated—medicinal
Water power companies—help
Water purifying companies—help
Water supply contractors
Wax figures—show windows
Weavers
Weighers
Well contractors—diggers
Whitewashing
Window cleaners
Window dressers
Wood carvers
Wood turners
Wood workers
Wrecking contractors—help

X-ray laboratories—operators

Yacht brokers

www.ingramcontent.com/pod-product-compliance
Lightning Source LLC
Chambersburg PA
CBHW030912050726
47498CB00003BA/699